GET THROUGH

MRCPsych
Paper A1: Mock
Examination Papers

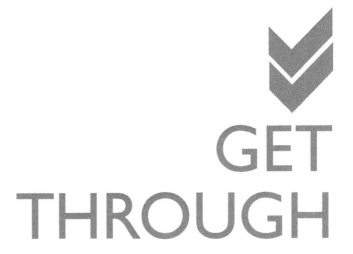

GET THROUGH

MRCPsych
Paper A1: Mock
Examination Papers

Melvyn WB Zhang MBBS, DCP, MRCPsych
National HealthCare Group, Singapore

Cyrus SH Ho MBBS, DCP, MRCPsych
National University of Singapore

Roger Ho MBBS, DPM, DCP, Gdip Psychotherapy,
MMed (Psych), MRCPsych, FRCPC
National University of Singapore

Ian H Treasaden MB, BS, LRCP, MRCS, FRCPsych, LLM
West London Mental Health NHS Trust,
Imperial College Healthcare NHS Trust, and
Bucks New University, UK

Basant K Puri MA, PhD, MB, BChir, BSc (Hons) MathSci,
DipStat, PG Dip Maths, MMath, FRCPsych, FSB
Hammersmith Hospital and Imperial College London, UK

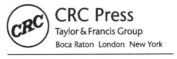

CRC Press
Taylor & Francis Group
Boca Raton London New York

CRC Press is an imprint of the
Taylor & Francis Group, an **informa** business

CRC Press
Taylor & Francis Group
6000 Broken Sound Parkway NW, Suite 300
Boca Raton, FL 33487-2742

© 2016 by Taylor & Francis Group, LLC
CRC Press is an imprint of Taylor & Francis Group, an Informa business

No claim to original U.S. Government works

Printed in Great Britain by Ashford Colour Press Ltd, Gosport, Hants
Version Date: 20160426

International Standard Book Number-13: 978-1-4822-4742-8 (Paperback)

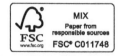

TABLE OF CONTENTS

INTRODUCTION

The two volumes that comprise this book consist of over 1800 questions. They correspond to the new format of Paper A of the Royal College of Psychiatrists' examinations, which has been revised recently. The questions (a mixture of both multiple choice questions [MCQs] as well as extended matching items [EMIs]) have been set so as to reflect the type and the current standard of the questions of the examinations, at the time of writing.

A good proportion of the questions featured in this book have been set so as to model against the core themes that have been commonly tested in the examinations in recent years. A good proportion of the questions are also being set based on the core domains of knowledge assessed in the examination. The authors have provided detailed explanation for each of the questions included in the mock examination paper. Readers are provided with references to which they could refer to, if they are in doubt with regards to any of the theoretical concepts. The format of the mock examination paper has been organized such that at least a third of the questions are EMIs, and the remaining two-thirds are MCQs.

We welcome any feedback from those of you who are using this book. Please also let us know further the type of questions you would like to see in the next edition of this book.

We wish to thank all the authors who have contributed to this revision guide-book and mock examination series.

Melvyn WB Zhang
Cyrus SH Ho
Roger CM Ho
Ian H Treasaden
Basant K Puri

Dr Melvyn Zhang, MBBS, DCP, MRCPsych, is a specialist registrar/senior resident at the National Healthcare Group, Singapore. He graduated from the National University of Singapore and received his postgraduate training with the Royal College of Psychiatrists (UK). He is currently working with the Institute of Mental Health, Singapore. He has a special interest in the application of web-based and smartphone technologies for education and research and has been published extensively in this field. He is a member of the Public Education and Engagement Board (PEEB), Royal College of Psychiatrists (UK), as well as a member of the editorial board of the *Journal of Internet Medical Research (Mental Health).* He has published extensively in the *British Medical Journal (BMJ), Lancet Psychiatry* and *BJPsych Advances.*

Dr Cyrus SH Ho, MBBS, DCP, MRCPsych, is an associate consultant psychiatrist and clinical lecturer from the National University Hospital, Singapore. He graduated from the National University of Singapore, Yong Loo Lin School of Medicine and subsequently obtained the Diploma of Clinical Psychiatry from Ireland and Membership of the Royal College of Psychiatrists from the United Kingdom. As a certified acupuncturist with the Graduate Diploma in Acupuncture conferred by the Singapore College of Traditional Chinese Medicine, he hopes to integrate both Western and Chinese medicine for holistic psychiatric care. He is actively involved in education and research work. His clinical and research interests include mood disorders, neuropsychiatry, pain studies and medical acupuncture.

Dr Roger Ho, MBBS, DPM, DCP, Gdip Psychotherapy, MMed (Psych), MRCPsych, FRCPC, is an assistant professor and consultant psychiatrist at the Department of Psychological Medicine, National University of Singapore. He graduated from the University of Hong Kong and received his training in psychiatry from the National University of Singapore. He is a general adult psychiatrist and in charge of the Mood Disorder Clinic, National University Hospital, Singapore. He is a member of the editorial board of *Advances of Psychiatric Treatment,* an academic journal published by the Royal College of Psychiatrists. His research focuses on mood disorders, psychoneuroimmunology and liaison psychiatry.

Dr Ian H Treasaden, MB, BS, LRCP, MRCS, FRCPsych, LLM, is currently an honorary consultant forensic psychiatrist at West London Mental Health NHS Trust and Imperial College Healthcare NHS Trust, as well as a visiting senior lecturer at Bucks New University.

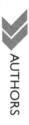

Until 2014, he was a consultant forensic psychiatrist at Three Bridges Medium Secure Unit, West London Mental Health NHS Trust, where he was also the clinical director, College and Coordinating Clinical Tutor for the Charing Cross Rotational Training Scheme in Psychiatry, and tutor in law and ethics and honorary senior clinical lecturer at Imperial College London.

He has authored papers on forensic and general psychiatry, and he is co-author of the books *Textbook of Psychiatry* (3 editions), *Mental Health Law: A Practical Guide* (2 editions), *Emergencies in Psychiatry, Psychiatry: An Evidence-Based Text* and *Revision MCQs and EMIs for the MRCPsych* and the forthcoming *Forensic Psychiatry: Fundamentals and Clinical Practice*.

He qualified in medicine from the London Hospital Medical College, University of London, in 1975 where he was awarded the James Anderson Prize in Clinical Medicine. He undertook training in forensic psychiatry at the Maudsley & Bethlem Royal Hospitals in London and Broadmoor Special Hospital, Berkshire, England between 1982 and 1984.

Basant K Puri, MA, PhD, MB, BChir, BSc (Hons) MathSci, DipStat, PG Dip Maths, MMath, FRCPsych, FSB, is based at Hammersmith Hospital and Imperial College London, United Kingdom. He read medicine at St John's College, University of Cambridge. He also trained in molecular genetics at the MRC MNU, Laboratory of Molecular Biology, Cambridge. He has authored or co-authored more than 40 books, including the second edition of *Drugs in Psychiatry* (Oxford University Press, 2013), third edition of *Textbook of Psychiatry* with Dr Ian Treasaden (Churchill Livingston, 2011) and, with the publisher of the present volume, the third edition of *Textbook of Clinical Neuropsychiatry and Neuroscience Fundamentals* with Professor David Moore (2012).

MRCPSYCH PAPER A1 MOCK EXAMINATION 1: QUESTIONS

GET THROUGH MRCPSYCH PAPER A1: MOCK EXAMINATION

Total number of questions: 194 (116 MCQs, 80 EMIs)
Total time provided: 180 minutes

Question 1
Vascular dementia has been known to be the second most common cause of dementia. A caregiver of a patient with vascular dementia is now worried about the risk of her acquiring the disorder. You would advise her that the most significant risk is
  a. Having an elevated lipid level
  b. Having poorly controlled blood pressure
  c. Having a previous smoking history
  d. Having an underlying heart disease
  e. Having a history of chronic alcohol abuse

Question 2
Which of the following would help to reduce the risk associated with acquiring vascular dementia?
  a. Low dose of aspirin daily
  b. Regular dose of multivitamins
  c. Regular dose of thiamine replacement
  d. Low dose of antipsychotics
  e. Anti-dementia medications

Question 3
Which of the following statements regarding the aetiology of alcoholism is false?
  a. Twin studies showed that monozygotic twins do have a higher concordance rate compared with dizygotic twins.
  b. Approximately half of the variance in regular drinking habits has been estimated to be genetic in origin for normal twins.
  c. Adoption studies support the hypothesis that there is a genetic transmission of alcoholism.

d. Sons of alcoholic parents have an increased risk (three to four times) of becoming alcoholics than the sons of non-alcoholics.
e. The rates of alcohol-related problems are not associated with the severity of the illness.

Question 4
During the lecture on ethics, the Tarasoff case was briefly mentioned. A student, new to psychiatry, has not heard of the key ruling made by the courts and the implications it has for psychiatrists. Which of the following statements about the implications is correct?
a. Psychiatrists now have a responsibility to inform and protect third parties who are at risk from their patients.
b. Psychiatrists should uphold the core principles of ethics and respect the rights of the patients.
c. Psychiatrists need to inform their seniors regarding issues pertaining to safety.
d. Psychiatrists are obliged to disclose information solely to the police for them to take necessary action in terms of protecting the welfare of others around.
e. Psychiatrists should remain focused and act on what is deemed to be in the best interest of their patients.

Question 5
Melanie Klein proposed the following, with the exception of
a. Depressive position
b. Paranoid-schizoid position
c. Projection
d. Introjection
e. Narcissism

Question 6
Which of the following statements is false with regards to the Present State Examination toolkit?
a. Information from the patients is used as a guide in questioning.
b. Information from the patients is used as a guide in scoring.
c. It has good validity.
d. It has good reliability.
e. It has good inter-related reliability.

Question 7
A medical student was puzzled as to why the old age consultant has asked his assistant to help administer the Clifton Assessment Procedures for the Elderly (CAPE). The consultant explains that the CAPE assessment scale is usually used in the assessment of the following:
a. Identification of dementia in the elderly
b. Identification of depression in the elderly

c. Identification of anxiety symptoms in the elderly
d. Identification of late-onset psychosis in the elderly
e. Identification of personality traits in the elderly

Question 8

A 35-year-old male recounts the feelings he has experienced when he lost his wife recently. He mentioned that he went through feelings of denial, anger and bargaining initially. The psychotherapist mentioned to him, 'I'm sorry to be hearing this. It is actually quite common for people to feel the same way as you do when dealing with losses of their loved ones'. This is an example of which interviewing technique?
a. Clarification
b. Encouragement
c. Rationalization
d. Summation
e. Validation

Question 9

The 'cocktail party phenomenon' best illustrates the Gestalt principle. From your understanding of this principle, which of the following would be true?
a. Figures that are separated apart tend not to be automatically visualized as a group.
b. There is a clear figure-ground differentiation and distinction.
c. The principle could only be applicable for visual objects.
d. The principle states that the sum of the whole cannot be greater than the sum of its corresponding parts.
e. The percept usually corresponds to the most complex simulation interpretation.

Question 10

According to the 10th Revision of *International Classification of Disease* (ICD-10) diagnostic classification, which of the following statement is part of the diagnostic criteria for persistent delusional disorder?
a. The delusions must be present for more than 3 months in duration.
b. The delusions are usually not congruent to the mood symptoms.
c. The delusions are not associated with any other psychopathologies.
d. There must be an identifiable stressor preceding the onset of the delusional beliefs.
e. The delusions usually involve multiple themes.

Question 11

Based on your understanding of first-rank symptoms, which of the following presentations is not characteristic of first-rank symptoms?
a. Voices making remarks about the patient
b. Voices performing a running commentary of the patient's symptoms

c. Voices commanding the patient
d. Voices talking amongst themselves
e. Voices addressing the patient in the third person

Question 12

A 30-year-old male, the chief executive manager of a multinational firm, was interested in the differences in leadership styles and how he could adopt them to manage his employees. He feels that laissez-faire leadership might be the most effective in management. You would recommend this if

a. His employees are known to have specialized knowledge of their tasks and could function by themselves independently.
b. His employees, though highly skilled, need constant monitoring to make sure that they would perform their assigned tasks.
c. His employees are not highly skilled.
d. His employees need constant monitoring to make sure that they achieve their assigned tasks.
e. His employees are good at suggesting solutions, but cannot come to a common agreement.

Question 13

A 50-year-old male has heard of genes being involved in Alzheimer's disease. He wonders what would be the increased incidence for an individual who is a heterozygote for apolipoprotein E4.

a. Two times
b. Three times
c. Four times
d. Five times
e. Six times

Question 14

Experiments performed previously by Asch on conformity in a group setting have illustrated that conformity is reduced by the presence of the following factors, with the exception of?

a. Presence of members who are self-reliant
b. Presence of intelligent members
c. Presence of expressive members
d. Presence of socially effective individuals
e. Presence of new members needing guidance from superiors

Question 15

Which of the following statements regarding the ICD-10 is false?
a. The ICD-10 is multi-axial.
b. The ICD-10 has separate categories for neurosis and psychosis.

c. The ICD-10 has a category for culture-bound syndromes.
d. The ICD-10 has a category for organic mental disorders.
e. The ICD-10 takes into account social functioning when establishing a
   diagnosis.

Question 16
When a 28-year-old female left her child in the clinic consultation room and
returned later, it was observed that her child did not cry during her absence and
even ignored her when she returned. This is an example of which particular type of
attachment?
a. Avoidant attachment
b. Anxious attachment
c. Insecure attachment
d. Secure attachment
e. Separation anxiety

Question 17
A child who is capable of understanding the laws of conservation belong to which
of the following stages?
a. Concrete operational
b. Formal operational
c. Operational
d. Preoperational
e. Sensorimotor

Question 18
Which of the following is considered to be a normal development milestone in a
child?
a. Tertiary circular reactions at 6 months
b. Constant babbling at 7 months
c. Development of colour vision at 8 months
d. Preoperational stage at 1 year
e. Fear of darkness at 3 years

Question 19
A 20-year-old medical student wondered how cognitive dissonance could affect
the dynamics of a group or even individuals in a normal population. It is found out
that cognitive dissonance would cause changes in
a. Baseline attitudinal perceptions
b. Degree of conformity to perspectives
c. Group-directed behaviours
d. Attributions within the group
e. Goal-targeted behaviours

Question 20

The four ethical principles (autonomy, beneficence, non-maleficence and justice) were recommended for use in medical ethics by
a. Beauchamp and Childress
b. Benjamin Rush
c. RD Laing
d. Thomas Percival
e. Thomas Szasz

Question 21

There has been increasing numbers of news reports regarding the association between cannabis use and schizophrenia. A 40-year-old mother knows that ever since her son got into university, he has started using cannabis on a regular basis due to the bad company that he mixes with now. What would be the chances of him developing schizophrenia?
a. No increased risk
b. Two times increased risk
c. Three times increased risk
d. Four times increased risk
e. Five times increased risk

Question 22

A 23-year-old male seemed much like a different person after the head injury which he sustained 1 year ago. He currently presents to the mental health specialist clinic and the consultant psychiatrist wishes to perform a detailed cognitive examination. He is intending to use the Wisconsin Card Sorting Test to test for the presence of impairments involving
a. Frontal lobe
b. Hippocampus
c. Parietal lobe
d. Occipital lobe
e. Temporal lobe

Question 23

The key worker, who has known a 25-year-old male, John, a patient with learning disability, has requested to speak to the psychiatrist, because John has been noted to have behavioural changes for the past 2 weeks or so after his scheduled home leave. She mentions to the psychiatrist that when John was well and less emotional, he was only able to communicate with nursing staff using sign language or one-word phrases. He also needed much assistance with his activities of daily living. From the aforementioned information, what level of learning disability would you say John has?
a. Mild
b. Moderate
c. Profound

d. Slightly below norms
e. Severe

Question 24
The following subtypes of schizophrenia could be found within the ICD-10 diagnostic criteria, with the exception of
a. Catatonic schizophrenia
b. Disorganized schizophrenia
c. Hebephrenic schizophrenia
d. Paranoid schizophrenia
e. Simple schizophrenia

Question 25
The consultant psychiatrist asked the core trainee to review a 70-year-old male who had been admitted last night due to behavioural difficulties at home. The core trainee had received some information from the nursing staff. The nursing staff reported based on observations that the patient had been having rapid changes in his consciousness levels. At times, he seemed to respond to both visual and auditory hallucinations. He had some rigidity and gait disturbances as well. Which one of the following might be a likely differential diagnosis for him?
a. Catatonia
b. Delirium
c. Delirium tremens
d. Frontotemporal dementia
e. Lewy body dementia

Question 26
The clinical diagnosis of atypical anorexia nervosa is made when an individual has the following symptoms:
a. Amenorrhea
b. Absence of significant weight loss
c. BMI less than 14
d. Massive and rapid weight loss
e. Marked body image disturbances

Question 27
A 21-year-old male, who was involved in a major road traffic accident, awoke finally after being unconscious for 7 days. The doctors in charge noted that he was unable to recognize familiar faces, like those of his relatives. This is termed as
a. Agnosia
b. Apraxia
c. Colour agnosia
d. Prosopagnosia
e. Visual object agnosia

Question 28
The college is aiming to develop a new programme to prevent suicide amongst patients with schizophrenia. What is the estimated risk of suicide in a patient with schizophrenia?
a. 0.01
b. 0.05
c. 0.08
d. 0.10
e. 0.20

Question 29
Ptosis is a common neurological sign that is present in all of the following clinical diagnoses, with the exception of
a. Myasthenia gravis
b. Horner's syndrome
c. Lambert Eaton syndrome
d. Third nerve palsy
e. Seventh nerve palsy

Question 30
Symptoms that are suggestive of benzodiazepine withdrawal include all of the following except
a. Autonomic hyperactivity
b. Pyrexia
c. Malaise and weakness
d. Tremors
e. Rigidity

Question 31
Pre-traumatic factors that predispose any individual to post-traumatic stress disorder (PTSD) include all the following except
a. Being female in sex
b. Having a previous psychiatric illness
c. Having an internal locus of control
d. Having received lesser education
e. Having experienced previous trauma

Question 32
A woman who has recently been diagnosed with depression is very concerned with regards to the antidepressant that the consultant psychiatrist is going to offer to her. She feels that with her mood symptoms, she is not capable of starting a family. Which of the following antidepressants might affect the efficacy of the oral contraceptive pills that she is taking at the moment?
a. Citalopram
b. Fluoxetine

c. St John's wort
d. Tricyclics
e. Venlafaxine

Question 33

A 22-year-old patient's father was shocked to be informed that his son has developed what seemed to be neuroleptic malignant syndrome (NMS) induced by olanzapine that was started. He wants to know more about NMS. Which of the following regarding NMS is not true?

a. The onset of NMS is much more rapid compared with serotonin syndrome.
b. Patients with NMS usually have an elevated temperature.
c. Patients with NMS might have rigidity and disturbances in gait.
d. Patients with NMS might have raised creatine kinase.
e. The contributing factor for NMS is usually antipsychotics, whereas the contributing factor for serotonin syndrome is usually antidepressants.

Question 34

After understanding the psychopathology of obsessive-compulsive disorder, a group of medical students were debating which would be the most common compulsive behaviour. The correct answer would be

a. Arranging things in a perfect symmetry
b. Checking things
c. Counting and performing rituals a fixed number of times
d. Cleaning things
e. Keeping items even when not needed

Question 35

Which of the following statements about the diagnosis of PTSD is not true?

a. Patients might complain of emotional numbing (inability to experience emotions).
b. Patients might complain of hyper-arousal and being easily startled.
c. Patients might complain of recurrent flashbacks and having nightmares of the previous incident.
d. Patients might have taken measures such as avoidance to prevent re-experiencing any aspect of the event.
e. The onset of symptoms is usually within 2 weeks after experiencing the trauma.

Question 36

An individual with bipolar affective disorder and long-term alcohol dependence develops haematemesis. He is advised by the gastroenterologist to go for an oesophago-gastro-duodenoscopy (OGD) to identify the bleeding site. On assessment, he appears to have the capacity to make that decision and he is not manic. The psychiatrist advises acceding to his wish not to have the OGD. This case illustrates which of the following?

a. The principle of respect for a person's autonomy
b. The principle of beneficence

c. The principle of non-maleficence
d. Paternalism approach
e. Utilitarian approach

Question 37
Which of the following regarding hormonal changes in anorexia nervosa is not correct?
a. Decrease in T3 levels
b. Increase in corticotrophin-releasing hormone (CRH)
c. Increase in cortisol
d. Decrease in growth hormone
e. Decrease in follicle-stimulating hormone

Question 38
A 30-year-old male has been increasingly concerned about his lower back pain. Despite having seen several specialists and having had a detailed investigation, he is still concerned that the doctors might have made a mistake. He is concerned that he might have a malignant tumour. The most likely diagnosis in this case would be
a. Depression with anxiety features
b. Generalized anxiety disorder
c. Hypochondriasis
d. Specific phobia
e. Somatization disorder

Question 39
A 24-year-old male has a long-standing history of alcohol dependence and is currently undergoing recovery. The addiction specialist has proposed that he be started on a course of a medication called acamprosate. Which of the following is not a side effect associated with this medication?
a. Changes in sexual drive
b. Diarrhoea
c. Nausea
d. Renal impairment
e. Rash

Question 40
A 32-year-old female has been started on citalopram 20 mg per day for her major depression following the death of her husband. After 2 weeks, she reports to the psychiatrist that she has noted improvements in the patient's biological symptoms. However, there are times when she still finds the patient's mood to be low. Which one of the following would be the next best approach with regards to the patient's management?
a. Continue the same dose of citalopram
b. Consider augmentation of the antidepressant with lithium
c. Consider electroconvulsive therapy (ECT)
d. Increase the dose of citalopram to 30 mg per day
e. Stop citalopram and consider venlafaxine

Question 41

A 30-year-old male was serving in the military in Syria. Around 6 months ago, he witnessed a traumatic incident in which his colleague was shot dead right beside him. He has seen the mental health specialist and has been diagnosed with PTSD. Which of the following statements is inconsistent with his diagnosis?

a. He reports that he has been experiencing repeated reliving of the trauma.
b. He reports that he has marked hyper-arousal and hyper-vigilance.
c. He reports that he has been sleeping more than usual to avoid thinking of the events.
d. He reports that he has been having intrusive memories of the event.
e. He reports that he feels an emotional detachment occasionally.

Question 42

Which of the following is considered to be the most common disorder of male sexual response?

a. Delayed ejaculation
b. Erectile dysfunction
c. Early ejaculation
d. Male hypoactive sexual desire disorder
e. Substance-/medication-induced sexual dysfunction

Question 43

Which of the following is the most useful tool to help in the diagnosis of dementia?

a. Clinical interview and examination
b. Cognitive assessment (Mini Mental State Examination [MMSE])
c. Cognitive assessment (frontal lobe assessment battery)
d. Computed tomography (CT) scan
e. Magnetic resonance imaging (MRI) scan

Question 44

It is not uncommon that some of the negative cognitions that depressed patients have involve that of learned helplessness. The one who was responsible for proposing the concept of learned helplessness was

a. Beck
b. Freud
c. Mahler
d. Seligman
e. Wolpe

Question 45

A 26-year-old female has been diagnosed with borderline personality disorder and she has been sectioned for admission to the ward following her active ideations of committing suicide. She has been inpatient for the past week, and the nurses are getting very upset with regards to nursing her. Which one of the following factors might be responsible for this?

a. Countertransference
b. Projective identification

c. Splitting
   d. Transference
   e. Reaction formation

Question 46
A 48-year-old female, the mother of a teenager daughter, is concerned when the consultant psychiatrist recommended antipsychotic treatment for her daughter. She heard that some antipsychotics might cause menstrual cycle disturbances as well as elevated levels of a hormone in the brain. From your understanding, which of the following might have a higher chance of causing the aforementioned?
   a. Clozapine
   b. Haloperidol
   c. Olanzapine
   d. Quetiapine
   e. Risperidone

Question 47
Bleuler introduced the concept of schizophrenia and further defined the symptoms that schizophrenic patients have. Which of the following did he identify as being of secondary status?
   a. Ambivalence
   b. Autism
   c. Affective incongruity
   d. Disturbance of association of thoughts
   e. Hallucinations

Question 48
A senior psychiatrist goes to work every day at least 30 minutes early and she needs to get the same parking spot every day. She would be frustrated and irritable if things do not go as she has planned. What is the most likely diagnosis?
   a. Anxiety disorder
   b. Depressive disorder with anxiety features
   c. No mental illness
   d. Obsessive-compulsive disorder
   e. Obsessive-compulsive personality disorder

Question 49
A psychology intern wonders which of the following would be the most effective in influencing and changing the general public's negative perspectives of mental health illness. The correct answer would be
   a. Using propaganda
   b. Using persuasive messages
   c. Using authority figures to disseminate messages
   d. Using authority figures to instill conformity
   e. Using authority figures to instill obedience

Question 50
A patient with a long-standing alcohol history has been recently admitted to the inpatient unit for an emergency back operation due to a herniated disc. He currently presents with Wernicke–Korsakoff syndrome. The medical student attempted a bedside cognitive examination, and the patient scored poorly on the MMSE. He wonders what form of memory loss the patient is currently experiencing.
a. Anterograde memory loss
b. Long-term memory loss
c. Procedural memory loss
d. Retrograde memory loss
e. Working memory deficits

Question 51
Which of the following is the diagnosis for a patient who makes up symptoms just to be in the sick role?
a. Conversion disorder
b. Factitious disorder
c. Hypochondriasis
d. Malingering
e. Somatization disorder

Question 52
A 30-year-old female tells her community psychiatric nurse that she has not been feeling good in her mood recently. She claims that she does not feel in control of her mood and shared that others are projecting unhappiness in her. This form of psychopathology is known as
a. Delusional feelings
b. Made emotions
c. Made impulse
d. Hallucinations
e. Somatic passivity

Question 53
A patient who is due for his routine outpatient review shares with the consultant that he does not feel safe in the clinic. He claims that those outside can freely access what he is thinking at the moment. What psychopathology does this refer to?
a. Thought insertion
b. Thought broadcasting
c. Thought block
d. Thought withdrawal
e. Delusional perception

Question 54
A 20-year-old male has been the star player on his team for the last three seasons. However, he missed a goal in the most crucial last match of the season, and now he

thinks and feels that he is a burden to the entire team. The specific cognitive error that he is having at the moment might be

a. Arbitrary inference
b. Magnification
c. Minimization
d. Rumination
e. Selective abstraction

Question 55

A trainee who has been working for the past 36 hours tells his colleague at 8 AM the next day that he is feeling depersonalized. Based on your understanding of the terminology 'depersonalization', it also refers to

a. The feeling of 'as if'
b. The feeling of 'if not'
c. The feeling of 'what if'
d. The feeling of 'what next'
e. The feeling of 'why me'

Question 56

You are interviewing the husband of a woman with personality disorder and invite the husband to talk about his feeling towards his wife. He replies, 'frustrated' and does not want to say more. Which of the following interview techniques is most likely to facilitate the interview to continue?

a. Closed-ended questions
b. Long pause
c. Prolonged eye contact
d. Summation
e. Transition

Question 57

A 25-year-old male told the police that he had broken into the house of his ex-girlfriend because people from his workplace had told him to do so. He claimed that he was not in control of his actions, and that his actions were not within his free will. This is an example of

a. Delusion
b. Hallucinations
c. Made impulse
d. Made actions
e. Thought process disorder

Question 58

The following are features of Ganser syndrome except

a. Approximate answers
b. Amnesia
c. Delusional beliefs
d. Pseudo-hallucinations
e. Somatic conversion

Question 59

A joint multidisciplinary team interview was being conducted for a 70-year-old male, named Mr Smith, as the team wanted to recommend to him home help services. During the interview, it was noted that Mr Smith made up false information when asked about the recent events, and he was not at all embarrassed by his lies. Which of the following statements is most likely to be true?
 a. He has underlying antisocial personality traits.
 b. He has anxious personality traits.
 c. He is having Ganser syndrome, and hence he is giving his best approximate answer.
 d. He is having memory difficulties, and hence he is confabulating.
 e. He is just trying to be funny and is joking with his team.

Question 60

This terminology is commonly used to describe the experience of having a stimulus in one sensory modality producing a sensory experience in another modality. Which of the following would be the most appropriate answer?
 a. Extracampine hallucination
 b. Functional hallucinations
 c. Reflex hallucinations
 d. Synaesthesia
 e. Visual hallucinations

Question 61

In which of the following personality disorders would one be extremely concerned about rejection and criticism?
 a. Anxious avoidant personality disorder
 b. Borderline personality disorder
 c. Obsessive-compulsive personality disorder
 d. Schizoid personality disorder
 e. Schizotypal personality disorder

Question 62

Emil Kraepelin was responsible for coining this term during a previous experiment that he had performed. In that experiment, he noted that some patients would repeatedly put out their tongue and allowed their tongues to be pricked, despite the fact that they knew of the consequences. This is an example of
 a. Automatic obedience
 b. Automatism
 c. Echolalia
 d. Echopraxia
 e. Stereotypies

Question 63

A 45-year-old male has persistent primary insomnia and his doctor has recommended a short course of benzodiazepines. He is very worried about next-day sedation. Which of the following benzodiazepine has the longest half-life and might not be suitable?

a. Alprazolam
b. Lorazepam
c. Nitrazepam
d. Oxazepam
e. Temazepam

Question 64

The mechanism of action of naltrexone, which might be helpful in people who are in abstinence, is by acting as which of the following?

a. Opioid agonist
b. Opioid antagonist
c. Gamma-aminobutyric acid (GABA) agonist
d. Glutamate antagonist
e. Glutamate agonist

Question 65

A core trainee, during his MRCPsych CASC examinations, asks the patient to help spell the word 'World' forwards and then backwards. This is an assessment of

a. Attention and concentration
b. Long-term memory
c. Language abilities
d. Short-term memory
e. Semantic memory

Question 66

Ganser previously described this syndrome that consists of all of the following except

a. Approximate answers
b. Auditory and visual hallucinations
c. Amnesia
d. Anhedonia
e. Clouding of consciousness

Question 67

Schizophrenia has been subclassified into different subtypes. Which of the following has the worst prognosis?

a. Catatonic schizophrenia
b. Hebephrenic schizophrenia
c. Paranoid schizophrenia
d. Simple schizophrenia
e. Undifferentiated schizophrenia

Question 68

A 30-year-old male has been increasingly concerned about his headache after his uncle recently passed away due to a brain tumour. He has been to several general practitioners (GPs) and neurologists, and the necessary investigation has been done. He seems to be reassured for a while thereafter, but gets worried about his headaches again. Recently, he has resorted to checking out the symptoms on the Internet, almost daily. The most likely clinical diagnosis is

a. Conversion disorder
b. Depression with anxiety features
c. Generalized anxiety disorder
d. Hypochondriasis
e. Somatoform pain disorder

Question 69

A 28-year-old female has decided to visit her GP as her mood has been anxious lately. For no reason, over the past 2 months or so, she has been able to listen to conversations from the post office in Manchester, despite the fact that she is living currently in London. This form of psychopathology is termed as

a. Pseudohallucination
b. Extracampine hallucination
c. Hypnopompic hallucination
d. Thought echo
e. Thought broadcasting

Question 70

A consultant psychiatrist was assessing a 20-year-old male in his depression clinic. When asked how his mood was, the patient claimed that he had much difficulty in expressing his current mood state. This form of psychopathology is termed as

a. Alexithymia
b. Apathy
c. Dysphoria
d. Euphoria
e. Affective blunting

Question 71

From your understanding about psychodynamic therapy and the works of Freud, which of the following is not classified as a mature defence mechanism?

a. Acting out
b. Anticipation
c. Altruism
d. Humour
e. Sublimation

Question 72

A 35-year-old female witnessed a fellow shopper being shot dead whilst shopping 3 weeks ago. Currently, she has been experiencing insomnia, poor concentration,

as well as tearfulness. She does have occasional nightmares too. Which would be the most appropriate clinical diagnosis?
a. Acute stress disorder
b. Adjustment disorder
c. Depression
d. Generalized anxiety disorder
e. PTSD

Question 73

A 30-year-old male has been admitted to the inpatient unit for first-episode psychosis. The social worker who accompanied him back from his Section 17 home leave noted that he had been tolerating critical comments from his family members for years. Which of the following psychological treatment might be suitable for him and his family in order to prevent a relapse of his underlying psychiatric disorder?
a. Cognitive analytical therapy
b. Cognitive behavioural therapy
c. Family therapy
d. Interpersonal therapy
e. Psychodynamic therapy

Question 74

Which of the following is true with regards to primary attribution error?
a. Making the inference that one is responsible primarily for his or her behaviour
b. Making the inference that other environmental factors are responsible
c. Making the inference that a combination of internal factors and external factors are responsible
d. It refers to a bias made when inferring the cause of another's behaviour – bias made towards situational attributions
e. It refers to a bias made when inferring the cause of another's behaviour – bias made towards internal factors

Question 75

A 55-year-old man is very concerned about dust in the environment. He was seen by various senior psychiatrists who suggested that he suffers from delusional disorder. You think that he may suffer from obsessive-compulsive disorder, and need to defend your diagnosis. Which of the following is expected in this patient if he indeed suffers from delusional disorder?
a. Anxiety
b. Depression
c. Hallucination
d. Normal functioning
e. Somatic passivity

Question 76
A core trainee was wondering which of the following medications would be the safest for treating a patient who is experiencing alcohol withdrawal symptoms, but also has a background of liver disease:
a. Alprazolam
b. Lorazepam
c. Zopiclone
d. Zolpidem
e. Diazepam

Question 77
Which of the following cognitive bias was not part of Aaron Beck's cognitive model of depression?
a. Arbitrary inference
b. Learned helplessness
c. Personalization
d. Magnification
e. Minimization

Question 78
Which of the following individuals proposed that the concept of mental illness has no validity?
a. Bentham
b. Fulford
c. Mil
d. Szasz
e. Williams

Question 79
A 14-year-old girl with Asperger syndrome is referred to the child and adolescent mental health service for quirky movements such as hair twisting. The psychopathology being described is
a. Ambitendency
b. Compulsion
c. Echopraxia
d. Mannerism
e. Stereotypy

Question 80
Which of the following statements about scapegoating is correct?
a. This usually occurs when members of the majority group tend to victimize members of the minority group simply out of frustration.
b. This usually occurs when members of the majority and the minority groups come into direct competition with each other.

c. This usually occurs when members of the minority group make negative remarks to downplay the position of the majority group.
d. This usually occurs when members of the majority group pick on the shortcomings of an individual of the minority group and generalize it to the entire group.
e. This usually occurs when there is a direct conflict of interest amongst members of the majority as well as the minority groups.

Question 81

A 30-year-old woman with a history of depression is in the last term of pregnancy. She complains of an irritating, non-painful sensation in her legs that give her an overwhelming urge to move them. The symptoms occur when she is resting, and get worse from evening onwards. She does not take psychotropic medication, and a recent full blood count shows anaemia. The psychopathology being described is
a. Akathisia
b. Antenatal anxiety
c. Catatonic excitement
d. Mannerism
e. Restless leg syndrome (Ekbom syndrome)

Question 82

An 18-year-old woman presents with auditory hallucination, delusional perception and thought interferences. Psychiatric evaluation established a diagnosis of schizophrenia. She has a history of asthma. She started treatment with haloperidol 10 mg per day because she cannot afford second-generation antipsychotics and cannot tolerate chlorpromazine. Shortly after taking haloperidol, she felt restless with inner tension. Later, her mother reports that she frequently is unable to remain seated, shifts in place and shuffles from foot to foot. The following are appropriate treatments that you might try in order to relieve her symptoms except
a. Reduce the dose of haloperidol
b. Start her on cryproheptadine
c. Start her on propranolol
d. Start her on a benzodiazepine
e. Start her on an antimuscarinic drug

Question 83

The sister of a man with schizophrenia has read about 'simple schizophrenia'. Which of the following symptoms found in her brother do not support a diagnosis of simple schizophrenia?
a. Failure to continue university studies
b. Florid third-person auditory hallucinations
c. Inability to maintain personal hygiene
d. Odd behaviour such as locking himself in the toilet and colouring the water in a bath tub
e. Progressive withdrawal and isolation

Question 84

A 30-year-old man complains that he hears voices from his late mother. Three months ago, his mother died in a car accident when he was driving his car. He feels very sad and guilty. He has not driven the car since the accident and he wants to sell the car. What is your diagnosis?

a. Delayed grief
b. Inhibited grief
c. Normal grief reaction
d. PTSD
e. Prolonged grief

Question 85

A patient is on treatment with psychotropic medications. He wonders which of the following would affect his medications, by acting as an enzyme inducer:

a. Caffeine
b. Grapefruit juice
c. Sertraline
d. Smoking
e. Valproate

Question 86

A 30-year-old man complains of chest pain after his late father died of myocardial infarction 6 months ago. His wife feels that he has become very angry and hostile to her after his father passed away. He has been drinking heavily in the last 3 months. When you ask him the reason of heavy drinking, he wants to be self-destructive. Which of the following abnormal grief reactions is the most accurate diagnosis for this man?

a. Chronic grief
b. Conflicted grief
c. Delayed grief
d. Distorted grief
e. Inhibited grief

Reference and Further Reading: Hooper M (2010). Multiple chemical sensitivity, in Puri BK, Treasaden I (eds), *Psychiatry: An Evidence-Based Text*. London: Hodder Arnold, pp. 811–817.

Question 87

Disorders of self-awareness (ego disorders) usually include the following disturbances except

a. Awareness of self-activity
b. Boundaries of self
c. Continuity of self
d. Immediate awareness of self-unity
e. Subconscious

Question 88

You are teaching depressive disorder to a group of medical students. They want to know the percentage of patients admitted to the university hospital who will have recurrence and require further admission in the long run without committing suicide. Your answer is

a. 20%
b. 30%
c. 40%
d. 60%
e. 80%

Question 89

During an experiment, participants were asked to listen to a speech made by a speaker that supported or opposed World War II. Participants were told that the speech they were about to hear was chosen at random by tossing a coin. After listening to the speech, the participants were asked whether they thought the speaker believed in what he or she said about the war. The results showed that the participants thought the speaker believed in what he or she said even when they knew the positions were chosen at random. Which heuristic best explains the aforementioned phenomenon?

a. Framing
b. Anchoring and adjustment heuristic
c. Availability heuristic
d. Representativeness heuristic
e. Counterfactual thinking

Question 90

A new psychiatric consultant has been appointed by the trust to head a community psychiatric team. He is known to be a 'hands-off' person and not available most of the time. He seldom gives feedback to his team members. Which of the following teams will be effective under his leadership?

a. Assertive team members who request major decisions to be made by voting and thorough discussion amongst the whole team.
b. Team members who are eager to learn and request constant supervision from the consultant psychiatrist.
c. Honest team members who are good at performing routine home visits repeatedly.
d. Humble team members who prefer the consultant psychiatrist to make major decisions.
e. Trustworthy team members who are experienced in community psychiatry and skilful in dealing with complicated issues. They require minimal supervision.

Question 91

A 24-year-old woman is admitted due to elated mood. A core trainee wants to know the differences between hypomania and mania. Which of the following statements is incorrect?

a. Patients with hypomania are not expected to have hallucinations.
b. Patients with hypomania are not expected to have mood-congruent delusions.

c. Patients with mania are expected to have reckless behaviour.

d. Patients with mania and hypomania are expected to have elated mood.

e. Patients with mania and hypomania are expected to have the same level of psychosocial functioning.

Question 92

A 33-year-old female has been diagnosed with PTSD after having witnessing a gun-shot incident in the supermarket that she was shopping at. She wants to get well as soon as possible and is keen on both pharmacological and psychological therapy. From your knowledge about PTSD management, which of the following would be contraindicated in her case?

a. Debriefing

b. Eye movement desensitization and reprocessing (EMDR)

c. Exposure therapy

d. Provision of social support

e. Trauma-focused cognitive behavioural therapy (CBT)

Question 93

A trainee passes the MRCPsych examination Paper 1 having based her revision on past examination questions but other trainees who have studied for long hours and based their revision on textbooks failed Paper 1 despite having gained vast knowledge. The phenomenon being described is

a. Barnum effect

b. Halo effect

c. Practice effect

d. Primacy effect

e. Recency effect

Question 94

A 30-year-old woman is a known case of schizophrenia. She presented to the Accident and Emergency Department with altered mental status, severe stiffness along with rapid eye blinking, unusual head and neck movements, and peculiar behaviour (simulating the doctor's movement). She is afebrile, and creatinine kinase is normal. Which of the following signs is not associated with her condition?

a. Ambitendency

b. Astasia-abasia

c. Automatic obedience

d. Echolalia

e. Gegenhalten

Question 95

The following is a condition that is common in Southeast Asia and China. A Chinese man has extreme anxiety and fear of impending death due to worries that his genitals might retract into his abdomen and would disappear. This condition is known as

a. Amok

b. Dhat

c. Frigophobia
d. Koro
e. Latah

Question 96
A 35-year-old pregnant woman develops depression during the second trimester. Which of the following symptoms is the least reliable in establishing the diagnosis of depression?
a. Anxiety
b. Guilt ruminations
c. Insomnia
d. Lack of interest in the baby
e. Social withdrawal

Question 97
A core trainee has determined that the patient he interviewed has moderate depression and would benefit from an antidepressant. The other medical problems the patient has include that of hypertension and seizure. The core trainee wonders which antidepressant he should avoid, as it might affect his seizure threshold. Which of the following medications should be avoided?
a. Bupropion
b. Citalopram
c. Fluoxetine
d. Mirtazapine
e. Paroxetine

Question 98
Based on the Holmes and Rahe Social Readjustment Rating Scale, which of the following events is considered to be the most stressful event contributing to illness?
a. Death of a close family member
b. Death of a spouse
c. Divorce
d. Marital separation
e. Imprisonment

Question 99
A 40-year-old man with schizophrenia is admitted to the psychiatric ward. The nurse informs you that he lies for hours on his bed with his head raised 10 cm off the mattress. The psychopathology being described is
a. Ambitendency
b. Gegenhalten
c. Mitgehen
d. Psychological pillow
e. Schnauzkrampf

Question 100
In an animal experiment, a rat pressed a lever in the cage and got an electric shock. The rat has never pressed the lever again ever since it was nearly electrocuted. The phenomenon being described is
a. Forward conditioning
b. Negative reinforcement
c. Positive reinforcement
d. Punishment
e. Stimulus discrimination

Question 101
The Nuremberg Code, which was formulated in 1947, is a very important piece of documentation regarding the ethics of medical research. Which of the following statements pertaining to the code is incorrect?
a. The trial involved conducting inquiries about doctors in wartime who performed human experiments in concentration camps.
b. The trial involved Japanese doctors who were deemed unethical.
c. The trial involved Nazi doctors who were deemed unethical.
d. As a result of the trial, this led to a set of 10 research principles.
e. The trial led to doctors recognizing the need to respect the human rights of subjects.

Question 102
In an animal experiment, a rat will get food after it presses a lever. The learning process being described is
a. Cognitive learning
b. Classical conditioning
c. Modelling
d. Operant conditioning
e. Social learning

Question 103
Which of the following can be used to prevent groupthink?
a. An authoritarian leader
b. Isolating the group members
c. A critical evaluator
d. An observer
e. Mindguards

Question 104
A 30-year-old male, Jordon, came to the emergency department, requesting to see Sarah, the psychiatric nurse who treated him 3 weeks ago. He is demanding to see her as he believes that she is in love with him, just from the way she smiled at him previously when he was undergoing treatment. He is keen to take her out for a

date and engage in sexual acts with her. Which of the following is the most likely diagnosis?

a. Grandiose delusion
b. Doppelganger
c. Cotard's syndrome
d. Erotomania
e. Couvade syndrome

Question 105

A 50-year-old man suffers from chronic schizophrenia. Three months ago, he developed shortness of breath, numbness, difficulty in handling tools and trouble in walking down the stairs. He came to the Accident and Emergency Department a few times, and the doctors felt that he presented with somatic complaints and then discharged him. His GP urged the doctors at the Accident and Emergency Department to admit this man for further evaluation. He turned out to suffer from cervical cord compression and required urgent operation. After the operation, he developed tetraplegia. His wife is very upset with the hospital. When the Chief Executive meets his wife, he says, 'It is quite acceptable to feel angry at the hospital and perhaps most people would feel angry as you do'. The Chief Executive demonstrates which of the following techniques?

a. Consideration
b. Explanation
c. Reflection
d. Legitimation
e. Negotiation

Question 106

A 29-year-old female has been diagnosed with rapid cycling bipolar disorder, as she has had more than four mood episodes per year. She is currently on pharmacological treatment with valproate. Which of the following factors might have an impact on her condition?

a. Hyperthyroidism
b. Hypertension
c. Usage of alcohol
d. Usage of antidepressants
e. Stressful life events

Question 107

A common cultural-bound syndrome described in North America, in which individuals believe that he or she might have undergone a transformation and become a monster that would practise cannibalism is known as

a. Amok
b. Brain fag syndrome
c. Dhat
d. Koro
e. Windigo

Question 108

Which one of the following terminologies best describes the ratio between the minimum plasma level that would cause a toxic effect and the minimum plasma level that would cause therapeutic effects?

a. Therapeutic index
b. Toxicity
c. Affinity
d. Potency
e. Volume of distribution

Question 109

A 50-year-old woman meets the diagnostic criteria for panic disorder with agoraphobia. Each time she leaves the house, she experiences high levels of anxiety. When she goes back home, her anxiety level goes down. After some time, she learns that by staying at home, she can avoid any possibility of a panic attack in public. This contributes to the maintenance of her disorder. Which of the following statements about the aforementioned phenomenon is incorrect?

a. The reinforcement is contingent upon the behaviour.
b. The behaviour is voluntary.
c. A negative reinforcer positively affects the frequency of response.
d. The reinforcement can occur before the behaviour.
e. An alteration in the frequency of behaviour is possible after reinforcement.

Question 110

A 24-year-old woman is diagnosed with agoraphobia. She attends psychotherapy sessions for the treatment of her agoraphobia. Which of the following statements about the aforementioned phenomenon is incorrect?

a. Shaping can lead to extinction.
b. Spontaneous recovery can occur after extinction.
c. Intermittent reinforcement diminishes the extinction rate.
d. Implosion cannot be used in extinction.
e. Reciprocal inhibition can be used in extinction.

Question 111

Which of the following concepts do not contribute to the aetiology of phobias?

a. Vicarious conditioning
b. Learned helplessness
c. Mowrer's two-factor theory
d. Classical conditioning
e. Biological preparedness

Question 112

Eugen Bleuler proposed the term 'schizophrenia' for what Emil Kraepelin had been calling 'dementia praecox'. The reason was

a. The term 'schizophrenia' refers to a disorder with onset in young adulthood that is different from dementia, which usually occurs in old age.
b. The term 'schizophrenia' refers to a chronic disorder comprising hallucinations and delusions with a downhill course.

c. The term 'schizophrenia' refers to the integration of functional psychiatric disorder and organic disorder (e.g. catatonia).

d. The term 'schizophrenia' refers to a significant deterioration of social functioning and poor long-term outcome that occurred in the era of asylums.

e. The term 'schizophrenia' refers to the 'splitting' of affect from other psychological functions leading to a dissociation between the social situation and the emotion expressed.

Question 113
During a routine physical examination for extra-pyramidal side effects, it was noted that the patient kept stretching out his hands, withdrawing them thereafter and repeating this several times, without allowing the examiner to check for the presence of Parkinson's features in the upper limbs. This form of psychopathology is termed as

a. Ambitendency
b. Automatic obedience
c. Catatonic posturing
d. Mitgehen
e. Perseveration

Question 114
In the United Kingdom, the determinants of social class are based on

a. Education
b. Financial status
c. Occupation
d. Type of residence
e. Geographic area of residence

Extended matching items (EMIs)

Theme: Memory

Lead in: Please identify the correct type of memory applicable to each one of the following situations. Each option may be used once, more than once or not at all.

Options:

a. Declarative memory
b. Working memory
c. Procedural memory
d. Episodic memory
e. Sensory memory
f. Anterograde memory
g. Retrograde memory

Question 115
A 30-year-old male was involved in a road traffic accident. When he awoke post-surgery, he realized that he is unable to recall events leading up to the accident.

Question 116
A MMSE assessment was conducted for a 70-year-old man. He was noted to be unable to recall the three items to which he was presented with.

Question 117
A 70-year-old female with dementia is still able to remember how to sew her dresses as she has been a tailor previously when she was younger.

Question 118
A 50-year-old male was asked to name the capital of the United Kingdom. Which type of memory is he using?

Question 119
A 70-year-old female has Alzheimer's dementia, but she is still able to remember personal events that happened when she was much younger and is still able to share her life story with her grandchildren. Which form of memory is she relying on?

Theme: Lab tests
Lead in: For the below-mentioned drugs please indicate the approximate duration that they could still be detected in the urine. Each option may be used once, more than once or not at all.
Options:
   a. 6–8 hours
   b. 12–24 hours
   c. 24 hours
   d. 48 hours
   e. 36–72 hours
   f. 6 days
   g. 8 days
   h. 2 weeks

Question 120
Amphetamines

Question 121
Barbiturates

Question 122
Cocaine

Question 123
Heroin

Question 124
Lysergic acid diethylamide (LSD)

Question 125
Methylene-dioxy-methamphetamine (MDMA)

Question 126
Phencyclidine (PCP)

Reference: Puri BK, Hall A, Ho R (2014). *Revision Notes in Psychiatry*. London: CRC Press, p. 529.

Theme: General psychiatry

Lead in: A 28-year-old man has suffered from schizophrenia for 5 years. He is currently stable and has recently got married. He and his wife are planning to have children. He consults you on the genetic risk of schizophrenia.

   Each option might be used once, more than once or not at all.

Options:
   a. 0%–4%
   b. 5%–9%
   c. 10%–14%
   d. 15%–19%
   e. 20%–24%
   f. 25%–29%
   g. 30%–34%
   h. 35%–50%
   i. 60%–65%
   j. 70%–75%
   k. 80%–85%

Question 127
The risk of schizophrenia for his child if his wife also suffers from schizophrenia. (Choose one option.)

Question 128
The risk of schizophrenia for his child if his wife does not suffer from schizophrenia. (Choose one option.)

Question 129
The risk of schizophrenia if he adopted a child with velocardiofacial syndrome. (Choose one option.)

Question 130
The risk of schizophrenia in his half-siblings. (Choose one option.)

Question 131
The risk of schizophrenia in his younger cousin. (Choose one option.)

Theme: Aetiology

Lead in: Match the given aetiological factors to the following clinical scenarios. Each option may be used once, more than once or not at all.

Options:
   a. Apolipoprotein E4 gene (homozygous for ε4)
   b. Cardiovascular disease

c. Cancer
d. Childhood sexual abuse
e. Death of the mother before the age of 11 years
f. Down syndrome
g. Dysbindin gene
h. Migration
i. Neuregulin gene
j. Old age
k. Streptococcal infection
l. Three children at home under the age of 14 years
m. Unemployment

Question 132
A 10-year-old boy develops obsessions and compulsive behaviour after a sore throat and fever. (Choose one option.)

Question 133
A 19-year-old woman presents with recurrent self-harm following the end of a transient and intense romantic relationship. She has a chronic feeling of emptiness and exhibits binge-eating behaviour. (Choose one option.)

Question 134
A 24-year-old man complains that MI5 is monitoring him and has tried to control his feelings and intentions. He heard the voices of two secret agents talking about him and they issued him with a command. (Choose three options.)

Theme: General adult psychiatry

Options:
a. Specific phobia
b. Adjustment disorder
c. Panic disorder
d. Generalized anxiety disorder
e. PTSD
f. Agoraphobia
g. Mixed anxiety/depression

Select the most appropriate answer for each of the following. Each option may be used once, more than once or not at all.

Question 135
A nurse was involved in a road traffic accident recently, about 3 months ago. Since then, she has been experiencing nightmare, flashbacks as well as irritable mood.

Question 136
A 21-year-old male has been recently enrolled into the military service and he has persistent low mood associated with loss of interest. He finds himself having much difficulty with coping with the demands of the military.

Question 137
A 23-year-old female finds that over the past 6 months she has been increasingly worried about everyday little things.

Theme: General adult psychiatry

Options:

  a. Hepatic encephalopathy
  b. Wilson's disease
  c. Hyperthyroidism
  d. Hypothyroidism
  e. Cushing's syndrome
  f. Addison's disease
  g. Syndrome of inappropriate anti-diuretic hormone hyper-secretion
  h. Hyperparathyroidism
  i. Hypoparathyroidism

Select the most appropriate answer for each of the following. Each option may be used once, more than once or not at all.

Question 138

Patients with this condition usually present with the disease during adolescence; however, the clinical onset may be detected as cognitive impairment, abnormal behaviour and personality change, and renal, haematological and endocrine symptoms.

Question 139

A 45-year-old female is no longer able to meet the demands of her job as she has been complaining of excessive tiredness, lethargy as well as constipation. She has no previous known medical history and has not been on long-term medications.

Question 140

A 25-year-old female has been feeling edgy quite recently and complaining that she has lost a huge amount of weight despite her good appetite.

Question 141

A 23-year-old female has long-standing irregular menses, and now presents with gradually worsening hirsutism and weight gain. She also has been having acnes on her face and feeling depressed.

Question 142

A 25-year-old female presents with weakness, dizziness, anorexia, weight loss and gastrointestinal disturbance. On physical examination, there is noted to be generalized hyper-pigmentation of the skin and mucous membrane. She also has postural hypotension and loss of pubic hairs.

Theme: Diagnostic classification

Options:

  a. Paranoid schizophrenia
  b. Hebephrenic schizophrenia
  c. Catatonic schizophrenia
  d. Undifferentiated schizophrenia
  e. Residual schizophrenia
  f. Simple schizophrenia

Select the most appropriate answer for each of the following. Each option may be used once, more than once or not at all.

Question 143
Based on the ICD-10, this is the most common subtype in which hallucinations and/or delusions are prominent.

Question 144
Based on the ICD-10, the age of onset of this condition is between 15 and 25 years. This particular subtype has been known to be associated with a poor prognosis.

Question 145
Based on the ICD-10 classification system, in this particular form of schizophrenia, psychomotor disturbances may alternate between extremes and violent excitement may occur.

Question 146
Based on the ICD-10 classification system, for individuals with this condition, there is an insidious onset of decline in functioning.

Question 147
In order to make this diagnosis, there must be the absence of depression, institutionalization or dementia or other brain disorders.

Theme: General adult psychiatry
Options:
  a. 20%
  b. 40%
  c. 60%
  d. 80%
  e. 85%
  f. 90%

Select the most appropriate answer for each of the following. Each option may be used once, more than once or not at all.

Question 148
For schizophrenia, the heritability estimate is around this value.

Question 149
For depressive disorder, the heritability estimate is around this value.

Question 150
For bipolar disorder, the heritability estimate is around this value.

Question 151
For panic disorders, the heritability estimate is around this value.

Theme: Basic psychopathology

Options:

a. Stupor
b. Depressive retardation
c. Obsessional slowness
d. Somnambulism
e. Compulsion
f. Psychomotor agitation
g. Ambitendency
h. Catalepsy
i. Cataplexy

Select the most appropriate answer for each of the following. Each option may be used once, more than once or not at all.

Question 152
In individuals with narcolepsy, this refers to the temporary loss of muscle tone.

Question 153
Patients with this psychopathology would make a series of tentative incomplete movements when expected to carry out a voluntary action.

Question 154
Patients with this psychopathology would maintain abnormal postures.

Question 155
Individuals with this psychopathology embark on a series of behaviours when they are asleep.

Question 156
This form of psychopathology is commonly referred to as the motor component of an obsessive thought.

Question 157
This form of psychopathology commonly refers to repeated doubts and compulsive rituals.

Question 158
This form of psychopathology might be seen in catatonic states, depressive states or even manic states.

Theme: Basic psychopathology

Amnesia refers to the inability to recall previous experiences.

Options:

a. Anterograde amnesia
b. Post-traumatic amnesia
c. Psychogenic amnesia
d. Retrograde amnesia
e. Transient global amnesia

f. Hypermnesia
g. Paramnesia

Select the most appropriate answer for each of the following. Each option may be used once, more than once or not at all.

Question 159

A 25-year-old male has just undergone six cycles of electroconvulsive therapy. He claimed to be having problems with his memories – forming new memories as well as recalling old memories. Which terminology correctly describes the pathology that James is experiencing?

Question 160

A 40-year-old male has just been involved in a major car accident. He lost consciousness immediately after the collision. He finds himself having major difficulties recollecting what has happened. Which terminology correctly describes the pathology that Tom is experiencing?

Question 161

A medical student was clerking a psychiatric inpatient, John. He realized that John was unable to recollect his own personal information, but appeared unconcerned about his memory loss. Which terminology best describes this psychopathology?

Question 162

A 25-year-old female's family members brought her into the emergency services. They were concerned about her having a sudden onset of disorientation and being unable to recollect immediate events. Which terminology best describes this psychopathology?

Question 163

A 28-year-old has been a chronic alcoholic. A medical student was assessing his memory and found that Thomas was confabulating at times. Which terminology best describes this psychopathology?

Theme: Neurology

Options:
a. Receptive aphasia
b. Agnostic alexia
c. Pure word deafness
d. Intermediate aphasia
e. Expressive aphasia
f. Global aphasia
g. Jargon aphasia
h. Semantic aphasia

Select the most appropriate answer for each of the following. Each option may be used once, more than once or not at all.

Question 164

In this condition, the person may have difficulties with naming objects or arranging words in the right sequences. Which condition is this?

Question 165

In this condition, the person may have difficulties with comprehending the meaning of words. Which condition is this?

Question 166

In this condition, the person may have difficulties in expressing thoughts in words but comprehension is normal. Which condition is this?

Question 167

In this condition, the person may have difficulties in expressing thoughts in words and also comprehending words. Which condition is this?

Theme: Basic psychology

Learning is defined as a change in behaviour as a result of prior experience. It does not include behavioural change due to maturation or other temporary conditions, such as that mediated by drug effects or fatigue. Two forms of learning have been recognized, which are classical conditioning and operant conditioning.

Options:
 a. Delayed conditioning
 b. Simultaneous conditioning
 c. Trace conditioning
 d. Backward conditioning
 e. Higher-order conditioning
 f. Extinction
 g. Generalization
 h. Discrimination
 i. Incubation
 j. Stimulus preparedness

Select the most appropriate answer for each of the following. Each option may be used once, more than once or not at all.

Question 168

This refers to the gradual increment in the strength of the condition response.

Question 169

This refers to a process whereby a response initially evoked by one stimulus could now be evoked by stimulus similar to the original.

Question 170

This refers to a process in which a conditioned stimulus is being paired with a second or third conditioned stimulus which, on presentation by itself, would elicit the original conditioned response.

Question 171

In this form of learning or conditioning, it has been noted that the learning and conditioning becomes less effective as the time interval between the two increases.

Question 172
This process of learning is considered to be optimal when the delay between the onsets of the two stimuli is around half a second.

Theme: Stages of development

Options:
a. Oral stage
b. Anal stage
c. Phallic stage
d. Latency stage
e. Genital stage
f. Trust/security
g. Autonomy
h. Initiative
i. Duty/accomplishment
j. Identity
k. Intimacy
l. Generativity
m. Integrity

Select the most appropriate answer for each of the following. Each option may be used once, more than once or not at all.

Question 173
The failure to negotiate this stage leads to hysterical personality traits.

Question 174
The failure to negotiate this stage leads to personality traits such as obsessive-compulsive personality, tidiness and rigidity.

Question 175
The failure to negotiate this stage might lead to generosity, depression and elation.

Question 176
Which of the aforementioned Erikson's stages is a 5-year-old child undergoing?

Theme: Social psychology

Options:
a. Autocratic
b. Democratic
c. Laissez-faire
d. Authority power
e. Reward power
f. Coercive power
g. Referent power
h. Expert power

Select the most appropriate answer for each of the following. Each option may be used once, more than once or not at all.

Question 177
Which of the aforementioned Erikson's stages is a teenager undergoing?

Question 178
This particular type of leadership is more appropriate for creative and open-ended tasks.

Question 179
For this particular type of leadership, there is a tendency for the tasks to be abandoned in the absence of the leader.

Question 180
This refers to the power derived from assignment to a specific role.

Question 181
This refers to the power derived from the ability to allocate resources.

Question 182
This refers to the power derived from skill, knowledge and experience.

Theme: Models of cognitive development

Options:
- a. Sensorimotor
- b. Preoperational
- c. Concrete operational
- d. Formal operational

Select the most appropriate answer for each of the following. Each option may be used once, more than once or not at all.

Question 183
Animism, in which life, thoughts and feelings are attributed to all objects, including inanimate ones, commonly develops during this stage.

Question 184
Primary, secondary and tertiary circular reactions develop during this stage.

Question 185
This is the stage that is characterized by the achievement of being able to think in the abstract.

Question 186
This is the stage in which an understanding of the laws of conservation, number and volume and then weight is normally achieved.

Theme: Psychological test

Options:
- a. Mini Mental State Examination
- b. Blessed Dementia Scale
- c. Geriatric Mental State Schedule

d. Cambridge Examination for Mental Disorders
e. Clifton Assessment Schedule
f. Present Behavioural Examination

Select the most appropriate answer for each of the following. Each option may be used once, more than once or not at all.

Question 187
This particular questionnaire is administered to a relative or friend who is asked to answer the questions on the basis of performance over the previous 6 months.

Question 188
This is an interview schedule that has three components: a structured clinical interview, a range of objective cognitive tests and a structured interview with a relative or informant.

Question 189
Amongst all of the options, this is considered to be a nursing-rated assessment.

Question 190
This particular questionnaire involves interviewing the carer more about the psychopathology associated with dementia.

Theme: Social sciences and stigma
Options:
  a. Death of spouse
  b. Divorce
  c. Marital separation
  d. Death of a close family member
  e. Marriage
  f. Pregnancy
  g. Minor legal violation

Select the most appropriate answer for each of the following. Each option may be used once, more than once or not at all.

Question 191
Which one of the aforementioned has the highest life change value based on the Holmes and Rahe (1967) life-change scale?

Question 192
Which one of the aforementioned has the second highest life-change value based on the Holmes and Rahe (1967) life-change scale?

Question 193
Which one of the aforementioned has a life-change value of approximately 50 based on the Holmes and Rahe (1967) life-change scale?

Question 194
Which one of the aforementioned has the lowest life-change value?

GET THROUGH MRCPSYCH PAPER A1: MOCK EXAMINATION

Question 1 Answer: b, Having poorly controlled blood pressure
Explanation: Hypertension has been known to be the most frequent risk factor among those with vascular dementia, and it contributes to as much as 50% of all patients with vascular dementia. Other risk factors known to increase the risk of stroke also increase the risk of vascular dementia, for example cigarette smoking, heart disease, homocystinuria, hyperlipidaemia, metabolic syndrome, low levels of high-density lipoprotein, moderate alcohol consumption, polycythaemia and sickle cell anaemia.

Reference: Puri BK, Hall A, Ho R (2014). *Revision Notes in Psychiatry*. London: CRC Press, p. 699.

Question 2 Answer: a, Low dose of aspirin daily
Explanation: The National Institute for Health and Care Excellence (NICE) guidelines do not recommend the usage of acetylcholinesterase inhibitors (AChEIs) or memantine for cognitive decline in vascular dementia. It is better to try to treat the underlying cardiovascular condition in order to slow down or even halt the progression of vascular dementia. The treatment of hypertension is particularly important. The common risk factors associated with the increased risk of stroke include homocystinuria, hyperlipidaemia, metabolic syndrome, low levels of high-density lipoprotein, moderate alcohol consumption, polycythaemia and sickle cell anaemia.

Reference: Puri BK, Hall A, Ho R (2014). *Revision Notes in Psychiatry*. London: CRC Press, p. 696.

Question 3 Answer: b, Approximately one half of the variance in drinking habits has been estimated to be genetic in origin for normal twins.
Explanation: (b) is wrong. It has been found that in normal twins, approximately one-third of the variance in the drinking habits have been estimated to be genetic in origin. Adoption studies do support the hypothesis of the genetic transmission of alcoholism. The sons of alcoholic parents are three to four times more likely

to become alcoholic than the sons of non-alcoholics, irrespective of the home environment.

Reference: Puri BK, Hall A, Ho R (2014). *Revision Notes in Psychiatry*. London: CRC Press, p. 520.

Question 4 Answer: a, Psychiatrists now have a responsibility to inform and protect third parties who are at risk from their patients.

Explanation: The duty to warn and protect follow Tarasoff's ruling. The duty to warn and protect is indicated when there are sufficient factual grounds for a high risk of harm to a third party, and the risk is sufficiently specified; the risk of danger to the public is imminent; the harm to a third party is not likely to be prevented unless the mental health professionals could make a disclosure; and the third party cannot reasonably be expected to foresee or comprehend the high risk of harm to himself or herself.

Reference: Puri BK, Hall A, Ho R (2014). *Revision Notes in Psychiatry*. London: CRC Press, p. 147.

Question 5 Answer: e, Narcissism

Explanation: Melanie Klein proposed all of the following concepts: object relations, paranoid-schizoid position, aggression and depressive position, and also proposed that the ego and superego developed during the first year of life. Klein believed that the infant was capable of object relations. The paranoid-schizoid position developed as a result of frustration during the first year of life with pleasurable contact with objects such as the good breast. The paranoid-schizoid position, characterized by isolation and persecutory fears, developed as a result of the infant viewing the world as part objects, using the following defence mechanisms: introjection, projective identification and splitting.

Reference: Puri BK, Hall A, Ho R (2014). *Revision Notes in Psychiatry*. London: CRC Press, p. 135.

Question 6 Answer: b, Information from the patients are used as a guide in scoring.

Explanation: The Present State Examination does not use information from patients as a guide in scoring. The Present State Examination has been previously used in the international pilot study of schizophrenia to generate diagnosis.

Reference: Puri BK, Hall A, Ho R (2014). *Revision Notes in Psychiatry*. London: CRC Press, pp. 353–460.

Question 7 Answer: a, Identification of dementia in the elderly

Explanation: The Clifton Assessment Procedures for the Elderly (CAPE) is commonly used to help predict survival, placement and decline in elderly people. The Kew Cognitive Map assesses for parietal lobe function and language functions in the dementing patient. This would help to predict the 6-month survival rates.

Reference: Puri BK, Hall A, Ho R (2014). *Revision Notes in Psychiatry*. London: CRC Press, p. 687.

Question 8 Answer: e, Validation
Explanation: This is an example of validation, which confirms the validity of a prior judgement or behaviour. Another example: 'I just say, if I were in your position, I might have a hard time dealing with those difficult people in your company'.

Reference: Puri BK, Hall A, Ho R (2014). *Revision Notes in Psychiatry*. London: CRC Press, p. 330.

Question 9 Answer: b, There is a clear figure-ground differentiation and distinction.
Explanation: The concept of Gestalt psychology states that the whole perception is different from the sum of its parts. The law of simplicity states that the percept corresponds to the simplest stimulation interpretation. The law of continuity states that interrupted lines are usually seen as continuous. The law of similarity states that like items are usually grouped together. The law of proximity states that adjacent items are grouped together. In figure-ground differentiation, figures are differentiated from their background with contours and boundaries.

Reference: Puri BK, Hall A, Ho R (2014). *Revision Notes in Psychiatry*. London: CRC Press, p. 31.

Question 10 Answer: a, The delusions must be present for more than 3 months in duration.
Explanation: Based on the 10th Revision of *International Classification of Disease* (ICD-10) diagnostic criteria, a delusional disorder is an ill-defined condition, manifesting as a single delusion or a set of related delusions, being persistent, sometimes lifelong and not having an identifiable organic basis. Delusions should be the most conspicuous or only symptom and they should be present for the past 3 months.

Reference: Puri BK, Hall A, Ho R (2014). *Revision Notes in Psychiatry*. London: CRC Press, p. 372.

Question 11 Answer: c, Voices commanding the patient
Explanation: Schneider was the one who proposed the concept of first-rank symptoms. It would include (a) auditory hallucinations – thought echo, in third person or in the form of a running commentary; (b) delusions of passivity – thought insertion, withdrawal, broadcasting, made feelings, impulses and action; (c) somatic passivity and delusional perception. The presence of the aforementioned first-rank symptom makes the diagnosis of schizophrenia highly likely.

Reference: Puri BK, Hall A, Ho R (2014). *Revision Notes in Psychiatry*. London: CRC Press, p. 351.

Question 12 Answer: a, His employees are known to have specialized knowledge of their tasks and could function by themselves independently.
Explanation: For laissez-faire leadership to be effective, it is expected that employees should have specialized knowledge in their tasks and are able to function independently.

Reference: Puri BK, Hall A, Ho R (2014). *Revision Notes in Psychiatry*. London: CRC Press, p. 59.

Question 13 Answer: c, Four times
Explanation: It is essential to note that genetic factors do account for disease only in some patients. In particular, genes such as the *APP* gene on chromosome 21, the Presenilin 1 gene on chromosome 14 and the Presenilin 2 gene on chromosome 1 have been found to be involved. Those who inherit just one allele on ApoE4 would have a two times increased incidence. In this case, given that the individual is a heterozygote, the estimated increased incidence is four times.

Reference: Puri BK, Hall A, Ho R (2014). *Revision Notes in Psychiatry*. London: CRC Press, p. 694.

Question 14 Answer: e, Presence of new members needing guidance from superiors.
Explanation: Self-reliant, intelligent, expressive and socially effective individuals are least vulnerable to group pressure. In addition, two types of conformity have been identified previously. Informational social influence refers to how an individual conforms to the consensual opinion and behaviour of the group both publicly and also in his or her own thoughts. Normative social influence refers to situations in which an individual publicly conforms to the consensual opinion and behaviour of the group, but has a different view in his or her own mind. The individual conforms to the group under social pressure in order to avoid social rejection.

Reference: Puri BK, Hall A, Ho R (2014). *Revision Notes in Psychiatry*. London: CRC Press, p. 60.

Question 15 Answer: e, The ICD-10 takes into account social functioning when establishing a diagnosis.
Explanation: The *Diagnostic and Statistical Manual of Mental Disorders*, 4th Edition, Text Revision (DSM-IV-TR) but not the ICD-10 takes into account social functioning when establishing a diagnosis.

Reference: World Health Organisation (1994). ICD-10 *Classification of Mental and Behavioural Disorders*. Edinburgh, UK: Churchill Livingstone.

Question 16 Answer: a, Avoidant attachment
Explanation: This is an example of an avoidant attachment style. When a child has this form of attachment, a distance is maintained usually from the mother, in

which case the child may sometimes feel ignored. Clinically, avoidant attachment caused by rejection by the mother may be a precursor to future poor social functioning. It might also predict aggression later in life. In contrast, for insecure attachment, there is chronic clinginess and ambivalence towards the mother. Separation anxiety refers to the fear shown by an infant of being separated from his or her caregiver.

Reference: Puri BK, Hall A, Ho R (2014). *Revision Notes in Psychiatry*. London: CRC Press, p. 64.

Question 17 Answer: a, Concrete operational
Explanation: The child is likely to be in the concrete operational stage. This is the third stage of development and usually occurs from the age of 7 years to around 12–14 years of age. During this stage, it is noted that the child is able to demonstrate and use logical thought processes and also make subjective moral judgments. In addition, he is also able to understand the laws of conservation, initially usually of number and volume and then weight.

Reference: Puri BK, Hall A, Ho R (2014). *Revision Notes in Psychiatry*. London: CRC Press, p. 68.

Question 18 Answer: b, Constant babbling at 7 months
Explanation: Tertiary circular reaction (part of sensorimotor stage, Piaget's cognitive model) occurs at 12–18 months. Development of colour vision occurs at 4–5 months. Development of fear of darkness occurs at 8–11 months. Preoperational stage (Piaget's cognitive model) occurs at 2 years.

Further Reading: Puri BK, Treasaden I (eds) (2010). *Psychiatry: An Evidence-Based Text*. London: Hodder Arnold, pp. 119–120, 280–281.

Question 19 Answer: a, Baseline attitudinal perceptions
Explanation: According to the theory on cognitive dissonance, discomfort will occur when two or more cognitions are held but are inconsistent with each other. The individual will be motivated to achieve cognitive consistency and may change one or more of these cognitions. Based on the attitude-discrepant theory, when the attitude and the behaviour are inconsistent, alteration of the attitude helps to bring about cognitive consistency.

Reference: Puri BK, Hall A, Ho R (2014). *Revision Notes in Psychiatry*. London: CRC Press, p. 52.

Question 20 Answer: a, Beauchamp and Childress
Explanation: Rush proposed less confining treatment in the United States. Laing was a psychiatrist who came to hold anti-psychiatry views. He was the author of *The Divided Self*. He saw schizophrenia as a sane response to an insane society. Percival established a code of ethics for Manchester Infirmary.

Szasz was both a professor of psychiatry and a leading proponent of anti-psychiatry. He identified psychiatrists as agents of social control. He also believed that it was unethical to restrict a patient's actions without his consent.

References: Musto DF (1998). A historical perspective, in Bloch S, Chodoff P, Green SA (eds), *Psychiatric Ethics* (3rd edition). Oxford, UK: Oxford University Press; Johnstone EC, Cunningham ODG, Lawrie SM, Sharpe M, Freeman CPL (2004). *Companion to Psychiatric Studies* (7th edition). London: Churchill Livingstone.

Question 21 Answer: b, Two times increased risk

Explanation: Cannabis does lead to a twofold increase in the associated risk of developing schizophrenia. It also leads to a fourfold increase in the associated risk of psychosis. It is important to note that not all cannabis users develop schizophrenia. It depends on the catechol-O-methyltransferase (COMT) genotype. People who have homozygous VAL/VAL alleles in the COMT genotype have a relatively higher risk. The usage of cannabis causes amotivational syndrome, flashback phenomena, changes in affect and heart rate, red eyes, motor incoordination, poor concentration and memory problems.

Reference: Puri BK, Hall A, Ho R (2014). *Revision Notes in Psychiatry*. London: CRC Press, p. 361.

Question 22 Answer: a, Frontal lobe

Explanation: The Wisconsin card sorting task is one of the neuropsychological assessment tests of frontal lobe function. Patients are usually given a pack of cards with symbols on them, which differ in form, colour and numbers. Four stimulus cards are available and the patient has to place each response card in front of one of the four stimulus cards. The person is required during the assessment to shift the set from one type of stimulus response to another as indicated by the psychologist.

Reference: Puri BK, Hall A, Ho R (2014). *Revision Notes in Psychiatry*. London: CRC Press, p. 111.

Question 23 Answer: e, Severe

Explanation: In severe mental intellectual disability, the intelligence quotient (IQ) score range is between 20 and 34. It accounts for 3% of all learning disabilities. There would be more marked motor impairment than that in moderate mental retardation, and achievements are at the lower end compared with that in moderate mental retardation. Moderate mental retardation refers to an IQ range of between 35 and 49. There would still be language use and development, and individuals could at least do simple practical work and live independently.

Reference: Puri BK, Hall A, Ho R (2014). *Revision Notes in Psychiatry*. London: CRC Press, p. 663.

Question 24 Answer: b, Disorganized schizophrenia
Explanation: The ICD-10 only includes the following subtypes for schizophrenia: paranoid, hebephrenic, catatonic, undifferentiated and residual. Paranoid schizophrenia is the commonest type with prominent hallucinations and delusions. Hebephrenic schizophrenia is associated with poor prognosis and characterized by marked affective changes. In catatonic schizophrenia, one or more of the following behaviours might be present: stupor, excitement, posturing, negativism, rigidity, waxy flexibility, command automatism and perseveration of words or phrases. For simple schizophrenia, there is an insidious onset of decline in functioning. Disorganized schizophrenia is named as hebephrenic schizophrenia in ICD-10.

Reference: Puri BK, Hall A, Ho R (2014). *Revision Notes in Psychiatry*. London: CRC Press, p. 353.

Question 25 Answer: e, Lewy body dementia
Explanation: The clinical features of Lewy body dementia usually include the following: (1) enduring and progressive cognitive impairment with impairments in consciousness, alertness and attention; (2) apathy, depression, hallucinations (usually complex visual hallucinations, 80%, and auditory hallucinations, 20%) and delusions (65%); (3) extrapyramidal signs and Parkinsonism; (4) neuroleptic sensitivity, falls, syncope and spontaneous loss of consciousness.

Reference: Puri BK, Hall A, Ho R (2014). *Revision Notes in Psychiatry*. London: CRC Press, p. 702.

Question 26 Answer: b, Absence of significant weight loss
Explanation: Based on the *Diagnostic and Statistical Manual of Mental Disorders, 5th Edition (DSM-5)* diagnostic criteria, in atypical anorexia nervosa, there is no significant weight loss but other criteria must be met. The DSM-5 states that for anorexia nervosa, there is restriction of energy and food intake, thus leading to a significantly low body weight in the context of age, sex, development and health status. Significantly low weight is defined as weight that is less than minimally normal. DSM-5 does not specify the percentage of weight loss (i.e. more than 15%) as in DSM-IV-TR. There must also be the presence of intense fear of weight gain or persistent behaviour that interferes with weight gain, even though the weight is significantly low. Body image disturbance is present, and this is a result of repetitive self-evaluation and poor insight of low body weight.

Reference: Puri BK, Hall A, Ho R (2014). *Revision Notes in Psychiatry*. London: CRC Press, p. 589.

Question 27 Answer: d, Prosopagnosia
Explanation: This refers to an inability to recognize faces. Associated with this is what is commonly known as the mirror sign, which may occur in advanced Alzheimer's disease, in which a person may misidentify his or her own mirrored

reflection. Agnosia is defined as the inability to interpret and recognize the significance of sensory information, which does not result from impairment of the sensory pathways, mental deterioration, disorders of consciousness and attention, or in the case of an object, a lack of familiarity with the object.

Reference: Puri BK, Hall A, Ho R (2014). *Revision Notes in Psychiatry*. London: CRC Press, p. 12.

Question 28 Answer: d, 0.10

Explanation: It has been estimated that around 10% of patients with schizophrenia commit suicide. For those who have been recently afflicted with the disorder, it usually happens early in this illness course. Suicide is more likely in the following cases: being male, being young, being unemployed, having chronic illness, relapses and remission, having a high educational attainment prior to onset, abrupt discontinuation of medications and recent discharge from inpatient care.

Reference: Puri BK, Hall A, Ho R (2014). *Revision Notes in Psychiatry*. London: CRC Press, p. 370.

Question 29 Answer: e, Seventh nerve palsy

Explanation: The seventh nerve, also known as the facial nerve, has the following components: the sensory component, the motor component and the autonomic component. None of them are responsible and will result in ptosis. The sensory component helps to detect taste on the anterior two-third of the tongue. The motor component is responsible for facial expression, elevation of the hyoid tension of stapes muscle and corneal reflex. The lesion affects reflex on the ipsilateral side of the face. The autonomic component would cause lacrimation and salivation from the sublingual and submandibular glands.

Reference: Puri BK, Hall A, Ho R (2014). *Revision Notes in Psychiatry*. London: CRC Press, p. 163.

Question 30 Answer: e, Rigidity

Explanation: Withdrawal symptoms might include that of somatic effects such as autonomic hyperactivity, malaise and weakness, tinnitus and grand mal convulsions. There are also cognitive effects with impaired memory and concentration as well as perceptual effects with hypersensitivity to sound, light and touch, besides depersonalization and de-realization. Delirium may develop within a week of cessation, and this is associated with visual, auditory, tactile hallucinations and delusions. It is also essential to note that the onset and intensity of withdrawal symptoms are related to the half-life of the drug used (shorter half-lives lead to a more abrupt and intense withdrawal syndrome). The withdrawal syndrome is also related to the dose used. Onset is usually within 1–14 days after drug reduction/cessation and may last for months.

Reference: Puri BK, Hall A, Ho R (2014). *Revision Notes in Psychiatry*. London: CRC Press, p. 548.

Question 31 Answer: c, Having an internal locus of control

Explanation: The following are psychosocial factors that are responsible for the development of post-traumatic stress disorder (PTSD). This includes female gender, low intelligence quotient at the age of 5 years, previous trauma history, previous psychiatric history: hyperactivity, anti-social behaviour, severity of trauma, perceived life threat, peri-traumatic dissociation, impaired social support and low socioeconomic status. Low education and social class, pre-existing psychiatric problems and female gender are vulnerability factors.

Reference: Puri BK, Hall A, Ho R (2014). *Revision Notes in Psychiatry*. London: CRC Press, p. 427.

Question 32 Answer: c, St. John's Wort

Explanation: It is an inducer of intestinal and hepatic CYP3A4, CYP2c and also intestinal P-glycoprotein, and the hyperforin content is responsible for this induction. According to several case reports, it could interact with other medicines, resulting in serious side effects. Some important drugs may be metabolized more rapidly and therefore become ineffective with serious consequences, for example, increased viral load in human immunodeficiency virus (HIV), failure or oral contraceptives leading to unwanted pregnancy and reduced anticoagulant effect with warfarin leading to thrombosis.

Reference: Taylor D, Paton C, Kapur S (2009). *The Maudsley Prescribing Guidelines* (10th edition). London: Informa Healthcare, p. 242.

Question 33 Answer: a, The onset of NMS is much more rapid as compared to serotonin syndrome.

Explanation: NMS is a life-threatening complication that can occur anytime during the course of antipsychotic treatment. The motor and behavioural symptoms include muscular rigidity and dystonia. The autonomic symptoms include high fever, sweating and increased pulse pressure and blood pressure. Laboratory findings include an increased white blood cell count and increased levels of creatinine phosphokinase. The symptoms usually evolve over 24–72 hours and, if not treated, would last for 10–14 days. Serotonin syndrome has a quicker rate of onset, in comparison.

Reference: Sadock BJ, Sadock VA (2008). *Kaplan and Sadock's Concise Textbook of Psychiatry* (3rd edition). Philadelphia, PA: Lippincott, Williams & Wilkins, p. 474.

Question 34 Answer: b, Checking things

Explanation: The most common compulsions are checking (60%), washing (50%) and counting (36%). Compulsions are defined as repetitive behaviours or mental acts in response to an obsession. The behaviours or mental acts are aimed at preventing or reducing anxiety or distress. Obsessions are defined as recurrent and intrusive thoughts, urges or images that cause marked anxiety or distress. Thus, an individual would resort to attempts to suppress such thoughts, urges or images or attempt to neutralize them using compulsive behaviour.

Reference: Puri BK, Hall A, Ho R (2014). *Revision Notes in Psychiatry*. London: CRC Press, p. 414.

Question 35 Answer: e, The onset of symptoms is usually within 2 weeks after experiencing the trauma.

Explanation: Based on the ICD-10 diagnostic criteria, PTSD arises within 6 months as a delayed and/or protracted response to a stressful event of an exceptionally threatening nature. The typical symptoms include that of repeated reliving of the trauma. Repetitive, intrusive memories (flashbacks), daytime imagery or dreams of the event must be present. Emotional detachment, persisting background numbness and avoidance of stimuli reminiscent of original event are often present, but not essential. Autonomic disturbances (hyper-arousal with hyper-vigilance, enhanced startle reaction and insomnia) and mood disorder contribute to the diagnosis but are not essential. Anxiety, depression and suicidal ideation are not common.

Reference: Puri BK, Hall A, Ho R (2014). *Revision Notes in Psychiatry*. London: CRC Press, p. 423.

Question 36 Answer: a, The principle of respect for a person's autonomy

Explanation: Although this man has a history of bipolar disorder, he has the capacity to make a decision. Hence, his autonomy is respected.

Reference: Puri BK, Treasaden I (eds) (2010). *Psychiatry: An Evidence-Based Text*. London: Hodder Arnold, p. 1231.

Question 37 Answer: d, Decreased in growth hormone

Explanation: The following are changes typically seen in anorexia nervosa. These included a decrease in T3, an increase in corticotrophin-releasing hormone (CRH), an increase in cortisol, an increase in growth hormone, a decrease in follicle-stimulating hormone (FSH), a decrease in luteinizing hormone (LH) and a decrease in oestrogen. The 24-hour pattern of secretion of LH resembles that normally seen in the pre-pubertal individuals. There might be a decrease in oestrogen in women or a decrease in testosterone in men. There are other abnormalities on the full blood count, in the electrolytes, in the arterial blood gas, in the renal and liver function tests as well as in the fasting blood. Radiological imaging such as computed tomography (CT) scan might show the presence of brain pseudo-atrophy, and the bone scan might reveal a reduction in bone mineral density.

Reference: Puri BK, Hall A, Ho R (2014). *Revision Notes in Psychiatry*. London: CRC Press, p. 579.

Question 38 Answer: c, Hypochondriasis

Explanation: In this case, the diagnosis would be hypochondriasis. Based on the ICD-10 diagnostic classification, there is a persistent belief of having at least one of several illness, despite the fact that multiple repeated investigations have not yielded anything of significance. The patient would not be amendable to the advice of different doctors that he has had previously consulted. Attention is usually focused on one or two organ systems only. Anxiety disorders such as generalized anxiety disorders, obsessive-compulsive disorder (OCD) and depressive disorder are common comorbidities. If depressive symptoms are prominent and precede the onset of hypochondriacal ideas, then depressive disorder may be primary.

Reference: Puri BK, Hall A, Ho R (2014). *Revision Notes in Psychiatry*. London: CRC Press, p. 471.

Question 39 Answer: d, Renal impairment
Explanation: Acamprosate, in combination with counselling, may be helpful in maintaining abstinence. It should be started as soon as possible after the achievement of abstinence. It should be maintained if a relapse occurs. An individual is only allowed to have one relapse while taking acamprosate. If there has been more than one relapse, the psychiatrist should advise the individual to stop the medication. The common side effects will include diarrhoea, nausea, rash, pruritus, bullous skin reactions and fluctuation in libido.

Reference: Puri BK, Hall A, Ho R (2014). *Revision Notes in Psychiatry*. London: CRC Press, p. 522.

Question 40 Answer: a, Continue the same dose of citalopram
Explanation: It would be the most appropriate to continue the current dose of citalopram as the medication has had some effect on the patient. The following are recommendations based on the NICE guidelines: If improvement is not noted with the first dose of antidepressant after 2–4 weeks, it is essential to check that the medication has been taken as prescribed. If the medication is taken as prescribed, then the dose could be titrated upwards. If there is improvement by 4 weeks, it is essential to continue the same treatment for another 2–4 weeks.

Reference: Puri BK, Hall A, Ho R (2014). *Revision Notes in Psychiatry*. London: CRC Press, p. 391.

Question 41 Answer: c, He reports that he has been sleeping more than usual to avoid thinking of the events.
Explanation: PTSD usually occurs within 6 months as a delayed response to an extremely stressful event. The symptoms that are typically experienced include repeated reliving of the trauma and repetitive, intrusive memories of the event. There might also be emotional detachment and avoidance of stimuli that are similar to the original event. There will also be autonomic disturbances such as hyper-arousal with hyper-vigilance. Patients usually present with insomnia.

Reference: Puri BK, Hall A, Ho R (2014). *Revision Notes in Psychiatry*. London: CRC Press, p. 427.

Question 42 Answer: c, Early ejaculation

Explanation: Early ejaculation or premature ejaculation is the most common disorder of the male sexual response. Studies with community samples indicate its prevalence to be around 36%–38%; 13% of attendees at a sexual disorder clinic presents with this problem. The ICD-10 diagnostic criteria state that premature ejaculation refers to the inability to delay ejaculation sufficiently to enjoy sexual intercourse. Ejaculation may occur in the absence of sufficient erection to make intercourse possible.

Reference: Puri BK, Hall A, Ho R (2014). *Revision Notes in Psychiatry*. London: CRC Press, p. 600.

Question 43 Answer: a, Clinical interview and examination

Explanation: A detailed clinical interview and examination is the most useful tool to help in the diagnosis of dementia. The following information should be assessed in a psychiatric interview for an old person: (1) description of the presenting complaints; (2) onset, frequency, intensity, duration and location; (3) antecedents and consequences; and (4) ameliorating and exacerbating factors.

Reference: Puri BK, Hall A, Ho R (2014). *Revision Notes in Psychiatry*. London: CRC Press, p. 687.

Question 44 Answer: d, Seligman

Explanation: Seligman found that dogs given unavoidable electric shocks suffered a number of phenomena, which he considered were similar to depression, such as reduced appetite, disturbed sleep and reduced sex drive. He called this learned helplessness. This is of importance as the cognitive theory of depression is based on this concept. Further studies have found that individuals who believe that they have no personal control over events are more likely to develop learned helplessness, whereas those who believe that nobody could have controlled the outcome are unlikely to do so. Hence, an individual's attribution of what is occurring would influence the likelihood of him developing major depression.

Reference: Puri BK, Hall A, Ho R (2014). *Revision Notes in Psychiatry*. London: CRC Press, p. 53.

Question 45 Answer: a, Countertransference

Explanation: The countertransference usually refers to the therapist's own feelings, emotions and attitudes towards his patient. In this case, the nurses are having countertransference towards the patient with borderline personality disorder. It is important to differentiate this from transference. Transference refers to an unconscious process in which the patient transfers to the therapist feelings, emotions and attitudes that were experienced and/or desired in the patient's childhood.

Reference: Puri BK, Hall A, Ho R (2014). *Revision Notes in Psychiatry*. London: CRC Press, p. 132.

Question 46 Answer: e, Risperidone

Explanation: Risperidone is the drug that causes the maximum elevation in the level of prolactin. This is due to the fact that dopamine would inhibit prolactin release, and hence dopamine antagonists can be expected to cause an increase in the plasma prolactin levels. Drugs such as clozapine, olanzapine, quetiapine and aripiprazole cause minimal change in the prolactin levels. Hyperprolactinaemia is often asymptomatic. However, persistent elevation in the plasma prolactin levels is associated with a number of adverse consequences. This might include sexual dysfunction, reductions in bone mineral density, menstrual disturbances, breast growth and galactorrhoea, suppression of the hypothalamic-pituitary-gonadal axis and a possible increase in the risk of breast cancer.

Reference: Taylor D, Paton C, Kapur S (2009). *The Maudsley Prescribing Guidelines* (10th edition). London: Informa Healthcare, p. 83.

Question 47 Answer: e, Hallucinations

Explanation: Ambivalence, autism, affective incongruity and disturbances of association of thoughts have been considered to be primary symptoms. He attributed hallucinations and delusions to be of secondary status.

Reference: Puri BK, Hall A, Ho R (2014). *Revision Notes in Psychiatry*. London: CRC Press, p. 351.

Question 48 Answer: e, Obsessive-compulsive personality disorder

Explanation: She is likely to have obsessive-compulsive personality disorder. Individuals with this disorder tend to have perfectionism that would interfere with completion of their tasks. In addition, they are extremely careful and are rigid and stubborn in their thinking. They also have excessive feelings of doubt and caution. Individuals with OCD usually present with clearly defined obsessions and compulsions. People with obsessive-compulsive personality disorder are more ego-syntonic with their behaviour, and hence they lend to be less anxious.

Reference: Puri BK, Hall A, Ho R (2014). *Revision Notes in Psychiatry*. London: CRC Press, p. 453.

Question 49 Answer: b, Usage of persuasive messages

Explanation: Attitudes can be modified either by central pathways, entailing the consideration of new information, or by peripheral pathways, involving the presentation of cues. In persuasive communication, the factors to be considered are concerned with those of the communicator, the recipient and also the message being communicated. It is key to note that message repetition can lead to a persuasive influence resulting in attitude change.

Reference: Puri BK, Hall A, Ho R (2014). *Revision Notes in Psychiatry*. London: CRC Press, p. 58.

Question 50 Answer: a, Anterograde memory loss
Explanation: Korsakoff's syndrome is an alcohol-induced amnestic disorder that is frequently preceded by Wernicke's encephalopathy. It has been described as an abnormal state in which memory and learning are affected out of proportion to the other cognitive functions in an otherwise alert and responsive patient. Clinical features would include retrograde amnesia, anterograde amnesia, sparing of immediate recall, disorientation to time, inability to recall the temporal sequence of events, confabulation and peripheral neuropathy.

Reference: Puri BK, Hall A, Ho R (2014). *Revision Notes in Psychiatry*. London: CRC Press, p. 513.

Question 51 Answer: b, Factitious disorder
Explanation: The diagnosis is that of factitious disorder. In this disorder, the patient intentionally produces the physical or psychological symptoms, but the patient is not conscious about his or her underlying motives. Common presenting signs might include bleeding, diarrhoea, hypoglycaemia, infection, impaired wound healing, vomiting, rashes and seizures. The patient often has poor prognosis and refuses to receive psychotherapy. Factitious disorder is different from malingering. In malingering, the patient intentionally produces physical or psychological symptoms and the patient is fully aware of his or her underlying motives. As a result, the patient does not want to cooperate for further assessment and evaluation due to the discrepancy between the severity of the symptoms reported and the objective physical findings revealed.

Reference: Puri BK, Hall A, Ho R (2014). *Revision Notes in Psychiatry*. London: CRC Press, p. 471.

Question 52 Answer: b, Made emotions
Explanation: Made emotions refer to the delusional belief that one's free will has been removed and an external agency is controlling one's feelings. Made impulse refers to the delusional belief that one's own free will has been removed and that an external agency is controlling one's impulses. Somatic passivity refers to the delusional belief that one is a passive recipient of somatic or bodily sensations from an external agency.

Reference: Puri BK, Hall A, Ho R (2014). *Revision Notes in Psychiatry*. London: CRC Press, p. 7.

Question 53 Answer: b, Thought broadcasting
Explanation: Thought broadcasting refers to the delusion that one's thought is no longer within one's own control, and that one's thoughts are being broadcast out loud so that others can freely access and understand. Thought broadcasting is a subset under thought alienation, in which the individual believes that his or her thoughts are under the control of an external agency or that others are participating in his or her thinking.

Reference and Further Readings: Puri BK, Hall A, Ho R (2014). *Revision Notes in Psychiatry*. London: CRC Press, p. 7; Sadock BJ, Sadock VA (2008). *Kaplan and Sadock's Concise Textbook of Psychiatry* (3rd edition). Philadelphia, PA: Lippincott, Williams & Wilkins, p. 31.

Question 54 Answer: b, Magnification

Explanation: Beck proposed the following cognitive triad in depressed patients. He stated that depressed patients tend to have a negative personal view, a tendency to interpret his or her on-going experience in a negative way and also a negative view of the future. Some of the common cognitive errors in depression include catastrophic thinking, dichotomous thinking, tunnel vision, selective abstraction, labelling, overgeneralization, personalization, should statements, magnification and minimization, arbitrary inference and emotional reasoning.

Reference: Puri BK, Hall A, Ho R (2014). *Revision Notes in Psychiatry*. London: CRC Press, p. 386.

Question 55 Answer: a, The feeling of 'as if'

Explanation: Depersonalization refers to a disturbance in the awareness of self-activity. In depersonalization, an individual might feel that he or she is altered or not real in some way. It also refers to the sensation of unreality concerning parts of oneself, or even one's environment, that occurs usually under extreme stress or fatigue. It is commonly seen in schizophrenia, depersonalization disorder, and also schizotypal personality disorder. This is in contrast to de-realization, to which the individual might feel that the surroundings do not appear real.

Reference and Further Readings: Puri BK, Hall A, Ho R (2014). *Revision Notes in Psychiatry*. London: CRC Press, p. 9; Sadock BJ, Sadock VA. (2008). *Kaplan and Sadock's Concise Textbook of Psychiatry* (3rd edition). Philadelphia, PA: Lippincott, Williams & Wilkins, p. 24.

Question 56 Answer: b, Long pause

Explanation: The husband has gone through a long difficult period by living with his wife and it is difficult to express his difficult feelings all at once. A long pause would be very helpful to give him a chance to organize his thoughts and facilitate the interview. Summation refers to a brief summary of what the person has said and this technique is irrelevant as he has not said much. Transition is a technique used gently to inform the person that the interview is moving on to another topic and it is irrelevant as the interview has not been progressing. Close-ended questions and prolonged eye contact would not facilitate a response from the husband.

Further Reading: Puri BK, Treasaden I (eds) (2010). *Psychiatry: An Evidence-Based Text*. London: Hodder Arnold, pp. 43, 75, 318–319, 1047–1048.

Question 57 Answer: c, Made impulse

Explanation: This is part of the passivity phenomenon. Made impulse refers to the delusional belief that one's free will has been removed and now is under the control of an external agency. In contrast, made actions refer to the delusional belief that one's own free will has been removed and an external agency is controlling one's actions. Made impulse is part of the passivity phenomenon. Other examples of passivity phenomenon includes thought alienation, made feelings, made actions and somatic passivity.

Reference: Puri BK, Hall A, Ho R (2014). *Revision Notes in Psychiatry*. London: CRC Press, p. 7.

Question 58 Answer: c, Delusional beliefs

Explanation: Ganser syndrome is considered and classified under dissociative disorders. It is known as a complex disorder, which is characterized by approximate answers and usually accompanied by several dissociative symptoms, often in circumstances that suggest psychogenic aetiology. The main features of Ganser syndrome include approximate answers, clouding of consciousness, somatic conversion, pseudo-hallucinations and subsequent amnesia.

Reference: Puri BK, Hall A, Ho R (2014). *Revision Notes in Psychiatry*. London: CRC Press, p. 434.

Question 59 Answer: d, He is having memory difficulties and hence is confabulating.

Explanation: He is likely to be having memory difficulties and is confabulating. In confabulation, the gaps in memory are being filled up with false memories. Confabulation is classified under paramnesia, which is a distorted recall thus leading to falsification of memory. Apart from confabulation, others include déjà vu, déjà entendu, déjà pense, jamais vu and retrospective falsification. Retrospective falsification refers instead to how false details are being added to the recollection of an otherwise real memory.

Reference: Puri BK, Hall A, Ho R (2014). *Revision Notes in Psychiatry*. London: CRC Press, p. 9.

Question 60 Answer: d, Synaesthesia

Explanation: Synaesthesia is commonly referred to as a condition in which a stimulation of one particular sensory modality leads to a perception of another sensation in a different sensory modality. A common example of this might be how a musical sound is being perceived as a colour instead. Extracampine hallucination refers to how a hallucination occurs outside an individual's sensory field. Functional hallucination refers to how the stimulus that is causing the hallucination is experienced in addition to the hallucination itself. Reflex hallucination is defined as a stimulus in one sensory field that leads to a hallucination in another sensory field. Visual hallucinations can be simple or complex in nature.

Reference and Further Readings: Sadock BJ, Sadock VA (2008). *Kaplan and Sadock's Concise Textbook of Psychiatry* (3rd edition). Philadelphia, PA: Lippincott, Williams & Wilkins, p. 31; Puri BK, Hall A, Ho R (2014). *Revision Notes in Psychiatry*. London: CRC Press, p. 8.

Question 61 Answer: a, Anxious avoidant personality disorder
Explanation: Individuals with anxious avoidant personality disorder usually avoid social or occupational activities that might involve significant interpersonal contact, as they are concerned about rejection and criticism. Based on the ICD-10 diagnostic criteria, they tend to have persistent and pervasive tension. They are unwilling to be involved with people unless they are certain of being liked. They have a restricted lifestyle due to the need for physical security. They tend to avoid social or occupational activities that involve significant interpersonal contact because of the fear of criticism, disapproval and rejection. They tend to believe that one is socially inept, personally unappealing and inferior as compared to others. They have excessive preoccupation with being criticized or rejected in social situations.

Reference: Puri BK, Hall A, Ho R (2014). *Revision Notes in Psychiatry*. London: CRC Press, p. 454.

Question 62 Answer: a, Automatic obedience
Explanation: Automatic obedience refers to a condition in which the person follows the examiner's instructions blindly without using his or her own judgement and resistance. For example, when the examiner asks the person to move his or her arm in a different direction and the individual is unable to resist doing it even if it is against his or her own will. Echopraxia refers to the automatic imitation by the individual of another person's movement. Stereotypies refer to repeated regular fixed patterns of movement (or even speech) that are not goal directed in nature.

Reference: Puri BK, Hall A, Ho R (2014). *Revision Notes in Psychiatry*. London: CRC Press, pp. 2–3.

Question 63 Answer: c, Nitrazepam
Explanation: Nitrazepam has the longest half-life and would not be suitable. The usual therapeutic dose is that of 5–10 mg per day, and the time to the onset of action is between 20 and 50 minutes. The guidelines recommend that short-acting hypnotics are better for people who have difficulty falling asleep, but it should be noted that tolerance and dependence would develop quite quickly. Long-acting hypnotics are more suitable for patients with frequent or early-morning awakening. However, it should be noted that for long-acting hypnotics, these drugs

could potentially cause much sedation the next day and there might be associated loss of coordination as well.

Reference: Taylor D, Paton C, Kapur S (2009). *The Maudsley Prescribing Guidelines* (10th edition). London, Informa Healthcare, p. 249.

Question 64 Answer: b, Opioid agonist
Explanation: Naltrexone is still not licensed to treat alcohol dependence in the United Kingdom due to the associated high risk of mortality after overdose and potential withdrawal associated with the usage of the medications. However, it could help people who are in abstinence from alcohol and who are highly motivated. It is known that the opioid receptors are responsible for reward and this would lead to increased craving. Naltrexone works by acting as an opioid antagonist. Hence, alcohol becomes less rewarding when those receptors are blocked.

Reference: Puri BK, Hall A, Ho R (2014). *Revision Notes in Psychiatry*. London: CRC Press, p. 526.

Question 65 Answer: a, Attention and concentration
Explanation: This is part of the Mini Mental State Examination and is largely a test of attention and concentration.

Reference: Puri BK, Hall A, Ho R (2014). *Revision Notes in Psychiatry*. London: CRC Press, p. 685.

Question 66 Answer: d, Anhedonia
Explanation: This is a complex syndrome that has been described by Ganser. It is characterized by approximate answers and usually accompanied by several dissociative symptoms, often in circumstances that suggest psychogenic aetiology. The five main core features of the syndrome include approximate answers, clouding of consciousness, somatic conversion, pseudo-hallucinations and subsequent amnesia. Ganser syndrome is classified as a dissociative disorder. Anhedonia refers to the loss in interest and withdrawal from activities that one usually enjoys.

Reference: Puri BK, Hall A, Ho R (2014). *Revision Notes in Psychiatry*. London: CRC Press, p. 434.

Question 67 Answer: b, Hebephrenic schizophrenia
Explanation: Amongst the various subtypes of schizophrenia, hebephrenic schizophrenia has been considered to have the worst prognosis. The age of onset is usually between 15 and 25 years. Affective changes are prominent. There might be fleeting and fragmentary delusions and hallucinations; irresponsible behaviour; fatuous, disorganized thought; rambling speech and mannerisms are common. Negative symptoms, particularly flattening of affect and loss of volition, are

common and prominent. Drive and determination are lost, goals are abandoned and behaviour becomes aimless and empty. The premorbid personality is usually shy and solitary.

Reference: Puri BK, Hall A, Ho R (2014). *Revision Notes in Psychiatry*. London: CRC Press, p. 353.

Question 68 Answer: d, Hypochondriasis
Explanation: The most likely clinical diagnosis is hypochondriasis. In this disorder, based on the ICD-10 classification system, there is a persistent belief in the presence of at least one serious physical illness, despite repeated investigations revealing no physical explanation of the presenting symptoms, or persistent preoccupation with presumed deformity. There is also persistent refusal to accept the advice of several different doctors that there is no physical illness underlying the symptoms.

Reference: Puri BK, Hall A, Ho R (2014). *Revision Notes in Psychiatry*. London: CRC Press, p. 471.

Question 69 Answer: b, Extracampine hallucination
Explanation: Extracampine hallucinations refer to hallucinations that occur outside of the person's sensory field, and this accounts for her experiences. Pseudo-hallucination refers to a form of imagery that arises from within the subjective inner space of the mind. Thought echo and thought broadcasting are both part of the thought alienation phenomenon, a passivity phenomenon.

Reference: Puri BK, Hall A, Ho R (2014). *Revision Notes in Psychiatry*. London: CRC Press, p. 8.

Question 70 Answer: a, Alexithymia
Explanation: This refers to the difficulty in the awareness of or description of one's emotion. Apathy refers to a loss of emotional tone and the ability to feel pleasure, associated with detachment or indifference. Dysphoria refers to the existence of an unpleasant mood. Euphoria refers to a personal or subjective feeling of unconcern and contentment, usually seen after taking opiates or as a late sequel to a head injury.

Reference: Puri BK, Hall A, Ho R (2014). *Revision Notes in Psychiatry*. London: CRC Press, p. 5.

Question 71 Answer: a, Acting out
Explanation: Acting out is not a mature defence mechanism. Acting out refers to the expression of unconscious emotional conflicts or feelings directly in actions without being consciously aware of their meaning. Sublimation refers to a process that utilizes the force of a sexual instinct in drives, affects and memories in order to motivate creative activities having no apparent connection with sexuality.

Reference: Puri BK, Hall A, Ho R (2014). *Revision Notes in Psychiatry*. London: CRC Press, p. 137.

Question 72 Answer: a, Acute stress disorder

Explanation: The diagnosis in this case is that of acute stress disorder. This is the diagnosis as the onset of symptoms is less than a month in duration. The diagnosis of an adjustment disorder is made when the onset is within 1 month of the stressor, and the duration is usually less than that of 6 months, except for prolonged depressive reaction.

Reference: Puri BK, Hall A, Ho R (2014). *Revision Notes in Psychiatry*. London: CRC Press, p. 432.

Question 73 Answer: c, Family therapy

Explanation: Psycho-educational family programmes to increase medication compliance and coping with stressors are successful in reducing the risk of relapse. Families with high EE were identified using the Camberwell Family Interview. Education and family sessions in the home run in parallel with a relative group. The programme is aimed at teaching problem-solving skills, lowering criticism and over-involvement, and reducing contact between patients while expanding social networks.

Reference: Puri BK, Hall A, Ho R (2014). *Revision Notes in Psychiatry*. London: CRC Press, p. 369.

Question 74 Answer: e, It refers to a bias made when inferring the cause of another's behaviour – bias made towards internal factors.

Explanation: Primary or fundamental attribution error is usually made when asked to infer the cause of another individual's behaviour. There is usually a bias towards dispositional rather than situational attribution.

Reference: Puri BK, Hall A, Ho R (2014). *Revision Notes in Psychiatry*. London: CRC Press, p. 59.

Question 75 Answer: d, Normal functioning

Explanation: If this man suffers from delusional disorder, his delusion is considered to be non-bizarre. Hence, he is expected to have normal functioning. The mean age of onset is 35 years for males and 45 years for females. The onset is gradual and unremitting in 62%. There might be a family history of psychiatric disorder but not of delusional disorder or schizophrenia.

Reference and Further Reading: Puri BK, Treasaden I (eds) (2010). *Psychiatry: An Evidence-Based Text*. London: Hodder Arnold, p. 677.

Question 76 Answer: b, Lorazepam

Explanation: Lorazepam would be the most appropriate medication to be given in this case. This is mainly because it has a short half-life with no active metabolites.

It is important to use low doses, as sedative drugs could potentially precipitate hepatic encephalopathy. Based on the NICE guidelines, both diazepam and chlordiazepoxide have marketing authorization for the management of acute alcohol withdrawal symptoms.

References: Puri BK, Hall A, Ho R (2014). *Revision Notes in Psychiatry*. London: CRC Press, p. 523; Taylor D, Paton C, Kapur S (2009). *The Maudsley Prescribing Guidelines* (11th edition). London: Informa Healthcare, p. 479.

Question 77 Answer: b, Learned helplessness

Explanation: Beck proposed a cognitive model from which cognitive therapy was developed. Based on the cognitive triad, the depressed person has a negative personal view, a tendency to interpret his or her ongoing experiences in a negative way and a negative view of the future. The proposed cognitive bias does not include that of learned helplessness. The common cognitive errors include that of catastrophic thinking, dichotomous thinking, tunnel vision, selective abstraction, labelling, overgeneralization, personalization, should statement, magnification, minimization, arbitrary inference and emotional reasoning.

Reference: Puri BK, Hall A, Ho R (2014). *Revision Notes in Psychiatry*. London: CRC Press, p. 384.

Question 78 Answer: d, Szasz

Explanation: Thomas Szasz (1930–2012), a prominent anti-psychiatrist, identified mental illness as problematic and somatic illnesses as unproblematic. In a society, bodily illness is a genuine illness, and genuine illness is defined as deviation from normal anatomy and physiology of a body organ. On the other hand, Szasz believed that mental illnesses are defined by deviation from social norms in terms of acceptable behaviours. Hence, mental illness is very different in its meaning and nature from a physical illness.

Reference: Puri BK, Hall A, Ho R (2014). *Revision Notes in Psychiatry*. London: CRC Press, p. 157.

Question 79 Answer: d, Mannerism

Explanation: Mannerisms are repeated involuntary movements that are goal-directed. An example would be 'A person repeatedly moving his hand when he talks and tries to convey his message to the examiner'. Stereotypy, on the other hand, refers to non-goal-directed repetitive movements (e.g. rocking forward and backward).

Reference and Further Reading: Rajagopal S (2007). Catatonia. *Advances in Psychiatric Treatment*, 13: 51–59.

Question 80 Answer: a, This usually occurs when members of the majority group tend to victimize members of the minority group simply out of frustration.
Explanation: Scapegoating usually involves members of a majority group targeting and displacing their aggression onto members of a minority group.

Reference: Ciccarelli SK, Meyer GE (2006). *Psychology*. Upper Saddle River, NJ: Pearson Education, p. 444.

Question 81 Answer: e, Restless leg syndrome (Ekbom's syndrome)
Explanation: Restless leg syndrome (Ekbom's syndrome) is an irresistible desire to move the legs when resting with unpleasant leg sensations. It is usually idiopathic. Secondary causes include iron deficiency, uraemia, pregnancy, diabetes, polyneuropathy and rheumatoid arthritis. Dopamine agonists and benzodiazepine such as clonazepam are commonly used for treatment. In psychiatry, Ekbom's syndrome also refers to delusional parasitosis.

Reference and Further Reading: Longmore M, Wilkinson I, Turmezei T, Cheung CK (2007). *Oxford Handbook of Clinical Medicine* (7th edition). Oxford, UK: Oxford University Press.

Question 82 Answer: c, Start her on propranolol
Explanation: This woman suffers from akathisia. Options (a)–(e) are recommended for the treatment of antipsychotic-induced akathisia. Propranolol is contraindicated in patients with asthma.

Reference and Further Reading: Taylor D, Paton C, Kapur S (2009). *The Maudsley Prescribing Guidelines* (10th edition). London: Inform Healthcare.

Question 83 Answer: b, Florid third-person auditory hallucinations
Explanation: Florid third-person auditory hallucinations do not support the diagnosis of simple schizophrenia in this case.

Reference and Further Reading: Puri BK, Treasaden I (eds) (2010). *Psychiatry: An Evidence-Based Text*. London: Hodder Arnold, pp. 593–609.

Question 84 Answer: c, Normal grief reaction
Explanation: This man suffers from normal grief reaction. Sadness, guilt and transient experience of hearing voices of the deceased are common among people with normal grief reaction. The accident occurred 3 months ago, and there is no evidence of prolonged grief. There is not enough clinical evidence to suggest that he suffers from post-traumatic stress disorder.

Reference and Further Reading: Puri BK, Treasaden I (eds) (2010). *Psychiatry: An Evidence-Based Text*. London: Hodder Arnold, pp. 811–817.

Question 85 Answer: d, Smoking

Explanation: Smoking is likely to affect the levels of his medication, as smoking would cause an induction of the CYP4501A2. This is mainly due to the polycyclic hydrocarbons that are present in the smoke itself. This particular enzyme is responsible for the metabolism of many of the common psychotropic drugs. Hence, smoking could thus result in a reduction in the blood levels of some drugs by as much as 50%. Some of the commonly affected drugs include clozapine, haloperidol, chlorpromazine, olanzapine, tricyclic antidepressants, mirtazapine, fluvoxamine and propranolol.

Reference: Taylor D, Paton C, Kapur S (2009). *The Maudsley Prescribing Guidelines* (10th edition). London: Informa Healthcare, p. 506.

Question 86 Answer: d, Distorted grief

Explanation: Distorted grief is associated with intense anger or guilt. The person may develop symptoms that the deceased had prior to death. Other signs of distorted grief are over-activity without a sense of loss hostility towards a specific person and taking self-destructive actions. Since the duration is only 6 months, he does not qualify for chronic grief. Conflicted grief refers to intense ambivalent feeling towards the deceased. Delayed grief refers to a bereaved person who does not show any grief reaction after the deceased person died but grief reaction only comes after a delayed period. Inhibited grief refers to some feelings towards the deceased, which is not expressed.

Question 87 Answer: e, Subconscious

Explanation: Disorders of self-awareness usually include disturbances to the awareness of self-activity, immediate awareness of self-unity, continuity of self and the boundaries of self. Disorders of self-awareness include depersonalization, which refers to the way one feels that one is altered or not real in some way, and de-realization, which refers to how the surroundings do not seem real.

Reference: Puri BK, Hall A, Ho R (2014). *Revision Notes in Psychiatry*. London: CRC Press, p. 9.

Question 88 Answer: d, 60%

Explanation: An old British study showed that approximately 60% of patients had been re-admitted at least once. Only 20% had recovered fully with no further episodes and 20% were incapacitated throughout or died of suicide.

Reference: Lee AS, Murray RM (1988). The long-term outcome of Maudsley depressives. *Br J Psychiatry*, 153: 741–751.

Question 89 Answer: b, Anchoring and adjustment heuristic

Explanation: In this experiment, participants knew that the speaker's position on the war was chosen at random, yet the speaker believed in what he had said. This is known as fundamental attribution error, defined as the tendency to overestimate the extent to which a person's behaviour is due to internal, dispositional factors and to underestimate the role of external, situational factors. The anchoring and adjustment heuristic is one explanation of fundamental attribution error. Participants use the speech as an initial 'anchor' to base their inference of the speaker's disposition. They then adjust their attributions to account for external, situational factors; this means that the position was chosen at random. Fundamental attribution error arises due to the tendency to insufficiently adjust the initial judgement or anchor.

Further Reading: Jones EE, Harris VA (1967). The attribution of attitudes. *Journal of Experimental Social Psychology*, 3: 1–24.

Question 90 Answer: e, Trustworthy team members who are experienced in community psychiatry and skilful in dealing with complicated issues. They require minimal supervision.
Explanation: This case refers to laissez-faire leadership. Option A is for democratic leadership. Option B applies to both autocratic and democratic leadership. Options C and D are suitable for autocratic leadership.

Further Reading: Puri BK, Treasaden I (eds) (2010). *Psychiatry: An Evidence-Based Text*. London: Hodder Arnold, pp. 292, 118.

Question 91 Answer: e, Patients with mania and hypomania are expected to have same level of psychosocial functioning.
Explanation: Patients with mania are expected to have a lower level of psychosocial functioning compared with patients with hypomania.

Reference and Further Reading: Puri BK, Treasaden I (eds) (2010). *Psychiatry: An Evidence-Based Text*. London: Hodder Arnold, pp. 610, 624–627.

Question 92 Answer: a, Debriefing
Explanation: Based on the NICE guidelines, with regards to the psychological treatment for PTSD, if the onset of the symptoms is less than 3 months after a trauma, it might be beneficial to offer trauma-focused psychological treatment. If the symptoms occur more than 3 months after a trauma, it might be better to offer trauma-focused psychological treatment, which might be trauma-focused cognitive-behavioural therapy (CBT) or eye movement desensitization and reprocessing (EMDR). Debriefing is a technique that is contraindicated for the management of PTSD.

Reference: Puri BK, Hall A, Ho R (2014). *Revision Notes in Psychiatry*. London: CRC Press, p. 424.

Question 93 Answer: d, Primacy effect
Explanation: Practice effect is the influence of test-taking performance due to prior exposure to a test. Practice effect usually results in improved scores.

Barnum effect is the tendency of people to endorse, as an accurate description of themselves. Halo effect is the influence of a positive or negative first impression on subsequent interpretations of a person's behaviour such that it is aligned with the first impression. Primacy and recency effects are the tendencies to remember information at the start and the end more accurately than information in the middle. This phenomenon is collectively known as serial position effect.

References and Further Readings: Collie A, Maruff P, Darby DG, McStephen M (2003). The effects of practice on the cognitive test performance of neurologically normal individuals assessed at brief test-retest intervals. *Journal of the International Neuropsychological Society*, 9: 419–428; Claridge G, Clark K, Powney E, Hassan E (2008). Schizotypy and the Barnum effect. *Personality and Individual Differences*, 44: 436–444; Puri BK, Treasaden I (eds) (2010). *Psychiatry: An Evidence-Based Text*. London: Hodder Arnold, p. 251.

Question 94 Answer: b, Astasia-abasia
Explanation: Her condition is catatonia. Clinical features of catatonia are all of the aforementioned options except astasia-abasia. Other signs of catatonia include stupor, posturing, negativism, stereotypy, mannerism, echolalia, echopraxia and logorrhoea. Causes of catatonia include schizophrenia, mood disorders, organic disorders (e.g. central nervous system [CNS] infection), epilepsy, recreational drugs (cocaine) and medications (ciprofloxacin). Astasia-abasia is a gait disturbance seen in conversion disorder.

Reference and Further Reading: Rajagopal S (2007). Catatonia. *Advances in Psychiatric Treatment*, 13: 51–59.

Question 95 Answer: d, Koro
Explanation: This condition is commonly referred to as Koro. It may occur in epidemic form. It involves the belief of genital retraction with disappearance into the abdomen and this is accompanied by intense anxiety and associated with fear of impending death. The development of Koro has been associated with psychosexual conflicts, personality factors and also cultural beliefs in the context of psychological stress. There have been cases of similar condition being described in non-Chinese subjects. In these cases, the syndrome is often only partial, such as the belief of genital shrinkage, not necessarily with retraction into the abdomen. It usually occurs within the context of another psychiatric disorder, and resolves once the underlying illness has been treated.

Reference: Puri BK, Hall A, Ho R (2014). *Revision Notes in Psychiatry*. London: CRC Press, p. 462.

Question 96 Answer: c, Insomnia
Explanation: Somatic symptoms of depression (e.g. sleep, appetite, energy and libido changes) are not reliable in establishing the diagnosis of depression in

antenatal period because non-depressed pregnant women also experience insomnia, poor appetite, nausea, tiredness and libido changes.

Reference and Further Reading: Puri BK, Treasaden I (eds) (2010). *Psychiatry: An Evidence-Based Text*. London: Hodder Arnold, pp. 715–732.

Question 97 Answer: a, Bupropion
Explanation: It would be recommended for the patient not to be started on bupropion due to the fact that it is contraindicated in seizure disorder. The guidelines state that most of the tricyclic antidepressants are epileptogenic, particularly at higher doses, as well as bupropion and hence should be avoided completely. If antidepressant treatment is necessary, moclobemide and selective serotonin reuptake inhibitors (SSRIs) are good choices. The use of mirtazapine, venlafaxine and duloxetine would require extra care.

Reference: Taylor D, Paton C, Kapur S (2009). *The Maudsley Prescribing Guidelines* (10th edition). London, Informa Healthcare, p. 421.

Question 98 Answer: b, Death of a spouse
Explanation: Death of a spouse is considered to be the most stressful event with 100 life change units (LCU), followed by divorce (73 LCU), marital separation (65 LCU), imprisonment (63 LCU) and death of a close family member (63 LCU).

Reference and Further Readings: Holmes TH, Rahe RH (1967). The Social Readjustment Rating Scale. *Journal of Psychosomatic Research*, 11: 213–218; Puri BK, Treasaden I (eds) (2010). *Psychiatry: An Evidence-Based Text*. London: Hodder Arnold, pp. 155–156; Puri BK, Treasaden I (eds) 2010: *Psychiatry: An Evidence-Based Text*. London: Hodder Arnold, pp. 309–318.

Question 99 Answer: d, Psychological pillow
Explanation: Psychological pillow is a feature of catatonia. The patient holds his or her head a few inches above the bed surface in a reclining posture, and is able to maintain this position for hours.

Reference and Further Reading: Rajagopal S (2007). Catatonia. *Advances in Psychiatric Treatment*, 13: 51–59.

Question 100 Answer: d, Punishment
Explanation: This phenomenon is punishment because it results in a reduction in behaviour. Punishment is any stimulus that is applied after a response and causes a weakening of that behaviour. Punishment is the opposite of reinforcement (both positive and negative). Reinforcement causes a strengthening of the behaviour, whereas punishment suppresses it. In negative reinforcement, an unpleasant stimulus is removed, hence resulting in an increased likelihood of the behaviour occurring again.

Reference and Further Reading: Puri BK, Treasaden I (eds) (2010). *Psychiatry: An Evidence-Based Text*. London: Hodder Arnold, pp. 200–205.

Question 101 Answer: b, The trial involved Japanese doctors who were deemed unethical.
Explanation: The code was developed by the war crimes tribunal against the Nazi German doctors and the main objective was to protect human subjects during experiment and research. An experiment should avoid suffering and injury. Experiments leading to death and disability should not be conducted. Proper preparations should be made to protect research subjects, and the experiments should be conducted by qualified personnel. During the experiment, the research subjects should have the liberty to withdraw at any time and the investigators should stop the experiments if continuation results in potential injury or death of research subjects. The design should be based on results obtained from animal experiments and natural history of the disease. Seeking consent from research subjects is absolutely necessary. Research should yield meaningful results for the good of mankind.

Reference: Puri BK, Hall A, Ho R (2014). *Revision Notes in Psychiatry*. London: CRC Press, p. 147.

Question 102 Answer: d, Operant conditioning
Explanation: Operant conditioning is the learning of voluntary behaviour (pressing the lever) through the effects of positive or negative consequences (obtaining food). This experiment is not an example of classical conditioning because classical conditioning involves involuntary or reflex responses.

Reference and Further Reading: Puri BK, Treasaden I (eds) (2010). *Psychiatry: An Evidence-Based Text*. London: Hodder Arnold, pp. 200–205.

Question 103 Answer: c, A critical evaluator
Explanation: Groupthink is a kind of thinking in which maintaining group cohesiveness and solidarity takes precedence over considering the facts in a realistic manner. This theory of group decision making was developed by Irving Janis. Antecedents to groupthink include options A and B. Option E is a symptom of groupthink. Mindguards are people who shield the group from contrary information. Irving Janis identified seven other symptoms of groupthink, which include illusion of unanimity, self-censorship and stereotyped views of out-group.

Groupthink style of decision making can be avoided by several methods, which include assigning each member the role of a critical evaluator, considering all alternatives and discussing ideas with external experts.

Reference and Further Reading: Aronson E, Wilson TD, Akert RM (2007). *Social Psychology*. Upper Saddle River, NJ: Prentice Hall, pp. 160–162.

Question 104 Answer: d, Erotomania

Explanation: The most likely clinical diagnosis is that of couvade syndrome. This refers to a form of delusion that another person, usually of higher status, might be deeply in love with the individual.

Reference: Puri BK, Hall A, Ho R (2014). *Revision Notes in Psychiatry*. London: CRC Press, p. 6.

Question 105 Answer: d, Legitimation

Explanation: Legitimation is a technique when the therapist allows the patient to describe his or her feelings and indicates to the patient that it is acceptable to feel the way he or she does.

Reference: Poole R, Higgo R (2006). *Psychiatric Interviewing and Assessment*. Cambridge, UK: Cambridge University Press.

Question 106 Answer: d, Usage of antidepressants

Explanation: Rapid cycling bipolar disorder refers to those individuals who have had experience with four or more affective episodes in the last 12 months. It is usually more common in women, and is predictive of poorer prognosis and poorer response to lithium and other treatments. It is known that as much as 20% are induced by antidepressants use. Antidepressants should be avoided and thyroid function tests should be performed 6-monthly. The NICE guidelines also recommend increasing the dose of the anti-manic drug or addition of lamotrigine. For long-term management, the NICE guidelines recommend a combination of lithium and valproate as first-line treatment. Lithium mono-therapy is the second-line treatment.

Reference: Puri BK, Hall A, Ho R (2014). *Revision Notes in Psychiatry*. London: CRC Press, p. 397.

Question 107 Answer: e, Windigo

Explanation: The culture-bound syndrome in this context is Windigo. It is most common amongst North American Indians and usually associated with depression, schizophrenia, hysteria and anxiety. It is a disorder in which the subject believes he or she has undergone a transformation and become a monster who practises cannibalism. It has been suggested that Windigo is in fact a local myth rather than an actual pattern of behaviour.

Reference: Puri BK, Hall A, Ho R (2014). *Revision Notes in Psychiatry*. London: CRC Press, p. 463.

Question 108 Answer: a, Therapeutic index

Explanation: Therapeutic index is the relative measure of the toxicity or safety of a drug and is usually defined as the ratio of the median toxic dose to the median effective dose. The median toxic dose is defined as the dose at which 50% of the patients would experience specific toxic effects. The median effective dose is defined as the dose at which 50% of the patients would have a specified therapeutic effect. A drug with a high therapeutic index implies that a wide range of dosages of the drug could be prescribed. Conversely, if the therapeutic index is low, closer monitoring of the prescribed medication would be essential.

Reference: Sadock BJ, Sadock VA (2008). *Kaplan and Sadock's Concise Textbook of Psychiatry* (3rd edition). Philadelphia, PA: Lippincott, Williams & Wilkins, p. 915.

Question 109 Answer: d, The reinforcement can occur before the behaviour.
Explanation: This phenomenon is known as operant conditioning, specifically negative reinforcement. Escape and avoidance learning are two examples of negative reinforcement. The removal of the unpleasant stimulus leads to reinforcement of the behaviour. In operant conditioning, the reinforcer (reduction in anxiety levels) is presented only after the behaviour (going home) is executed, which is why Option D is incorrect.

Reinforcements, both positive and negative, work to increase the frequency of the conditioned behaviour. In operant conditioning, this conditioned response is voluntary, whereas in classical conditioning, the conditioned response is involuntary (e.g. salivating in the Pavlov's dogs).

Reference and Further Reading: Puri BK, Treasaden I (eds) (2010). *Psychiatry: An Evidence-Based Text*. London: Hodder Arnold, pp. 200–205.

Question 110 Answer: d, Implosion cannot be used in extinction.
Explanation: Implosion is a behaviour technique used in the treatment of phobias, where the patient is exposed to the feared stimulus all at once, through imagination or visualization. Unlike flooding, implosion does not involve direct contact with the feared stimulus. Reciprocal inhibition is a technique used in systematic desensitization, where the antagonistic response to anxiety (i.e. relaxation) is maintained when the feared stimulus is presented. Shaping involves reinforcement of small approximations to achieve a desired behaviour. It has been used in reducing undesired behaviours such as cocaine addiction.

Reference and Further Readings: Puri BK, Treasaden I (eds) (2010). *Psychiatry: An Evidence-Based Text*. London: Hodder Arnold, pp. 199, 655, 990–991; Preston KL, Umbricht A, Wong CJ, Epstein DH (2001). Shaping cocaine abstinence by successive approximation. *Journal of Consulting Clinical Psychology*, 69: 643–654.

Question 111 Answer: b, Learned helplessness
Explanation: Learned helplessness does not contribute to the aetiology of phobias but can exacerbate the condition of a person with specific phobia. Vicarious conditioning is also known as observational learning. It involves the learning of fear responses by watching the reaction of another person. The concept of

preparedness suggests that fear of certain objects may be evolutionarily adaptive to increase survival and this would make phobias more difficult to treat.

Reference and Further Reading: Puri BK, Treasaden I (eds) (2010). *Psychiatry: An Evidence-Based Text*. London: Hodder Arnold, pp. 195–200, 206, 207, 654.

Question 112 Answer: e, The term 'schizophrenia' refers to the 'splitting' of affect from other psychological functions leading to a dissociation between the social situation and the emotion expressed.
Explanation: Eugene Bleuler proposed the term schizophrenia which refers to the 'splitting' of affect from other psychological functions leading to a dissociation between the social situation and the emotion expressed.

References and Further Readings: Charlton B (2000). *Psychiatry and the Human Condition*. Oxford, UK: Radcliffe Publishing; Shorter E (1997). *A History of Psychiatry*. New York: John Wiley & Sons; Puri BK, Treasaden I (eds) (2010). *Psychiatry: An Evidence-Based Text*. London: Hodder Arnold, pp. 11, 593, 614, 624.

Question 113 Answer: a, Ambitendency
Explanation: In this condition, the person makes a series of tentative incomplete movements when expected to carry out a voluntary action. For example, a woman offers a handshake, then withdraws, and then offers it again 10 times. The examiner cannot make a handshake with her at the end.

Reference: Puri BK, Hall A, Ho R (2014). *Revision Notes in Psychiatry*. London: CRC Press, p. 1.

Question 114 Answer: c, Occupation
Explanation: The determinants of social class include education, financial status, occupation, type of residence, geographic area of residence and leisure activities. In British psychiatry, the Office of Population Censuses and Surveys has traditionally based their classification using occupation. Social class I includes professional, higher managerial and landowners. Social class II includes those with intermediate skills. Social class III includes those who are skilled, or who are doing manual or clerical work. Social class IV includes those who are semiskilled. Social class Y refers to those who are unskilled. Social class 0 refers to those who are unemployed, or who are students.

Reference: Puri BK, Hall A, Ho R (2014). *Revision Notes in Psychiatry*. London: CRC Press, p. 115.

Extended matching items (EMIs)

Theme: Memory
Question 115 Answer: g, Retrograde memory
Explanation: Also known as retrograde amnesia, this refers to the loss of memory for events that occurred prior to an event or condition.

Question 116 Answer: b, Working memory
Explanation: His working memory or short-term memory is clearly affected. The anatomical correlate of auditory verbal short-term memory is the left dominant parietal lobe, while that of the visual verbal short-term memory is the left temporo-occipital area.

Question 117 Answer: c, Procedural memory
Explanation: This is also known as implicit memory. It is recalled automatically without much effort and is learned slowly through repetition. Its storage requires the functioning of the cerebellum, the amygdala, and specific sensory and motor systems used in the learned task.

Question 118 Answer: a, Declarative memory
Explanation: Declarative memory belongs to the subset of explicit memory. Declarative memory involves memory of autobiographical events.

Question 119 Answer: d, Episodic Memory
Explanation: Both declarative memory and episodic memory belong to the sub-set of explicit memory. It is possible to lose one type of memory while retaining the other. Episodic memories involve memories of autobiographical events.

Reference: Puri BK, Hall A, Ho R (2014). *Revision Notes in Psychiatry*. London: CRC Press, p. 103.

Theme: Lab tests
Question 120 Answer: d, 48 hours
Explanation: The length of time for detection of amphetamines in the urine is approximately 48 hours.

Question 121 Answer: c, 24 hours
Explanation: For short-acting barbiturates, the length of time for detection is approximately 24 hours. For long-acting ones, the length of time for detection is approximately 3 weeks.

Question 122 Answer: a, 6–8 hours
Explanation: The duration of detection of cocaine is approximately 6–8 hours.

Question 123 Answer: e, 36–72 hours
Explanation: The duration of detection of heroin is approximately 36–72 hours.

Question 124 Answer: b, 12–24 hours
Explanation: The duration of detection is 12–24 hours.

Question 125 Answer: d, 48 hours
Explanation: The duration of detection is 48 hours.

Question 126 Answer: g, 8 days
Explanation: It could be detected up until 8 days.

Theme: General psychiatry

Question 127 Answer: h, 35%–50%
Explanation: The estimated lifetime expectancy rate when both parents have schizophrenia has been estimated to be around 46%.

Question 128 Answer: c, 10%–14%
Explanation: In this case, given that only one parent has schizophrenia, the rate has been estimated to be around 13%.

Question 129 Answer: e, 20%–24%
Explanation: The estimated incidence should be around 23%. This is a condition that is caused by a micro-deletion in chromosome 22q11.2. More than 50% of patients have mild-to-moderate learning disability. In addition, there is an increased incidence of schizophrenia.

Question 130 Answer: a, 0%–4%
Explanation: The estimated increase in incidence for half-siblings is 4%.

Question 131 Answer: a, 0%–4%
Explanation: The risk of schizophrenia has been estimated to be around 2.4%.

Reference and Further Reading: Puri BK, Treasaden I (eds) (2010). *Psychiatry: An Evidence-Based Text*. London: Hodder Arnold, pp. 474–475, 597, 599.

Theme: Aetiology

Question 132 Answer: k, Streptococcal infection
Explanation: This patient suffers from paediatric autoimmune neuropsychiatric disorders associated with streptococcal infections (PANDAS).

Reference and Further Reading: Puri BK, Treasaden I (eds) (2010). *Psychiatry: An Evidence-Based Text*. London: Hodder Arnold, p. 551.

Question 133 Answer: d, Childhood sexual abuse
Explanation: This patient suffers from borderline personality disorder, and childhood sexual abuse is an important aetiological factor.

Reference and Further Reading: Puri BK, Treasaden I (eds) (2010). *Psychiatry: An Evidence-Based Text*. London: Hodder Arnold, pp. 707, 709.

Question 134 Answer: g, Dysbindin gene, h, Migration, i, Neuregulin gene
Explanation: This patient suffers from schizophrenia, and dysbindin, neuregulin and migration may be the aetiological factors.

Reference and Further Reading: Puri BK, Treasaden I (eds) (2010). *Psychiatry: An Evidence-Based Text*. London: Hodder Arnold, pp. 593–609.

Theme: General adult psychiatry

Question 135 Answer: e, PTSD

Explanation: Based on the current ICD-10 diagnostic criteria, PTSD arises within 6 months as a delayed and/or protracted response to a stressful event of an exceptionally threatening nature. Symptoms include that of repeated reliving of the trauma, emotional detachment and autonomic disturbances.

Question 136 Answer: b, Adjustment disorder

Explanation: These symptoms usually occur within 1 month of exposure to an identifiable psychosocial stressor. The ICD-10 has four sub-classifications, which are brief depressive reaction, prolonged depressive reaction, mixed anxiety and depressive reaction and predominant disturbance of emotions and/ or conduct.

Question 137 Answer: d, Generalized anxiety disorder

Explanation: Patients usually report uncontrollable worry. A negative response to the question, 'Do you worry excessively over minor matters?' virtually rules out GAD as a diagnosis. Symptoms of muscle and psychic tension are the most frequently reported by people with GAD.

Reference and Further Reading: Puri BK, Hall A, Ho R (2014). *Revision Notes in Psychiatry*. London: CRC Press, p. 409.

Theme: General adult psychiatry

Question 138 Answer: b, Wilson's disease

Explanation: Wilson's disease is an autosomal recessive disorder of hepatic copper metabolism. The incidence is 1 in 200,000. The gene responsible for this disorder has been located on chromosome 13 and encodes a copper-binding, membrane-spanning ATPase that regulates meta I transport protein. Cirrhosis and fulminant hepatic failure are known complications.

Question 139 Answer: d, Hypothyroidism

Explanation: Hypothyroidism is one of the most common conditions in the United Kingdom with a prevalence of 1.4% in females, but it is less common in males. Thyroxine replacement therapy may help to reverse psychiatric symptoms.

Question 140 Answer: c, Hyperthyroidism

Explanation: This is a condition that affects 2%–5% of all women mostly between the age of 20 and 45 years with a female-to-male ratio of 5:1. Anti-thyroid medication, radioactive thyroxine or thyroid surgery might be able to reverse the psychiatric symptoms.

Question 141 Answer: e, Cushing's syndrome
Explanation: This is a syndrome that is most commonly caused by exogenous administration of steroids. Other causes include ACTH-dependent causes, non-ACTH–dependent causes and alcohol-dependent pseudo-Cushing's syndrome.

Question 142 Answer: f, Addison's disease
Explanation: The aforementioned clinical symptoms are consistent with those of Addison's disease. Fatigue, weakness and apathy are common in the early stage. Around 90% of patients with adrenal disorders present with psychiatric symptoms.

Reference: Puri BK, Hall A, Ho R (2014). *Revision Notes in Psychiatry*. London: CRC Press, p. 477.

Theme: Diagnostic classification

Question 143 Answer: a, Paranoid schizophrenia
Explanation: This is known to be the most common subtype. Auditory, olfactory, gustatory and somatic hallucinations and visual hallucinations may occur. There may also be delusions of control, influence, passivity and persecution.

Question 144 Answer: b, Hebephrenic schizophrenia
Explanation: The aforementioned is true with regards to hebephrenic schizophrenia. The age of onset is generally between 15 and 25 years, and affective changes are usually prominent.

Question 145 Answer: c, Catatonic schizophrenia
Explanation: In this form of schizophrenia, one or more of the following behaviours may dominate: stupor, excitement, posturing, negativism, rigidity, waxy flexibility and command automatism and preservation of words or phrases.

Question 146 Answer: f, Simple schizophrenia
Explanation: There is an insidious onset of decline in functioning. Negative symptoms develop without preceding positive symptoms. Diagnosis requires changes in behaviour over at least 1 year, with marked loss of interest, idleness and social withdrawal.

Question 147 Answer: e, Residual schizophrenia
Explanation: This is a form of schizophrenia that is characterized largely by negative symptoms. There is past evidence of at least one schizophrenic episode and a period of at least 1 year in which the frequency of the positive symptoms has been minimal and negative schizophrenic symptoms have been present.

Reference: Puri BK, Hall A, Ho R (2014). *Revision Notes in Psychiatry*. London: CRC Press, p. 354.

Theme: General adult psychiatry

Question 148 Answer: e, 85%
Explanation: Based on the studies by Farmer et al. (1987) and Cardno et al. (1999), the heritability estimates have been around 80%–85%.

Question 149 Answer: b, 40%
Explanation: Based on key studies by Kendler et al. (1992) and McGulffin et al. (1996), the estimates are around 40%.

Question 150 Answer: d, 80%
Explanation: Based on key studies, the heritability estimates are between 79% and 93%.

Question 151 Answer: b, 40%
Explanation: Based on key studies (Kendler et al., 1992), the estimates are around 44%.

Reference: Puri BK, Hall A, Ho R (2014). *Revision Notes in Psychiatry*. London: CRC Press, p. 290.

Theme: Basic psychopathology

Question 152 Answer: i, Cataplexy
Explanation: This refers to the loss of muscle tone in narcolepsy. For example, a person develops temporary paralysis after emotional excitement.

Question 153 Answer: g, Ambitendency
Explanation: In this condition, the person makes a series of tentative incomplete movements when expected to carry out a voluntary action. For example, a woman offers a handshake, then withdraws and then offers it again for 10 times. The examiner is unable to make a handshake with her even at the end of the interview.

Question 154 Answer: h, Catalepsy
Explanation: Catalepsy refers to the abnormal maintenance of postures. For example, a person holds his or her arm in the air for a long time like a wax statue.

Question 155 Answer: d, Somnambulism
Explanation: This refers to a complex sequence of behaviours carried out by a patient who rises from sleep and is not fully aware of his or her surroundings.

Question 156 Answer: e, Compulsion
Explanation: This refers to a repetitive and stereotyped seemingly purposeful behaviour. It is commonly referred to as the motor component of an obsessional thought. Examples of compulsions include checking, cleaning, counting, dipsomania and dressing rituals.

Question 157 Answer: c, Obsessional slowness
Explanation: Obsessional slowness usually occurs secondary to repeated doubts and compulsive rituals.

Question 158 Answer: a, Stupor
Explanation: The key features of stupor include mutism, immobility, occasional periods of excitement and over-activity. Stupor is commonly seen in catatonic states, depressive states, manic states and also epilepsy and hysteria.

Reference: Puri BK, Hall A, Ho R (2014). *Revision Notes in Psychiatry*. London: CRC Press, pp. 1–2.

Theme: Basic psychopathology

Question 159 Answer: a, Anterograde amnesia and d, Retrograde amnesia
Explanation: Anterograde amnesia refers to the inability to form new memories due to the failure to consolidate or inability to retrieve. Retrograde amnesia refers to the loss of the memory for events that occurred prior to the events (such as intoxication or head injury). It tends to improve with some distant events in the past recovering first. In general, the retrograde amnesia is shorter than the post-traumatic amnesia.

Question 160 Answer: b, Post-traumatic amnesia
Explanation: This refers to the memory loss from the time of the accident to the time that the person can give a clear account of the recent events. It tends to remain unchanged.

Question 161 Answer: c, Psychogenic amnesia
Explanation: This is part of the dissociative disorder consisting of a sudden inability to recall important personal data. It is associated with la belle indifference (lack of concern) of the memory difficulties.

Question 162 Answer: e, Transient global amnesia
Explanation: In this condition, the person presents with a sudden onset of disorientation, loss of ability to encode recent memories and retrograde amnesia for a variable duration. This episode lasts for a few hours and is never repeated. The cause is the transient ischaemia of the hippocampus–fornix–hypothalamus system.

Question 163 Answer: g, Paramnesia
Explanation: Paramnesia refers to a distorted recall leading to falsification of memory. Paramnesias include confabulation, déjà vu, deja extend, dejapense, jamais vu and retrospective falsification.

Reference: Puri BK, Hall A, Ho R (2014). *Revision Notes in Psychiatry*. London: CRC Press, p. 9.

Theme: Neurology

Question 164 Answer: d, Intermediate aphasia
Explanation: Intermediate aphasia includes central aphasia and nominal aphasia. Central aphasia refers to the difficulty in arranging words in their proper sequence.

Nominal aphasia refers to the difficulty in naming objects. The person may use circumlocutions to express certain words, for example the person cannot name the clock but can label the clock as a thing that tells the time.

Question 165 Answer: a, Receptive aphasia, b, agnostic alexia, c, Pure word deafness.
Explanation: Receptive aphasia refers to the difficulty in comprehending the meaning of words. Types of receptive aphasia might include agnostic alexia, which means that words can be seen but cannot be read; pure word deafness, which means that words can be heard but cannot be comprehended and visual asymbolia, which means that words can be transcribed but cannot be read.

Question 166 Answer: e, Expressive aphasia
Explanation: Expressive aphasia is also known as Broca's non-fluent aphasia. This refers to difficulty in expressing thoughts in words whilst comprehension remains.

Question 167 Answer: f, Global aphasia
Explanation: In this condition, both receptive aphasia and expressive aphasia are present at the same time.

Reference: Puri BK, Hall A, Ho R (2014). *Revision Notes in Psychiatry*. London: CRC Press, p. 10.

Theme: Basic psychology

Question 168 Answer: i, Incubation
Explanation: Incubation refers to the gradual increment in the strength of the conditioned response following repeated brief exposure to the conditioned stimulus.

Question 169 Answer: g, Generalization
Explanation: This process refers to generalization. This is a process whereby once a CR has been established to a given stimulus, that particular response could in turn be evoked by other stimuli that are similar to the original conditioned stimulus.

Question 170 Answer: e, Higher-order conditioning
Explanation: In higher-order conditioning, the conditioned stimulus is paired with a second or even a third conditioned stimulus, which on presentation by itself would elicit the original conditioned response. It should be noted that higher-order conditioning is weaker than first-order conditioning, and the higher the order, the much weaker is the conditioning.

Question 171 Answer: c, Trace conditioning
Explanation: In trace conditioning, the conditioned stimulus ends before the onset of the unconditioned stimulus and the conditioning becomes less effective as the delay between the two increases.

Question 172 Answer: a, Delayed conditioning

Explanation: In delayed conditioning, the onset of the conditioned stimulus precedes that of the unconditioned stimulus, and the conditioned stimulus continues until the response occurs. Delayed conditioning is only optimal if the delay between the onset of the two stimuli is around half a second.

Reference: Puri BK, Hall A, Ho R (2014). *Revision Notes in Psychiatry*. London: CRC Press, p. 25.

Theme: Stages of development

Question 173 Answer: c, Phallic stage

Explanation: Phallic stage occurs between the ages of 3 and 5 years. Genital interest relates to own sexuality. The failure to negotiate leads to hysterical personality traits such as competitiveness and ambitiousness.

Question 174 Answer: b, Anal stage

Explanation: This stage occurs between the ages of 1 and 3 years. The anus and defecation are sources of sensual pleasure. Failure to negotiate leads to anal personality traits such as obsessive-compulsive personality, tidiness, parsimony, rigidity and thoroughness.

Question 175 Answer: a, Oral stage

Explanation: This stage occurs between the ages of 0 and 1 year. The failure to negotiate this stage leads to oral personality traits such as moodiness, generosity, depression, elation, talkativeness, greed, optimism, pessimism, wishful thinking and narcissism.

Question 176 Answer: h, Initiative

Explanation: The child is undergoing Erikson's stage of initiative. From the age of 0–1 year, the stage is that of trust and security and from the age of 1–4 years, the stage is that of autonomy.

Question 177 Answer: k, Intimacy

Explanation: The stage that lasts from the age of 15 years to adulthood is that of intimacy.

Reference: Puri BK, Hall A, Ho R (2014). *Revision Notes in Psychiatry*. London: CRC Press, p. 48.

Theme: Leadership and social power

Question 178 Answer: c, Laissez-faire

Explanation: Laissez-faire leadership is more appropriate for creative, open-ended and person-oriented tasks.

Question 179 Answer: a, Autocratic

Explanation: For autocratic leadership, there is a tendency for members to abandon the tasks in the leader's absence. It is good for situations of urgency.

Question 180 Answer: d, Authority power
Explanation: Authority power refers to power derived from a specific role.

Question 181 Answer: e, Reward power
Explanation: Reward power refers to power derived from ability to allocate resources.

Question 182 Answer: h, Expert power
Explanation: Expert power refers to power that is derived from skill, knowledge and experience.

Reference: Puri BK, Hall A, Ho R (2014). *Revision Notes in Psychiatry*. London: CRC Press, p. 59.

Theme: Models of cognitive development

Question 183 Answer: b, Preoperational
Explanation: This is considered to be the second stage of Piaget's cognitive model and occurs from the ages of 2 to 7 years. During this stage, the child learns to use the symbols of language. Thought processes exhibited during this stage include animism, artificialism, authoritarian morality, creationism, egocentrism and finalism.

Question 184 Answer: a, Sensorimotor
Explanation: This is considered to be the first stage and occurs from birth to 2 years of age. Circular reactions are repeated voluntary motor activities, for example, shaking a toy, occurring from around 2 months. Primary circular reaction occurs from 2 to 5 months, and they have no apparent purpose. Secondary circular reaction occurs from 5 to 9 months, and experimentation and purposeful behaviour are gradually manifested. Tertiary circular reactions occur from 1 year to 18 months and include the creation of original behaviour patterns and the purposeful quest for novel experiences.

Question 185 Answer: d, Formal operational
Explanation: Formal operational stage is the final stage and occurs from the age of around 12–14 years. It is characterized by the achievement of being able to think in the abstract, including the ability systematically to test hypotheses.

Question 186 Answer: d, Formal operational
Explanation: This is the third stage and occurs from the age of 7 to around 12–14 years of age. During this stage, the child demonstrates logical thought processes and more subjective moral judgements. An understanding of the laws of conservation of, initially, number and volume and the weight is normally achieved. Reversibility and some aspects of classifications are mastered.

Reference: Puri BK, Hall A, Ho R (2014). *Revision Notes in Psychiatry*. London: CRC Press, p. 68.

Theme: Psychological test

Question 187 Answer: b, Blessed Dementia Scale
Explanation: This particular questionnaire is administered to a relative or a friend of the subject who is asked the questions on the basis of performance over the previous 6 months. There are three sets of questions. The first set deals with activities of daily living, the second set deals with further activities of daily living and the third set is concerned largely with changes in personality, interest and drive.

Question 188 Answer: d, Cambridge Examination for Mental Disorders
Explanation: This is an interview schedule that consists of three sections: (1) a structured clinical interview with the patient to obtain systematic information about the present state, past history and family history; (2) a range of objective cognitive tests that constitute a mini-neuropsychological battery, commonly known as the Cambridge Cognitive Examination; (3) a structured interview with a relative or other informant to obtain independent information about the respondent's present state, past history and family history.

Question 189 Answer: e, Clifton Assessment Schedule
Explanation: This is a nursing rated assessment. Other nursing-rated assessments include the Stockton Geriatric Rating Scale.

Question 190 Answer: f, Present Behavioural Examination
Explanation: The Present Behavioural Examination involves interviewing carers and rates psychopathological and behavioural changes in dementia.

Reference: Puri BK, Hall A, Ho R (2014). *Revision Notes in Psychiatry*. London: CRC Press, p. 99.

Theme: Social sciences and stigma

Question 191 Answer: a, Death of spouse
Explanation: The death of spouse is associated with a life-change value of 100.

Question 192 Answer: b, Divorce
Explanation: Divorce is associated with a life-change value of 73.

Question 193 Answer: f, Pregnancy
Explanation: Pregnancy is associated with a life-change value of 50, with the birth of a child associated with a life-change value of 39.

Question 194 Answer: g, Minor legal violation
Explanation: Minor legal violation is associated with the lowest life-change value of 11.

Reference: Puri BK, Hall A, Ho R (2014). *Revision Notes in Psychiatry*. London: CRC Press, p. 122.

MRCPSYCH PAPER A1 MOCK EXAMINATION 2: QUESTIONS

GET THROUGH MRCPSYCH PAPER A1: MOCK EXAMINATION

Total number of questions: 185 (118 MCQs, 67 EMIs)
Total time provided: 180 minutes

Question 1
A 20-year-old male has been brought to the mental health service by his parents as he has been complaining that he has been hearing voices. During the interview with the psychiatrist, he was noted to be repeating particular words with increasing frequency. This form of psychopathology is known as
  a. Palilalia
  b. Logoclonia
  c. Neologism
  d. Metonym
  e. Punning

Question 2
A dentist proudly mentions that patients in his dental clinic are provided with a relaxing chair, ice cream and magazines to read after that they receive stressful dental procedures. Which of the following best describes the arrangement in his clinic?
  a. Avoidance learning
  b. Classical conditioning
  c. Extinction
  d. Operant conditioning
  e. Reciprocal inhibition

Question 3
You are posted to work in a new UK-based medical school in Singapore. A nurse is not certain how to keep the following psychotropic drugs in the ward and comes to consult you. The bioavailability of which of the following psychotropic drugs is most likely to be affected by exposure to humid atmosphere?
  a. Haloperidol
  b. Gabapentin

c. Lithium carbonate

d. Phenobarbital sodium

e. Risperidone

Question 4

A 25-year-old male has been referred by his general practitioner (GP) for a psychiatric assessment. He shared with the psychiatrist that he has been uncomfortable with his gender and is determined to have a gender re-assignment operation to become a woman. Which of the following would be the most appropriate clinical diagnosis?

a. Obsessive-compulsive disorder (OCD)

b. Body dysmorphic syndrome

c. Fetishistic transvestism

d. Transexualism

e. Delusional disorder

Question 5

A medical student asks you the specific type of epilepsy most commonly associated with olfactory hallucination. Your answer should be

a. Medial frontal lobe lesions and complex partial seizure

b. Medial parietal lobe lesions and complex partial seizure

c. Medial parietal lobe lesions and simple partial seizure

d. Medial temporal lobe lesions and complex partial seizure

e. Medial temporal lobe lesions and simple partial seizure

Question 6

Based on your understanding about neurosis and anxiety disorders in general, which of the following phobias has a strong underlying genetic linkage?

a. Agoraphobia

b. Social phobia

c. Blood injection phobia

d. Animal phobia

e. Illness phobia

Question 7

You are posted to work in Kenya. There is a lot of sunlight in the daytime and the hospital does not have an air-conditioned room to keep the psychotropic medications. The bioavailability of which of the following psychotropic drugs is most likely to be affected by exposure to air and light?

a. Carbamazepine

b. Gabapentin

c. Phenobarlatone

d. Topiramate

e. Zonisumide

Question 8
Paramnesia refers to a distorted recall leading to falsification of memory. The feelings of 'being there before' is best described by which of the following terms?
a. Déjà vu
b. Déjà entendu
c. Déjà pense
d. Jamais vu
e. Retrospective falsification

Question 9
A 37-year-old woman is diagnosed with depression. She feels miserable and thinks that her job requires her working long, stressful hours with brash and unfriendly colleagues. Although she is aware of the poor working environment, she does not do anything to better her situation and remains in the same job for many years. Which of the following statements about the above phenomenon is incorrect?
a. This phenomenon occurs when reinforcement is not contingent on behaviour.
b. This phenomenon is the result of a history of repeated failures.
c. This phenomenon is an example of classical conditioning.
d. There is a feeling of having no personal control over events.
e. This phenomenon was described by Seligman.

Question 10
A 25-year-old man suffers from treatment-resistant schizoaffective disorder and takes clozapine. Which of the following psychotropic drugs is contradicted as an augmentation?
a. Carbamazepine
b. Fluoxetine
c. Lithium
d. Valproate
e. Risperidone

Question 11
Which of the following risk factors is associated with the highest risk of developing agranulocytosis in schizophrenic patients taking clozapine?
a. Afro-Caribbean descent
b. Young age
c. Female gender
d. High dose of clozapine
e. Long duration of clozapine use

Question 12
A 45-year-old female has been very concerned about her son Thomas. She has received feedback from his teachers at school that he has been very rigid in his duties and is not able to participate in group work as he cannot delegate tasks.

He consistently seeks perfectionism in all that he does. Which of the following is the most likely clinical diagnosis?
a. OCD
b. Obsessive-compulsive personality disorder
c. No mental illness
d. Schizoid personality disorder
e. Antisocial personality disorder

Question 13
Which of the following is a good prognostic factor for an individual with anorexia nervosa (AN)?
a. Onset younger than the age of 15
b. Lower weight at onset and at presentation
c. Frequent vomiting and the presence of bulimia
d. Long duration of symptoms
e. Male gender

Question 14
A 40-year-old woman complains about generalized headache which has gotten worse over the past 3 weeks. Her GP thought that she suffers from tension headache. Which of the following symptoms suggest an underlying serious pathology?
a. Headache which bands around the head
b. Headache getting worse when lying down
c. Headache and giddiness
d. Pain at the occipital
e. Severity of the headache

Question 15
A 5-year-old boy is brought by his parents for assessment. His parents complain that he has abnormalities in reciprocal social interaction and restricted interest in buses. He was speaking fluently at the age of 2. Physical examination shows stereotyped movement and motor clumsiness. Which of the following is the most likely diagnosis?
a. Autism
b. Asperger's syndrome
c. Attention deficit and hyperkinetic disorder
d. Childhood disintegrative disorder
e. Rett's syndrome

Question 16
Which of the following is true with regards to the psychopathology that a patient is experiencing when he keeps repeating everything that the examiner has been saying?
a. Approximate answers
b. Cryptolalia
c. Circumstantiality

d. Echolalia

e. Flight of ideas

Question 17
Which of the following statements is false?
a. Second-order conditioning is the basis for single-object phobia.
b. Animal phobias have the best prognosis among the various phobias.
c. Punishment is a component of aversion therapy.
d. Second-order conditioning is more easily demonstrated than classical conditioning
e. Forward conditioning is more used than backward conditioning.

Question 18
A 24-year-old man suffers from treatment-resistant schizophrenia and has started clozapine for 1 week. He refuses to have the weekly full blood count but is keen to continue clozapine. His GP is concerned that he will develop agranulocytosis and wants to find out when is the peak period for developing agranulocytosis. Your answer is
a. First month of treatment
b. Second month of treatment
c. Third month of treatment
d. Fourth month of treatment
e. Fifth month of treatment

Question 19
A 1-year-old child should be fearful of
a. Animals
b. Loud noises
c. Death
d. Darkness
e. 'Monsters'

Question 20
A newborn baby possesses all of the following visual characteristics except
a. Ability to discriminate the level of brightness
b. Ability to focus on an object at a distance of 0.2 m
c. Ability to scan objects
d. Depth perception
e. Figure-ground differentiation

Question 21
A 50-year-old man has an infarct in the anterior cerebral artery. Which of the following neurological signs is most likely to be found?
a. Broca's aphasia
b. Ipsilateral lower limb paralysis

c. Contralateral lower limb weakness
d. Contralateral III nerve palsy
e. Nystagumus

Question 22

A concerned mother brought her 5-year-old son for assessment because she worries he has developmental delay. Which of the following development tasks is mainly achieved at 5 years but not in earlier years?
a. The child is able to count age on hand.
b. The child is able to imitate a drawing of a circle and a cross.
c. The child is able to name items at home.
d. The child is able to run on tiptoes.
e. The child knows his name.

Question 23

Which of the following statements regarding the diagnostic criteria for post-schizophrenic depression is false?
a. Based on the *Diagnostic and Statistical Manual of Mental Disorders* (DSM)-IV-TR criteria, post-schizophrenic depression is not a diagnostic entity.
b. Based on the International Classification of Diseases (ICD)-10 criteria, the general criteria for schizophrenia must have been met within the previous 12 months prior to onset of depressive episode.
c. Based on the ICD-10 criteria, a depressive episode instead of post-schizophrenic depression should be diagnosed if the patient no longer has any schizophrenic symptoms for a long time.
d. Based on the ICD-10 criteria, dysthymia is severe enough to meet diagnostic criteria of post-schizophrenic depression.
e. The post-schizophrenic depressive episodes are associated with an increased risk of suicide.

Question 24

Which of the following types of schizophrenia is not found in the DSM-IV-TR?
a. Catatonic type
b. Disorganized type
c. Hebephrenic type
d. Paranoid type
e. Residual type

Question 25

Which of the following is not a bad prognostic factor for individuals with AN?
a. Onset at an older age
b. Long duration of AN
c. Previous hospitalization

d. Extreme resistance to treatment
e. Female gender

Question 26

A 40-year-old woman reports that she is the prime minister's sister. When asked what makes her think this, she replies that it is true without further elaboration. Her affect was flat without pressure of speech. Collateral history of her family reveals that she has no relationship with the prime minister and the realization came to her 'out of the blue'. The psychopathology being described is
a. Autochthonous delusion
b. Delusional memory
c. Delusional mood
d. Delusional perception
e. Delusion of grandeur

Question 27

Gestalt principle is based on the following, with the exception of
a. Proximity
b. Similarity
c. Continuity
d. Closure
e. Three-dimensional similarity

Question 28

A 30-year-old schizophrenia man is prescribed with clozapine and the daily dose is 700 mg per day. The consultant psychiatrist worries about the high risk of seizure. Which of the following anticonvulsants is the most appropriate prophylactic agent against clozapine-induced epilepsy?
a. Carbamazepine
b. Lamotrigine
c. Phenytoin
d. Topiramate
e. Valproate

Question 29

A 30-year-old man suffers from third-person auditory hallucination, thought interference and delusion of control for 3 months. Which of the following statements is correct?
a. He fulfils the diagnostic criteria for schizophrenia based on the ICD-10.
b. He fulfils the diagnostic criteria for schizophrenia based on DSM-IV-TR.
c. He fulfils the diagnostic criteria for schizophrenia based on both the DSM-IV-TR and the ICD-10.
d. He does not fulfil diagnostic criteria for schizophrenia based on both the DSM-IV-TR and the ICD-10.
e. None of the aforementioned options.

Question 30
Based on research into conformity and group behaviour, which of the following statements is incorrect?
a. Within the group, member's individual opinions were distorted based on the opinions of others in the group.
b. Conformity was greater in groups that had individuals who were less self-reliant.
c. Conformity was greater in groups that had individuals who were less intelligent.
d. Conformity was greater in groups that had individuals who were less self-expressive.
e. Conformity to the group's decision on a line judgement experiment was greater in a group of 25 members as compared to a group of four.

Question 31
Which of the following statements about the theory of mind is incorrect?
a. In primate research, theory of mind refers to the abilities of primates to mentalize their fellows.
b. In humans, the theory of mind refers to the ability of most normal people to comprehend the thought processes (such as attention, feelings, beliefs and knowledge) of others.
c. At the age of 3, normal human children do not acknowledge the false belief as they have a difficulty in differentiating belief from the world.
d. Cognitive changes occur at the age of 5 for children to adopt the theory of mind.
e. It has been suggested that a failure to acquire a theory of mind is associated with disorders such as autism.

Question 32
Based on the DSM-5 diagnostic criteria, a patient who drinks more than what amount of caffeine is considered to be intoxicated?
a. 80 mg
b. 100 mg
c. 120 mg
d. 150 mg
e. 250 mg

Question 33
The psychological therapy that deals with traps, snags and dilemmas would be
a. Cognitive behavioural therapy
b. Cognitive analytical therapy
c. Interpersonal therapy
d. Psychodynamic psychotherapy
e. Rational emotive therapy

Question 34
There have been multiple aetiologies accounting for the development of personality disorders. In particular, which of these personality disorders has the strongest genetic relationship?
a. Schizoid personality disorder
b. Schizotypal personality disorder

c. Borderline personality disorder
d. Dependent personality disorder
e. Obsessive-compulsive personality disorder

Question 35
A 70-year-old man has a tumour in the frontal lobe. Which of the following neurological signs is most likely to be found?
a. Amusia
b. Anosmia
c. Anterograde amnesia
d. Apraxia
e. Bitemporal hemianopia

Question 36
Previous research has demonstrated that when there are more people around during an emergency, the participants are less likely to help. Which of the following best describes this?
a. Social dilemma
b. Moral dilemma
c. Bystander effect
d. Groupthink
e. Conformity to the norm

Question 37
A 25-year-old male has treatment-resistant schizophrenia and has been sectioned for inpatient hospitalization on multiple occasions. He has just been started on clozapine, but he has been complaining of a change in the tone of his upper limbs. Which of the following terminology best describes the psychopathology that he has been experiencing?
a. Cenesthesia
b. Delusional perception
c. Made feelings
d. Somatic passivity
e. Visceral hallucinations

Question 38
A 40-year-old African man is referred to you for psychiatric assessment after he attempted to attack his wife. He believes that his wife has been unfaithful to him and she is having an affair with a Caucasian man. He has been trying for 1 year to prove this belief despite her repeated denial and reassurance from friends and relatives. His attempts included following her, searching her mobile phone, confronting her and checking her clothes. Which of the following aetiological factors is least likely to be associated with his condition?
a. Alcohol dependence
b. Amphetamine misuse

c. Delusional misidentification
d. Depression
e. Paranoid schizophrenia

Question 39
Based on Bandura model of learning, all of the following are crucial steps in the modelling process, with the exception of which of the following?
a. Attention
b. Retention
c. Reproduction
d. Motivation
e. Insight

Question 40
Which of the following is not considered to be a theory of interpersonal attraction?
a. Reinforcement theory
b. Conditioning theory
c. Social exchange theory
d. Equity theory
e. Proxemics

Question 41
An examiner asks a person to move his arm in different directions and the person is unable to resist even if it is against her will. This phenomenon is known as
a. Automatic obedience
b. Gegenhalten
c. Mitmachen
d. Mitgehen
e. Waxy flexibility

Question 42
A 32-year-old female has just given birth to a baby boy 5 days ago. She has been afraid to care for her newborn, as she has been hearing voices of the devil telling her nasty things about her child. She believes that the child has been placed under a curse by the devil. Which of the following would be the most appropriate clinical diagnosis for her?
a. Postnatal depression
b. Postnatal psychosis
c. Postnatal blues
d. Depression with psychotic features
e. Schizophrenia

Question 43
A voluntary organization is attempting to recruit more volunteers to help them. They first started by asking the new volunteers to help out in a once-off charity

event. Thereafter, they started to ask the volunteers to commit more of their time in helping out the organization. Which of the following techniques best describes this?

a. Door in the face technique
b. Foot in the door technique
c. Reinforcement technique
d. Conditioning technique
e. Gradual approximation technique

Question 44

When the examiner is attempting passively to move the arm of an 80-year-old man with dementia, the examiner feels that the patient is applying the same amount of force in resisting the passive movement. This phenomenon is known as

a. Ambitendency
b. Gegenhalten
c. Mitmachen
d. Mitgehen
e. Waxy flexibility

Question 45

A medical student was asked to examine a patient and determine what pathology he has. On neurological examination, it was noted that the patient is unable to cooperate and looks downwards and laterally. He complains of double vision when attempting to do so. This is most likely due to a lesion involving

a. Second cranial nerve
b. Third cranial nerve
c. Fourth cranial nerve
d. Fifth cranial nerve
e. Sixth cranial nerve

Question 46

Aggression has been described as a behaviour intended to harm others. There are various explanations for aggressive behaviours. Which of the following is incorrect?

a. Aggression is perceived to be a learnt response, from previous observation, imitation and operant conditioning.
b. Victim suffering and material gains will reinforce subsequent aggressive behaviour.
c. The consequences of aggression usually play a role in determining future aggression.
d. Behaviours such as maintaining a distance, evoking a social response incompatible with aggression and familiarity will help to inhibit aggression.
e. Emotional arousal might or might not increase aggression.

Question 47

A 30-year-old man was brought to the Accident and Emergency Department. He suddenly fell down after hearing a loud sound at a party. There was no loss of consciousness. The psychopathology being described is

a. Catalepsy

b. Cataplexy

c. Catatonia

d. Posturing

e. Waxy flexibility

Question 48

Which of the following movement disorders is not typically associated with schizophrenia?

a. Ambitendency

b. Mannerism

c. Mitgehen and mitmachen

d. Negativism

e. Stupor

Question 49

A 50-year-old man suffers from schizophrenia and he has been taking chlorpromazine for the past 20 years. You are the consultant psychiatrist and reviewing his drug list because you are concerned of drug interaction. Which of the following drug interaction is the most significant?

a. Amitriptyline decreases the serum concentration of chlorpromazine.

b. Chlorpromazine decreases the serum concentration of amitriptyline.

c. Chlorpromazine increases the serum concentration of amitriptyline.

d. Chlorpromazine decreases the serum concentration of valproate.

e. Chlorpromazine increases the serum concentration of valproate.

Question 50

A 28-year-old female has been diagnosed with a previous psychiatric condition. Her symptoms have remitted over the past 2 years, but recently due to increased stress at work, she has been resorting to measures to cope with stress. One of the methods she has been using is to restrict her diet, in order to reduce her body mass index from the current of 20 to 15. What form of psychological therapy would be the most useful and beneficial for her?

a. Cognitive behavioural therapy

b. EDMR

c. Trauma-focused therapy

d. Dialectic behavioural therapy

e. Supportive therapy

Question 51

Which of the following aphasia resembles speech disturbances that schizophrenic patients have?

a. Intermediate aphasia
b. Expressive aphasia
c. Global aphasia
d. Jargon aphasia
e. Semantic aphasia

Question 52
Schemas help to influence the way people organize knowledge about the social world and also help them to interpret new situations. All of the following about schemas are incorrect with the exception of
a. Schemas tend to slow down the rate of mental processing.
b. Schemas are not likely to be helpful when dealing with an ambiguous situation.
c. Schemas usually require more effortful thinking.
d. Schemas tend to persist even after evidence for the schema has been discredited.
e. Schemas play a part in maintaining prejudice.

Question 53
A 40-year-old man with schizophrenia is admitted to the psychiatric ward. The nurse informs you that he always protrudes his lips, which resemble a snout. The psychopathology being described is
a. Ambitendency
b. Gegenhalten
c. Pout
d. Rooting
e. Schnauzkrampf

Question 54
A 30-year-old male, Thomas, was at his father's funeral, helping to carry his father's coffin when he developed an acute onset of bilateral blindness. The medical team doctors have seen him, and they have found nothing medically wrong. He has also been seen by the on-call psychiatrist, to which he reports feeling indifferent to the blindness. What is the most likely clinical diagnosis?
a. Somatoform disorder
b. Conversion disorder
c. Body dysmorphic disorder
d. Generalized anxiety disorder
e. Malingering

Question 55
All of the following are known clinical features of Wernicke's encephalopathy, with the exception of
a. Ophthalmoplegia
b. Nystagmus
c. Hypothermia

d. Ataxia
e. Clouding of consciousness

Question 56
Which of the following correctly describes fundamental attribution error?
a. Attributing others mistakes to the context in which the mistakes occur
b. Attributing one's own mistakes to one's character and personality
c. Refusing to accept one's own errors
d. Denying the fundamental flaws behind one's own negative behaviour
e. Attributing others' mistakes to their personal dispositions

Question 57
A 60-year-old man suffers from prostate cancer and was admitted to the hospital for chemotherapy. He developed nausea and vomiting after chemotherapy. Whenever he sees the hospital building, he feels nauseated. He has completed chemotherapy and is not required to return to the hospital. The nausea feeling disappears. The disappearance of nausea feeling is known as
a. Discrimination
b. Extinction
c. Generalization
d. Inhibition
e. Recovery

Question 58
A 60-year-old man suffers from prostate cancer and he was admitted to the hospital for chemotherapy. He developed nausea and vomiting after chemotherapy. Two months later, he feels nausea when he sees the hospital building. The nausea feeling associated with the hospital building is known as
a. Conditioned response
b. Conditioned stimulus
c. Unconditioned response
d. Unconditioned stimulus
e. Second order conditioning

Question 59
A 35-year-old man sets a daily alarm on his mobile phone to remind him to take his medication, Drug A. He constantly experiences side effects whenever he takes Drug A, which includes nausea. After some time, when he hears a similar alarm from his alarm clock, he also experiences nausea. This phenomenon is known as
a. Discrimination
b. Extinction
c. Generalization
d. Inhibition
e. Recovery

Question 60

A 25-year-old woman meets the diagnostic criteria for schizophrenia and exhibits first-rank symptoms. First-rank symptoms include the following except

a. Delusional perception
b. Delusion of passivity
c. Delusion of persecution
d. Thought insertion
e. Thought withdrawal

Question 61

A 65-year-old woman with a history of depression presents with bilateral ptosis. Which of the following condition is least likely?

a. Levator palpebrae muscle paralysis
b. Myasthenia gravis
c. Myotonic dystrophy
d. Ocular dystrophy
e. Guillain–Barre syndrome

Question 62

Which of the following is not true about fundamental attribution error?

a. Seen in adults in western societies
b. Primarily an attribution error
c. Overestimation of personal factors
d. Bias towards attributing a behaviour to situational causes
e. Overestimation of dispositional factors

Question 63

A public health official wants to consult you on the use of APOE alleles as a screening test to identify individuals with a high chance to develop Alzheimer's disease and offer early intervention. Which of the following is true about APOE screening test?

a. Low positive predictive value; low negative predictive value; low sensitivity and low specificity
b. Low positive predictive value; high negative predictive value; low sensitivity and low specificity
c. Low positive predictive value; high negative predictive value; high sensitivity and low specificity
d. Low positive predictive value; high negative predictive value; high sensitivity and high specificity
e. High positive predictive value; high negative predictive value; high sensitivity and high specificity

Question 64

A medical student attached to the Consultation–Liaison team asked the consultant psychiatrist which of the following would be the earliest and most reliable sign to differentiate between dementia and delirium. The correct answer would be

a. Presence of focal neurological signs on clinical examination
b. Presence of short-term memory deficits

c. Presence of long-term memory deficits
d. Presence of hallucinations
e. Presence of altered consciousness

Question 65

Which of the following is the best way to prevent dementia?
a. Offer genetic testing to older adults
b. Prescribe oestrogen to older women
c. Prescribe nonsteroidal anti-inflammatory drugs
d. Supplement with vitamin E
e. Treat systolic hypertension (>160 mm Hg) in older people (age >60 years)

Question 66

The consultant psychiatrist shows his medical students a video on interviewing a schizophrenic patient, and mentions to them that the patient in the video has the full set of all the first-rank symptoms. Which of the following should the consultant psychiatrist clarify with the students and tell them that it is not considered as a first-rank symptom?
a. Thought insertion
b. Thought block
c. Thought broadcast
d. Thought withdrawal
e. Auditory hallucinations

Question 67

Peri-trauma factors that predispose and cause an individual to develop post-traumatic stress disorder (PTSD) include all the following except
a. Being female in sex
b. Perceived lack of social support during the trauma
c. Perceived threat to life
d. Peri-trauma dissociation
e. Severity of the trauma

Question 68

Which of the following best defines social psychology?
a. The scientific study of the way in which people's thoughts, feelings and behaviours are influenced by the real, imagined or implied presence of other people
b. The scientific study of how people's behaviours, thoughts and feelings are influenced by the social environment
c. The scientific study of how people's behaviours, thoughts and feelings are influenced by society
d. The scientific study of behaviour and mental processes
e. The scientific study of how behaviours are influenced by mental processes

Question 69

A 30-year-old woman is referred by her dermatologist to see you. She complains of pruritus as a result of an infestation with parasites. She shows you her debris contained in plastic wrap and claims that it contains the parasites. The patient is most likely suffering from

a. Capgras syndrome
b. Cotard syndrome
c. De Clerambault's syndrome
d. Ekbom syndrome
e. Fregoli syndrome

Question 70

A 35-year-old man sets a daily alarm on his mobile phone to remind him to take his medication, Drug A. He constantly experiences side effects whenever he takes Drug A, which includes nausea. After some time, when he hears a similar alarm from his alarm clock, he also experiences nausea. However, this phenomenon disappears after a few days. This phenomenon is known as

a. Discrimination
b. Extinction
c. Generalization
d. Inhibition
e. Recovery

Question 71

A 35-year-old man sets a daily alarm on his mobile phone to remind him to take his medication, Drug A. He constantly experiences side effects whenever he takes Drug A, which includes nausea. After changing his medication to Drug B, he stops experiencing nausea. However, after a few days, he again starts to feel nauseated when he hears his mobile phone alarm. This phenomenon is known as

a. Discrimination
b. Extinction
c. Generalization
d. Inhibition
e. Recovery

Question 72

A 50-year-old man has a lesion in the left occipital lobe. Which of the following sign is most likely to be found?

a. Dyslexia without agraphia
b. Homonymous hemianopia
c. Left eye papilloedema
d. Loss of pupillary reflex
e. Quadrantanopia

Question 73
Which of the following trails or tests led to public outrage and request from Queen Victoria to clarify the legal standard in the 1840s?
a. Bifurcated trial
b. First right versus wrong test
c. Daniel M'Naghten trial
d. The irresistible impulse test
e. Wild beast test

Question 74
A 25-year-old male presented to the mental health services as he has been feeling low for the past 2 months. The low mood is associated with diminished interests, feelings that life is not worth going on and biological symptoms such as poor sleep and appetite. Which of the following descriptors best describes the severity of his underlying depression?
a. No depression
b. Mild
c. Moderate
d. Severe
e. Prolonged

Question 75
A 38-year-old father is diagnosed with schizophrenia. His wife does not have any psychiatric illness. He wants to know the risk of his son developing the disorder. Your answer is
a. 5%
b. 10%
c. 15%
d. 20%
e. 25%

Question 76
A 55-year-old male is extremely upset that his son has been sectioned for admission for psychosis. He knows that it might be due to the drugs – cannabis which his son has been using. Cannabis is known to increase the incidences of psychosis by approximately how much percent?
a. No increased risk
b. Two times increased risk
c. Three times increased risk
d. Four times increased risk
e. Six times increased risk

Question 77
A 40-year-old female Sally is concerned whether her brother who has Down's syndrome would develop psychosis. Based on the current research evidence, the risk of her brother developing schizophrenia has been estimated to be

a. Two percent increased risk.
b. Four percent increased risk.
c. Six percent increased risk.
d. The same as the normal population.
e. There has been found to be an association, but there is no strong evidence to support the estimated increment in risk.

Question 78

A 6-year-old girl has a fear of injections but requires frequent injections. She has to consult with a doctor before getting her injection. She recognizes her doctor by his white coat. After her consultation with the doctor, she has to wait for her turn in the waiting area before proceeding to another room for her injection. Soon, whenever she sees a doctor's white coat, she reports feeling scared and anxious. This phenomenon is known as
a. Backward conditioning
b. Delayed conditioning
c. Simultaneous conditioning
d. Temporal conditioning
e. Trace conditioning

Question 79

The term 'schizoaffective psychosis' was introduced by Kasanin in which of the following decades?
a. 1910s
b. 1920s
c. 1930s
d. 1940s
e. 1950s

Question 80

Based on the Driver and Vehicle Licensing Agency (DVLA) guidelines in the UK, how long must a bipolar patient be stable and well before being allowed to drive again?
a. 2 weeks
b. 1 month
c. 3 months
d. 6 months
e. 1 year

Question 81

The relative risk of developing Alzheimer's disease in a 55-year-old patient with Down's syndrome has been estimated to be
a. 10%–15%
b. 20%–25%
c. 35%–40%
d. 45%–50%
e. More than 50%

Question 82
Deinstitutionalization peaked in the 1970s. Which of the following statements is not associated with deinstitutionalization?
a. Availability of antipsychotic medications.
b. People with mental illnesses are not at a higher risk of offending compared to general population.
c. Increase in awareness of civil rights of people with mental illnesses.
d. Increase in costs of institutionalization care.
e. Reduction in availability of hospital beds.

Question 83
An 8-year-old girl has a phobia of spiders. When she is presented with a spider, it elicits high levels of fear and anxiety. The experimenter plays a ringing sound at the same time and for the duration of the presentation of the spider. The experimenter is hoping to elicit similar feelings of fear and anxiety when the girl hears the ringing sound without the presentation of the spider. This phenomenon is known as
a. Backward conditioning
b. Delayed conditioning
c. Simultaneous conditioning
d. Temporal conditioning
e. Trace conditioning

Question 84
Based on your understanding about the history of schizophrenia, the concept that schizophrenia developed from a split mind was proposed by
a. Bleuler
b. Kraeplin
c. Morel
d. Hecker
e. Kahlbarum

Question 85
Schizoaffective disorder was a disorder introduced by the following individual:
a. Hecker
b. Sommer
c. Kurt Schneider
d. Kasanin
e. Cooper

Question 86
Which of the following statements is false with regards to the consequentialist approach?
a. An action is moral if it makes the greatest number of people happy.
b. Different treatment options can be measured by foreseeable consequences such as quality-adjusted life years (QALYs).

c. In managed mental health care, the consequentialist approach may lead to discrimination of individual patients and moral dilemmas owing to factual uncertainties.
d. It is based on an obligation of fidelity (including a pledge for confidentiality), deontological theory and virtue ethics.
e. Under the consequentialist approach, confidentiality is an absolute condition in psychiatric practice.

Question 87

You are assigned to provide tutorial to four medical students. Each student needs to write a case report for a psychiatric patient. One student is confused about the meaning of mental state examination (MSE). Which of the following statements is true?
a. The Mini Mental State Examination (MMSE) is a shorter version of the Mental State Examination.
b. MSE provides important information in establishing a psychiatric diagnosis.
c. MSE should be conducted after history taking.
d. The student does not need to report any physical finding because MSE has replaced physical examination in psychiatry.
e. When there is a discrepancy between information from the history and findings at the MSE, the student should establish the diagnosis based on the information from the history.

Question 88

You are interviewing a woman who was diagnosed with schizophrenia. You think that she may suffer from other psychiatric disorders as her first-rank symptoms are inconsistent. Which of the following features is not typically associated with schizophrenia?
a. Catatonia
b. Delusional perception
c. Emotional liability
d. Passivity
e. Negativism

Question 89

A 50-year-old man with chronic schizophrenia says, 'The community psychiatric nurse syringerisperidone me fortnightly'. This psychopathology is known as
a. Asyndesis
b. Cryptolalia
c. Metonym
d. Neologism
e. Vorbeigehen

Question 90

Based on the ICD-10 diagnostic and classification criteria, the diagnosis of delusional disorder could be made only if the symptoms have lasted for at least the past
a. 1 week
b. 1 month

c. 3 months
d. 6 months
e. 1 year

Question 91
Which of the following statements about the genetics of AN is correct?
a. Heritability of AN is around 50%.
b. Less than 5% of first-degree relatives are usually affected.
c. Linkage genes on chromosome 3 have been found.
d. The ratio for monozygotic (MZ) to dizygotic (DZ) concordance is around 56:5.
e. Research has found the concordance rates for monozygotic twins to be the same as that for dizygotic twins.

Question 92
The mother of a 21-year-old male, who has just been diagnosed with OCD, wonders which of the following compulsions is the most common amongst adults. Which of the following is true?
a. Checking
b. Counting
c. Doubting
d. Symmetry
e. Washing

Question 93
A 45-year-old female has been dependent on medications to help her with her anxiety condition. Recently, her psychiatrist removed one of the chronic medications that she used to be taking. This has resulted in the following withdrawal symptoms: autonomic hyperactivity, malaise and weakness, tinnitus and grand mal convulsions. Which of the following is the most likely clinical diagnosis for her?
a. Neuroleptic malignant syndrome
b. Serotonin syndrome
c. Serotonin discontinuation syndrome
d. Benzodiazepine withdrawal syndrome
e. Organic causes

Question 94
The Folstein's MMSE includes all of the following items except
a. Drawing an intersecting pentagon
b. Drawing the face of a clock, indicating 10 past 11
c. Orientation to time, place and person
d. Serial subtraction or spelling 'WORLD' backwards
e. Three-stage command

Question 95
A Greenland Inuit woman suddenly strips off her clothes and rolls in the snow followed by echolalia and echopraxia. She has no recollection of the episode

afterwards. This woman suffers from which of the following culture-bound syndromes?
a. Amok
b. Latah
c. Pibloktoq
d. Uqamairineq
e. Windigo

Question 96
What was the implication of Tarasoff I (1974)?
a. Duty to assess
b. Duty to protect
c. Duty to respect
d. Duty to treat
e. Duty to warn

Question 97
What was the implication of Tarasoff II (1976)?
a. Duty to assess
b. Duty to protect
c. Duty to respect
d. Duty to treat
e. Duty to warn

Question 98
An Inuit living in the Arctic Circle complains of sudden paralysis when he slept. He recalls that he was very agitated during the paralysis. The day before the attack, he could hear transient and unusual sound in his neighbourhood. He attributes the unusual experience to spirit possession. This man suffers from which of the following culture-bound syndromes?
a. Amok
b. Latah
c. Pibloktoq
d. Uqamairineq
e. Windigo

Question 99
A 6-year-old boy has phobia of snakes. When he is presented with a snake, it elicits high levels of fear and anxiety. The experimenter plays a ringing sound after the presentation of the snake. The experimenter is hoping to elicit similar feelings of fear and anxiety when the boy hears the ringing sound without the presentation of the snake. This phenomenon is known as
a. Backward conditioning
b. Delayed conditioning
c. Simultaneous conditioning

d. Temporal conditioning
e. Trace conditioning

Question 100
Which of the following is not a feature of pseudobulbar palsy?
a. Donald Duck speech
b. Emotional incontinence
c. Normal jaw jerk
d. Spastic tongue
e. Upper motor neuron lesions as a result of bilateral lesions above the mid-pons

Question 101
Which of the following statements regarding Montreal Cognitive Assessment (MoCA) is correct?
a. A score of 21 or above is considered normal.
b. MoCA has lower sensitivity compared to the MMSE in identifying mild cognitive impairment.
c. MoCA is available in English and French only.
d. The short-term memory recall task involves two learning trials of ten nouns and delayed recall after approximately 20 minutes.
e. Visuospatial abilities are assessed using a clock-drawing task and a three-dimensional cube copy.

Question 102
A 20-year-old African university student has been preparing for a pharmacology examination and presents with a burning headache, blurred vision, difficulty in understanding the meaning of the textbook and an inability to remember the drugs he studied. This man suffers from which of the following culture-bound syndromes?
a. Amok
b. Brain fag
c. Dhat
d. Koro
e. Latah

Question 103
The most common defence mechanism seen in paranoid personality disorder is
a. Denial
b. Projection
c. Reaction formation
d. Sublimation
e. Undoing

Question 104
The case *Tarasoff v. Regents of the University of California* is related to which of the following ethical principles:

a. Autonomy
b. Capacity
c. Confidentiality
d. Consent
e. Equality

Question 105

A 20-year-old Chinese national serviceman in Singapore is referred by the army doctor. He complains that his penis is getting shorter and that it will continue to retract into his abdomen. He measures his penis every day and he cannot concentrate on his work. This man suffers from which of the following culture-bound syndromes?
a. Amok
b. Brain fag
c. Dhat
d. Koro
e. Latah

Question 106

A 22-year-old female has had a previous episode of depression 2 years ago. Currently, she presents to the mental health service with hypomania. Which one of the following clinical diagnosis would you label her with?
a. Bipolar disorder type I
b. Bipolar disorder type II
c. Bipolar disorder type III
d. Rapid cycling bipolar disorder
e. Cyclothymia

Question 107

A core trainee wants to know more about the Addenbrooke's Cognitive Examination—Revised (ACE-R). Which of the following statements is correct?
a. The ACE-R does not incorporate MMSE.
b. The ACE-R is available in Cantonese for Hong Kong patients.
c. The cut-off score gives rise to high sensitivity and 100% specificity for diagnosing dementia.
d. The cut-off score gives rise to high specificity and 100% sensitivity for diagnosing dementia.
e. It is a cognitive test commonly used for screening delirium.

Question 108

A 50-year-old woman was admitted to the ward and the nurses are having difficulty with her. She appears to be arrogant, refuses to follow ward rules and insists to drink alcohol in the ward. She believes that she is a 'special' patient and requests first-class treatment. Her husband mentions that she tends to exploit

others and that most people try to avoid her. Which defence mechanism is the least commonly used by people with such a disorder?
a. Denial
b. Distortion
c. Projection
d. Rationalization
e. Suppression

Question 109
A 60-year-old man suffers from prostate cancer and was admitted to the hospital for chemotherapy. He developed nausea and vomiting after chemotherapy. Whenever he sees the hospital building, he feels nausea. Today he needs to see an oncologist in the clinic. When he sees the doctor's white coat, he feels nausea. The nausea feeling associated with white coat is known as
a. Conditioned response
b. Conditioned stimulus
c. Unconditioned response
d. Unconditioned stimulus
e. Second order conditioning

Question 110
Based on the ACE-R scale, which of the following cut-off scores is the most specific?
a. 80
b. 82
c. 84
d. 86
e. 88

Question 111
A 43-year-old man is angry at being caught speeding by the traffic police. He goes home and yells at his wife and children. Which of the following defence mechanisms best describes the aforementioned phenomenon?
a. Denial
b. Reaction formation
c. Displacement
d. Projection
e. Sublimation

Question 112
Based on previous research studies, it has been demonstrated that patients with schizophrenia would relapse if they were discharged back to their families with high expressed emotions for more than
a. 20 hours per week
b. 23 hours per week
c. 30 hours per week

d. 33 hours per week

e. 50 hours per week

Question 113

The anatomical correlate of this form of memory is either in the visual association cortex or in the auditory association cortex. Which of the following terminologies best describes this form of memory?

a. Declarative memory

b. Episodic memory

c. Implicit memory

d. Sensory memory

e. Short-term memory

Question 114

A 50-year-old businessman was killed in a road traffic accident when he crossed the road. His son turns his anger and plans to take revenge on the negligent driver into the energy of taking over his father's business. Which of the following defence mechanisms best describes the aforementioned phenomenon?

a. Denial

b. Reaction formation

c. Displacement

d. Projection

e. Sublimation

Question 115

A 5-year-old girl is scared of monkeys. When she goes to the zoo, she behaves aggressively on seeing a monkey, as if she is about to attack the monkey. Which of the following defence mechanisms best describes the aforementioned phenomenon?

a. Denial

b. Reaction formation

c. Displacement

d. Projection

e. Sublimation

Question 116

You are seeing a 60-year-old woman who is referred by her GP for depression. She complains of 6-month history of worsening progressive dysphagia and there has been no improvement. Her husband confirms her history. This patient is most likely suffering from

a. Cerebrovascular accident

b. Moderate depressive episode with somatic complaints

c. Myasthenia gravis

d. Motor neuron disease

e. Hypochondriasis

Question 117

When a 25-year old female was asked to describe her premorbid personality, she claimed that she is someone who always finds it tough to make decision. Which particular personality disorder is she likely to have?

a. Schizoid personality disorder
b. Schizotypal personality disorder
c. Borderline personality disorder
d. Dependent personality disorder
e. OCD

Question 118

Patients with catatonia tend to present with the following symptoms, with the exception of

a. Ambitendency
b. Echopraxia
c. Specific mannerisms
d. Echopraxia
e. De-personalization

Extended matching items (EMIs)

Theme: Cognitive testing

Lead in: Please select the most appropriate answer for each one of the following. Each option may be used once, more than once or not at all.

Options:

a. Mini Mental State Examination
b. Cambridge Neuropsychological Test Automated Battery
c. Blessed Dementia Scale
d. Geriatric Mental State Schedule
e. Clifton Assessment Schedule
f. Vineland Social Maturity Scale

Question 119

This is a test which could be used for the assessment of dementia as well as in the assessment of childhood development and learning disability.

Question 120

This is a nursing rated assessment scale.

Question 121

This is a questionnaire that is usually administered to a relative or friend of the patient.

Question 122

This is a semi-structured interview that assesses the subject's mental state.

Question 123
This is a questionnaire that consists of 13 computerized tasks.

Question 124
This is a brief test that could be used to rapidly detect possible dementia, to follow up on the course of cognitive changes over time and to differentiate between delirium and dementia.

Theme: Executive function tests

Lead in: Please select the most appropriate answer for each one of the following. Each option may be used once, more than once or not at all.

Options:
a. Stroop Test
b. Verbal fluency test
c. Tower of London Test
d. Wisconsin Card Sort Test
e. Cognitive Estimates Test
f. Six elements test
g. Multiple errands task
h. Trail making test

Question 125
Some frontal lobe damaged patients may occasionally give grossly incorrect answers to known phenomena.

Question 126
This is a strategy application test that helps to uncover evidence of organization difficulty that might have occurred as a result of frontal lobe damage.

Question 127
The following abilities are tested in this test: sequencing, cognitive flexibility, visual scanning, spatial analysis, motor control, alertness and concentration.

Question 128
This is a test that helps to pick up perseverative errors.

Question 129
Left frontal lobe lesions are usually associated with poor performance on this particular test that tests for planning ability.

Question 130
This is a test that involves asking the subject to articulate as many words as possible over a fixed duration of time.

Question 131
This is a test that tests the interference that may occur between reading words and naming colours.

Theme: Clinical interview

Options:

a. Acting-out
b. Ambivalence
c. Anger
d. Disinhibition
e. Dysphoric mood
f. Euphoric mood
g. Failure of empathy
h. Fatuousness
i. Flat affect
j. Good rapport
k. Guardedness
l. Humour
m. Humiliation
n. Incongruous affect
o. Labile affect
p. Resistance
q. Restricted affective range

Lead in: A 30-year-old woman was admitted to the neurosurgical ward after she was hit on her head after a fight in the pub. The neurosurgeon refers her for psychiatric assessment. When a male trainee interviews her, she exhibits the following phenomenon. Identify which of the aforementioned terminology resembles her clinical presentation. Each option might be used once, more than once or not at all.

Question 132

She copes with her memory impairment by making jokes. (Choose one option.)

Question 133

She laughs and jokes with the trainee. Then she suddenly bursts into tears and asks for forgiveness. (Choose one option.)

Question 134

When a male trainee interviews her, she touches his inner thigh and wants to take off her blouse. (Choose one option.)

Theme: Basic psychology

Options:

a. Context-dependent forgetting
b. Cue-dependent forgetting
c. Decay theory
d. Displacement theory
e. Motivated forgetting
f. Proactive interference
g. Retrieval failure
h. Retroactive interference

i. State-dependent forgetting
   j. Storage failure

Lead in: Identify which of the above terms best explains the following scenarios. Each option might be used once, more than once or not at all.

Question 135
A patient is busy sending a SMS message while the psychiatrist is talking to him. When the psychiatrist asks the patient to recall what he has just said, the patient cannot recall. (Choose one option.)

Question 136
A 50-year-old man hears a gunshot when he is walking in a city centre park. He suddenly remembers a long forgotten memory of witnessing an armed robbery. (Choose one option.)

Question 137
A 25-year-old woman from Canada visits her brother who lives in the UK. When she is about to get in his car, she always finds herself getting into the driver side despite multiple reminders from her brother. (Choose one option.)

Theme: Classification systems
Options:
   a. ICD-6
   b. ICD-11
   c. DSM-1
   d. DSM-II
   e. DSM-III
   f. DSM-III-R
   g. DSM-IV

Lead in: Select the most appropriate answer for each of the following. Each option may be used once, more than once or not at all.

Question 138
This was a classification system developed and based upon the mental disorders section of ICD-6.

Question 139
This was considered to be an innovative psychiatric classification system that tried not to appear to favour any theories and included the multi-axial classification.

Question 140
Revisions were done and this was published in 1987.

Theme: Learning theories and behavioural change
Options:
   a. Positive reinforcer
   b. Negative reinforcer

c. Punishment
d. Primary reinforcement
e. Secondary reinforcement
f. Continuous reinforcement
g. Fixed interval schedule
h. Variable interval schedule
i. Fixed ratio schedule
j. Variable ratio schedule

Lead in: Select the most appropriate answer for each of the following. Each option may be used once, more than once or not at all.

Question 141
Escape conditioning is an example of this.

Question 142
This refers to a situation in which an aversive stimulus is presented whenever a given behaviour occurs.

Question 143
This refers to reinforcement that is occurring through reduction of needs driving from basic drives.

Question 144
This refers to reinforcement that is derived from association with primary reinforcers.

Question 145
In this particular schedule of reinforcement, reinforcement occurs only after a fixed interval of time.

Question 146
In this particular schedule of reinforcement, reinforcement occurs only after variable intervals.

Question 147
This particular schedule of reinforcement is generally considered to be good with regards to maintaining a high response rate.

Theme: Attachment abnormalities
Options:
a. Insecure attachment
b. Avoidant attachment
c. Separation anxiety
d. Acute separation reaction
e. Stranger anxiety
f. Maternal deprivation

Lead in: Select the most appropriate answer for each of the following. Each option may be used once, more than once or not at all.

Question 148
This form of attachment would predispose individuals towards childhood emotional disorders and disorders such as agoraphobia.

Question 149
This form of attachment would predispose individuals towards poor social functioning in later life, which might include aggression.

Question 150
As a result of this, an infant may hold a comfort object or a transitional object.

Question 151
Developmental language delay, shallow relationships and lack of empathy might arise due to this.

Theme: Clinical assessment and neuropsychological processes
Options:
   a. Lexical dysgraphia
   b. Deep dysgraphia
   c. Neglect dysgraphia
   d. Dyspraxic dysgraphia
   e. Alexia without agraphia
   f. Alexia with agraphia

Lead in: Select the most appropriate answer for each of the following. Each option may be used once, more than once or not at all.

Question 152
A patient breaks down the word's spelling and has much difficulty in writing irregular words. This is an example of

Question 153
A patient is unable to spell non-existent words. This is an example of

Question 154
A patient tends to misspell the initial part of words. This is an example of

Question 155
Three months after suffering a stroke, a patient develops a new technique to help himself recognize words. He reads letter by letter and spells the word out loud. Then he recognizes the word after hearing himself spell it out. This is an example of

Theme: Psychology
Options:
   a. Aversive conditioning
   b. Chaining
   c. Flooding

d. Habituation
  e. Insight learning
  f. Latent learning
  g. Penalty
  h. Premack's principle
  i. Reciprocal inhibition
  j. Shaping
  k. Systematic desensitization
  l. Token economy

Lead in: Select the aforementioned behavioural techniques to match the following examples. Each option might be used once, more than once or not at all.

Question 156
The staff of a hostel for learning disability patients wants to train her clients to clean up the tables after meals. She develops a successive reinforcing schedule to reward her clients. The clients will be rewarded successively over time for putting their utensils away from the dining table back to the pantry. Then they need to clean the utensils and put them back to the cupboard. (Choose one option.)

Question 157
A 2-year-old son of a woman is scared of dogs. His mother tries to reduce his fear by bringing him to see the dogs in the park. The fear-provoking situation is coupled and opposed by putting him on her lap and allowing him to drink his favourite juice. (Choose one option.)

Question 158
A 40-year-old woman staying in London develops fear of the tube and she sees a psychologist for psychotherapy. The psychologist has drafted a behavioural programme where the patient is advised to start with travelling between two tube stations with her husband and gradually increase to more stations without her husband. At the end of the hierarchy, she will travel from the Heathrow terminal station to the Cockfosters Station along the Piccadilly line. (Choose one option.)

Question 159
A 40-year-old woman staying in London develops fear of the tube. She is instructed to start with the most fearful situation by taking a train from the Heathrow terminal station to the Cockfosters Station along the Piccadilly line on her own. (Choose one option.)

Question 160
An 11-year-old girl is referred to the Child and Adolescent Mental Health Service (CAMHS) as she refuses to do her homework. She prefers to stay in her room and plays piano for the whole day. The team has advised the parents to adopt the following plan: The girl is allowed to play her piano for 30 minutes only after spending 1 hour on her homework. (Choose one option.)

Question 161
A 9-year-old girl is referred to the CAMHS as she refuses to do her homework. The case manager advises the mother to reward her child with a sticker every time she has completed her homework. Once she gets 20 stickers, she can use them to exchange for a present. (Choose one option.)

Question 162
In the prison, the psychologists have developed an *in vivo* exposure programme for the prisoners to expose themselves to the images of being arrested and other social sanctions on their criminal behaviour. Some prisoners find that their urge to commit crime reduces after repeated exposures. (Choose one option.)

Theme: Psychology
Options:
   a. Aversive conditioning
   b. Chaining
   c. Flooding
   d. Habituation
   e. Insight learning
   f. Latent learning
   g. Penalty
   h. Premack's principle
   i. Reciprocal inhibition
   j. Shaping
   k. Systematic desensitization
   l. Token economy

Lead in: Select the above behavioural techniques to match the following examples. Each option might be used once, more than once or not at all.

Question 163
A 6-year-old boy is put in a maze to look for the toy box. After a few trials, he learns the cognitive map of the maze and getting shorter time to find the toy box. (Choose one option.)

Question 164
A 2-year-old child is undergoing toilet training. The complex behaviour is broken down into simpler steps. She is rewarded with a sticker if she informs her mother of her urge to urinate. The positive reinforcement continues until she can inform her mother reliably without failures. Then the contingencies are altered and she needs to go to the toilet on her own before the sticker is given. (Choose one option.)

Question 165
A patient with moderate learning disability has aggressive tendency and tends to assault the other residents in the hostel. The staff has devised a plan in response to his aggressive behaviour. His main pleasurable activity is watching television. He

will be removed from the TV room and put in a single room for a 2-hour time-out period if he assaults any resident. (Choose one option.)

Question 166
A 14-year-old anorexia nervosa patient with body mass index (BMI) of 11 was admitted to the eating disorder unit for inpatient treatment. Initially, she was hostile to the staff and resistant to feeding. She did not like the ward environment. She has decided to comply with the treatment programme. She also wants to reach the target weight as soon as possible as she wants to get out of the ward. (Choose one option.)

Question 167
A 10-year-old boy was taught by his parents not to respond to the TV sound when he is doing homework as the stimulus is not significant. (Choose one option.)

Question 168
A 20-year-old man was sacked by his company. His partner had criticized him. He suddenly realized that he had been lazy and irresponsible. He decided to change and wanted to demonstrate his competency to his partner. The next day, he went to the career centre to look for a job. (Choose one option.)

Theme: History of psychiatry
Options:
   a. Bleuler
   b. Kahlbaum
   c. Kasanin
   d. Kraepelin
   e. Langfeldt
   f. Leonard
   g. Hecker
   h. Griesinger
   i. Kane
   j. Andreasson
   k. Crow
   l. Liddle
   m. Mayer–Gross
   n. Kendler

Lead in: Select one person who is associated with each the following terms.

Question 169
Catatonia. (Choose one option.)

Question 170
Cycloid psychosis. (Choose one option.)

Question 171
Dementia praecox. (Choose one option.)

Question 172
Hebephrenia. (Choose one option.)

Question 173
Schizophrenia. (Choose one option.)

Question 174
Schizoaffective disorder. (Choose one option.)

Theme: General adult psychiatry

Options:
  a. 0%–4%
  b. 5%–9%
  c. 10%–14%
  d. 15%–19%
  e. 20%–24%
  f. 25%–29%
  g. 30%–34%
  h. 35%–50%
  i. 60%–65%
  j. 70%–75%
  k. 80%–85%

Lead in: A 28-year-old man has suffered from schizophrenia for 5 years. He is currently stable and recently got married. He and his wife are planning to have children. He consults you on the genetic risk on schizophrenia.
  Each option might be used once, more than once, or not at all.

Question 175
The risk of schizophrenia in his child if his wife also suffers from schizophrenia. (Choose one option.)

Question 176
The risk of schizophrenia in his child if his wife does not suffer from schizophrenia. (Choose one option.)

Question 177
The risk of schizophrenia if he adopted a child with velocardiofacial syndrome. (Choose one option.)

Question 178
The risk of schizophrenia in his half siblings. (Choose one option.)

Question 179

The risk of schizophrenia in his younger cousin. (Choose one option.)

Theme: Basic pharmacolog

Options:

a. 1

b. 2

c. 5

d. 15

e. 25

f. 35

g. 45

h. 55

i. 65

j. 75

Lead in: A 17-year-old man was referred to the early psychosis team for the first episode of schizophrenia. You gave him risperidone 1 mg nocte. His mother requests an answer from you on the following questions. Each option might be used once, more than once or not at all.

Question 180

His psychotic symptoms are not controlled. His mother wants to know the minimum effective dose (in mg) of risperidone in his case. (Choose one option.)

Question 181

His psychotic symptoms are under control. His mother wants to know the duration of antipsychotic treatment (in months) in his case. (Choose one option.)

Question 182

After 18 months of treatment, the patient has decided to stop the medication. His mother wants to know the risk of relapse in percentage. (Choose one option.)

EMI on aetiology

a. Apolipoprotein E4 gene (homozygous for ε4)

b. Cardiovascular disease

c. Cancer

d. Childhood sexual abuse

e. Death of mother before the age of 11 years

f. Down syndrome

g. Dysbindin gene

h. Migration

i. Neuregulin gene

j. Old age

k. Streptococcal infection
l. Three children at home under the age of 14 years
m. Unemployment

Lead in: Match the aforementioned aetiological factors to the following clinical scenarios. Each option may be used once, more than once or not at all.

Question 183
A 10-year-old boy develops obsessions and compulsive behaviour after a sore throat and fever. (Choose one option.)

Question 184
A 19-year-old woman presents with recurrent self-harm following the end of a transient and intense romantic relationship. She has a chronic feeling of emptiness and exhibits binge eating behaviour. (Choose one option.)

Question 185
A 24-year-old man complains that MI5 is monitoring him and has tried to control his feelings and intentions. He heard the voices of two secret agents talking about him and they issued him with a command. (Choose three options.)

MRCPSYCH PAPER A1 MOCK EXAMINATION 2: ANSWERS

GET THROUGH MRCPSYCH PAPER A1: MOCK EXAMINATION

Question 1 Answer: a, Palilalia
Explanation: This is known as palilalia, which means that a patient repeats a word with increasing frequency. It is important to differentiate this with logoclonia, which occurs when the person repeats just the last syllable of the last word. Both of these terms are examples of preservation of speech. In perseveration, mental operations are continued beyond the point at which they are relevant.

Reference: Puri BK, Hall A, Ho R (2014). *Revision Notes in Psychiatry*. London: CRC Press, p. 4.

Question 2 Answer: e, Reciprocal inhibition
Explanation: Reciprocal inhibition is a technique used in systematic desensitization, where the antagonistic response to anxiety (i.e. relaxation) is maintained when the feared stimulus is presented.

Reference and Further Reading: Puri BK, Treasaden I (eds) (2010). *Psychiatry: An Evidence-Based Text*. London: Hodder Arnold, pp. 655, 990.

Question 3 Answer: d, Phenobarbital sodium
Explanation: This question is asking which of the aforementioned psychotropic drugs is hygroscopic. A hygroscopic drug is one which attracts moisture from the atmosphere. Phenobarbital sodium is hygroscopic. Even in the absence of light, phenobarbital sodium is gradually degraded on exposure to a humid atmosphere. The other psychotropic medications are coated and they are very stable compounds because no degradation is observed by the action of heat and light.

Reference: Church C, Smith J (2006). How stable are medicines moved from original packs into compliance aids? *Pharmaceutical Journal*, 276: 75–81.

Question 4 Answer: d, Transsexualism
Explanation: The clinical diagnosis is that of transsexualism. In this condition, there is the desire to live as a member of the opposite sex, with marked discomfort

with one's own anatomic sex and with an intense desire to change the body into that of the preferred sex. It is important to differentiate this from transvestism, which refers to the wearing of the clothes of the opposite sex to obtain sexual excitement. More than a single item is worn, often an entire outfit. It is clearly associated with sexual arousal; there is no wish to continue cross-dressing once orgasm occurs, distinguishing this from dual-role transvestism.

Reference: Puri BK, Hall A, Ho R (2014). *Revision Notes in Psychiatry.* London: CRC Press, p. 603.

Question 5 Answer: d, Medial temporal lobe lesions and complex partial seizure

Explanation: Seizures are associated with medial temporal lobe lesions, and complex partial seizures are known as uncinate seizures which can give rise to olfactory hallucinations.

Reference and Further Reading: Cummings JL, Mega MS (eds) (2003). *Neuropsychiatry and Behavioural Neuroscience.* New York: Oxford University Press; Puri BK, Treasaden I (eds) (2010). *Psychiatry: An Evidence-Based Text.* London: Hodder Arnold, p. 532.

Question 6 Answer: c, Blood injection phobia

Explanation: The blood injection phobia (usually associated with needles, injections, medical procedures) has a strong underlying genetic linkage. In defining a phobia, the following need to be considered: It is considered to be out of proportion to objective risks; it cannot be reasoned or explained away; it is beyond voluntary control and it leads to avoidance behaviour.

Reference: Puri BK, Hall A, Ho R (2014). *Revision Notes in Psychiatry.* London: CRC Press, p. 406.

Question 7 Answer: a, Carbamazepine

Explanation: This is another version of a multiple-choice question (MCQ) about storage of psychotropic medications. Among all the options, carbamazepine is most likely to be affected by exposure to air and light. In these circumstances, the psychiatrist should recommend the nurses to keep carbamazepine in a sealed container and avoid sunlight.

Reference and Further Reading: Puri BK, Treasaden I (eds) (2010). *Psychiatry: An Evidence-Based Text.* London: Hodder Arnold, pp. 532, 538, 910.

Question 8 Answer: a, Déjà vu

Explanation: This refers to déjà vu, which is when the individual feels that the current situation has been seen or experienced before. Option (b) refers to the illusion of an auditory recognition. Option (c) refers to the illusion of recognition of a new thought. Option (d) refers to the illusion of failure to recognize a familiar situation. Option (e) refers to how false details are being added to the recollection of an otherwise real memory.

Reference: Puri BK, Hall A, Ho R (2014). *Revision Notes in Psychiatry*. London: CRC Press, p. 9.

Question 9 Answer: c, This phenomenon is an example of classical conditioning.
Explanation: This phenomenon is learned helplessness. It is the tendency to fail to escape from a situation due to repeated failures in the past. Seligman first described learned helplessness. The classic experiment involved delivering electric shocks to dogs that were harnessed so that they could not escape the shock. Subsequently, these dogs did not try to escape the shocks even when unharnessed. Learned helplessness was applied to the cognitive theory depression. One's vulnerability to depression is dependent on one's attribution style, that is one's habitual pattern of explaining life events. Learned helplessness is not an example of classical conditioning.

Reference and Further Reading: Puri BK, Treasaden I (eds) (2010). *Psychiatry: An Evidence-Based Text*. London: Hodder Arnold, pp. 206, 298, 614.

Question 10 Answer: a, Carbamazepine
Explanation: Combination of clozapine and carbamazepine will lead to blood dyscrasia. Lithium is sometimes added to clozapine to treat clozapine-induced neutropenia. Risperidone is sometimes added to clozapine in patients who do not respond to clozapine alone. There is no contraindication to add fluoxetine or valproate onto clozapine.

Reference and Further Reading: Puri BK, Treasaden I (eds) (2010). *Psychiatry: An Evidence-Based Text*. London: Hodder Arnold, pp. 425–457, 603.

Question 11 Answer: c, Female gender
Explanation: Female gender, Ashkenazi Jewish descent and older age are associated with a high risk of developing agranulocytosis. The risk of developing agranulocytosis is not directly proportional to dose and duration of treatment.

Reference: Alvir JMJ, Lieberman JA, Safferman AZ, Schwimmer JL, Schaaf JA (1993). Clozapine-induced agranulocytosis. Incidence and risk factors in the United States. *N Engl J Med*, 329:162–167. http://www.nejm.org/toc/nejm/329/3/.

Question 12 Answer: b, Obsessive-compulsive personality disorder
Explanation: The clinical diagnosis is as aforementioned. Individuals with this disorder tend to have feelings of excessive doubt and caution. They are obsessed with perfectionism that would interfere with tasks. They tend also to be very rigid and stubborn in their cognitions.

Reference: Puri BK, Hall A, Ho R (2014). *Revision Notes in Psychiatry*. London: CRC Press, p. 453.

Question 13 Answer: a, Onset younger than the age of 15
Explanation: The earlier onset, especially below the age of 15, is indicative of a good prognostic factor. The good prognostic factors include that of onset prior to the age of 15, higher weight at onset and at presentation, those who have received treatment within 3 months after the onset of the illness, those who recovered within 2 years after the initiation of treatment, those with supportive family, good motivation to change and good childhood social adjustment.

Reference: Puri BK, Hall A, Ho R (2014). *Revision Notes in Psychiatry*. London: CRC Press, p. 581.

Question 14 Answer: b, Headache getting worse when lying down
Explanation: Postural trigger of headache may suggest raised intracranial pressure.

Reference: Fuller G, Manford M (2003). *Neurology – A Illustrated Colour Text*. Edinburgh, UK: Churchill Livingstone.

Question 15 Answer: b, Asperger's syndrome
Explanation: Autism and Asperger's syndrome are similar except that delayed speech is found in autism but not in Asperger's syndrome. In autism, performance IQ is higher than verbal IQ. In contrast, verbal IQ is higher than performance IQ in Asperger's syndrome. Rett's syndrome occurs in girls with sudden arrest of development at 6 months. Children with childhood disintegrative disorder have normal development up to 2 years and have loss of skills in language, play, social skills, bladder or bowel controls and motor skills.

Reference and Further Reading: Puri BK, Treasaden I (eds) (2010). *Psychiatry: An Evidence-Based Text*. London: Hodder Arnold, pp. 1066–1067, 1088–1090.

Question 16 Answer: d, Echolalia
Explanation: Echolalia refers to the automatic imitation by the person of another person's speech. Approximate answers refer to an approximate answer that, although clearly incorrect, does demonstrate that the is known. Cryptolalia refer to speech in a language that no one could understand. Circumstantiality refers to thinking that appears slow with the incorporation of unnecessary trivial details. The goal of thought is finally reached, however. Flight of ideas refers to speech that consists of a stream of accelerated thoughts with no central direction.

Reference: Puri BK, Hall A, Ho R (2014). *Revision Notes in Psychiatry*. London: CRC Press, p. 3.

Question 17 Answer: d, Second-order conditioning is more easily demonstrated than classical conditioning.
Explanation: Option (d) is false. Classical conditioning is more easily demonstrated than second-order conditioning because second-order conditioning requires an initial learning of associations between conditioned and unconditioned stimuli

before learning an extra association, which would constitute second-order conditioning. Option (a) is true. Objects resembling fear-provoking stimuli can elicit fear themselves through second-order conditioning. Option (b) is true. Animal phobias have the best prognosis, social phobias are likely to improve gradually and agoraphobia has the worst prognosis. Option (e) is true. Forward conditioning is also known as delayed conditioning. Backward conditioning produces little learning.

Reference and Further Reading: Puri BK, Treasaden I (eds) (2010). *Psychiatry: An Evidence-Based Text*. London: Hodder Arnold, pp. 198–199, 653–656.

Question 18 Answer: c, Third month of treatment
Explanation: The hazard rate for agranulocytosis peaked during the third month of treatment.

Reference: Alvir JMJ, Lieberman JA, Safferman AZ, Schwimmer JL, Schaaf JA (1993). Clozapine-induced agranulocytosis. Incidence and risk factors in the United States. *N Engl J Med*, 329: 162–167. http://www.nejm.org/toc/nejm/329/3/.

Question 19 Answer: b, Loud noises
Explanation: From 6 months, children develop a fear of loud noises. Fears of animals, darkness and 'monsters' begin at 3–5 years. The fear of death begins in adolescence.

Reference and Further Reading: Puri BK, Hall AD (2002). *Revision Notes in Psychiatry*. London: Arnold, p. 73; Puri BK, Treasaden I (eds) (2010). *Psychiatry: An Evidence-Based Text*. London: Hodder Arnold, pp. 119–120.

Question 20 Answer: d, Depth perception
Explanation: Depth perception is developed at 2 months.

Reference and Further Reading: Berk LE (2006). *Child Development* (7th edition). Boston: Pearson, pp. 152–160.

Question 21 Answer: c, Contralateral lower limb weakness
Explanation: The neurological signs and lesions of specific branches of anterior cerebral arteries are summarized as follows:

- Orbital branch: apathy and memory impairment
- Medial striate artery (supplying cranial V, VII and XII nerves): dysarthria and dysphagia
- Callosomarginal brain (supplying the supplementary motor area): contralateral hemiparesis (leg > arm), incontinence as a result of weakness in pelvic floor and mutism
- Pericallosal branch (suppling corpus callosum): ideomotor apraxia and tactile anomia

- Left anterior cerebral artery: mixed aphasia
- Right anterior cerebral artery: dysapraxia
- Bilateral anterior cerebral artery: akinetic mutism

Lesions in unilateral posterior cerebral artery cause contralateral III nerve palsy. Lesions in vertebral and basilar arteries cause nystagmus.

Reference: Malhi GS, Malhi S (2006). *Examination Notes in Psychiatry: Basic Sciences* (2nd edition). London: Hodder Arnold.

Question 22 Answer: d, The child is able to run on tiptoes.
Explanation: A child is able to walk a few steps on tiptoe by age two, 10 feet by age four and run on tiptoes by age five. Option (c) and (e) are achieved by age two. Options (a) and (b) are achieved by age three.

Reference and Further Reading: Berk LE (2006). *Child Development* (7th edition). Boston: Pearson, p. 175.

Question 23 Answer: d, Based on the ICD-10 criteria, dysthymia is severe enough to meet diagnostic criteria of post-schizophrenic depression.
Explanation: The depressive symptoms must be severe and extensive to meet criteria for at least a mild depressive episode.

References: American Psychiatric Association (2000). *Diagnostic Criteria from DSM-IV-TR*. Washington, DC: American Psychiatric Association; World Health Organisation (1994). *ICD-10 Classification of Mental and Behavioural Disorders*. Edinburgh, UK: Churchill Livingstone.

Question 24 Answer: c, Hebephrenic type
Explanation: Both hebephrenic and simple schizophrenia are found in the ICD-10 but not in the DSM-IV-TR. Hebephrenic schizophrenia is characterized by flattening of affect, aimless behaviour, disjointed thought and less prominent hallucinations and delusions. Simple schizophrenia has a slow but progressive development over a period of at least 1 year. There is a significant change in the overall quality of personal behaviour, deepening of negative symptoms and a marked decline in performance.

References: American Psychiatric Association (2000). *Diagnostic Criteria from DSM-IV-TR*. Washington, DC: American Psychiatric Association; World Health Organisation (1994). *ICD-10 Classification of Mental and Behavioural Disorders*. Edinburgh, UK: Churchill Livingstone.

Question 25 Answer: e, Female gender
Explanation: All of the aforementioned are considered to be bad prognostic factors for anorexia nervosa (AN), with the exception of female gender. The other bad prognostic factors include onset at an older age, lower weight at onset and at presentation, very frequent vomiting and presence of bulimia, very severe weight loss, long duration of anorexia nervosa (AN), previous hospitalization, extreme resistance to treatment, continued family problems, neurotic personality and male gender.

Reference: Puri BK, Hall A, Ho R (2014). *Revision Notes in Psychiatry*. London: CRC Press, p. 581.

Question 26 Answer: a, Autochthonous delusion
Explanation: Primary delusion is a fully formed delusion that arises without any discernible connection with previous events. Primary delusions (e.g. delusional perception and delusional memory) do not start with an idea and can occur out of the blue or may be preceded by delusional mood, which is a feeling that something unusual and threatening is about to happen.

Reference and Further Reading: Puri BK, Hall AD (2002). *Revision Notes in Psychiatry*. London: Arnold, p. 152.

Question 27 Answer: e, Three-dimensional similarity
Explanation: All of the aforementioned are based on the principles of Gestalt psychology, with the exception of option (e). It proposes that the whole perception is different from the sum of its parts. It also proposes the law of simplicity, the law of continuity, the law of similarity, and the law of proximity and figure-ground differentiation. The law of simplicity states that the percept would correspond to the simplest stimulation interpretation. The law of continuity refers to how interrupted lines are being perceived as continuous. The law of similarity refers to how like items are being grouped together. The law of proximity refers to how adjacent items are grouped together.

Reference: Puri BK, Hall A, Ho R (2014). *Revision Notes in Psychiatry*. London: CRC Press, p. 31.

Question 28 Answer: e, Valproate
Explanation: An audit performed in the South London and Maudsley National Health Service (NHS) Trust in 2007 suggests that valproate actually prevents clozapine-induced seizures. Carbamazepine is contraindicated in this case.

Reference: Sparshatt A, Whiskey E, Taylor E (2008). Valproate as prophylaxis for clozapine induced seizures: Survey of practice. *Psychiatric Bulletin*, 32: 262–265.

Question 29 Answer: a, He fulfils the diagnostic criteria for schizophrenia based on the ICD-10.
Explanation: Based on the ICD-10, a period of at least 1 month is required before a diagnosis of schizophrenia could be made. Based on the DSM-IV-TR, a period of at least 6 months is required.

Reference and Further Reading: American Psychiatric Association (2000). *Diagnostic Criteria from DSM-IV-TR*. Washington, DC: American Psychiatric Association; World Health Organisation (1994). *ICD-10 Classification of Mental and Behavioural Disorders*. Edinburgh, UK: Churchill Livingstone; Puri BK, Treasaden I (eds) (2010). *Psychiatry: An Evidence-Based Text*. London: Hodder Arnold, pp. 594–596.

Question 30 Answer: e, Conformity to the group's decision on a line judgement experiment was greater in a group of 25 members as compared to a group of four.

Explanation: Previous research has demonstrated that as the size of the group increases, the impact of one's decision decreases, thus leading to lesser pressure to conform. It should be noted that self-reliant, intelligent, expressive, socially effective individuals are least vulnerable to group pressure.

Reference: Puri BK, Hall A, Ho R (2014). *Revision Notes in Psychiatry*. London: CRC Press, p. 60.

Question 31 Answer: d, Cognitive changes occur at the age of five for children to adopt the theory of mind.

Explanation: Cognitive changes usually occur at the age of four for children to acquire a theory of mind. It has been suggested that a failure to acquire such a theory of mind is associated with disorders such as autism.

Reference: Puri BK, Hall A, Ho R (2014). *Revision Notes in Psychiatry*. London: CRC Press, p. 59.

Question 32 Answer: e, 250 mg

Explanation: Based on the DSM-5, individuals who consume more than 250 mg per day of caffeine is considered to be intoxicated. This might result in anxiety, restlessness, nausea, muscle twitching and facial flushing. It is important to note that at levels of intake in excess of 600 mg per day, dysphoria will replace euphoria, anxiety and mood disturbances become prominent, and insomnia, muscle-twitching, tachycardia and sometimes cardiac arrhythmias might occur.

Reference: Puri BK, Hall A, Ho R (2014). *Revision Notes in Psychiatry*. London: CRC Press, p. 544.

Question 33 Answer: b, Cognitive analytical therapy

Explanation: Cognitive analytical therapy is a combination of cognitive and analytical therapy. It helps in the identification of faculty procedures such as traps (which are repetitive cycles of behaviour and their consequences that become perpetuation), dilemma (false choice or unduly narrowed options) and snag (extreme pessimism about the future and halt a plan before it even starts).

Reference: Puri BK, Hall A, Ho R (2014). *Revision Notes in Psychiatry*. London: CRC Press, p. 337.

Question 34 Answer: b, Schizotypal personality disorder

Explanation: Schizotypal disorder has been demonstrated to have the strongest genetic linkage. Almost all the studies of the families of schizophrenic pro-bands have found an excess of both schizophrenia and schizotypal personality disorder among relatives (22% in the biological relatives of schizophrenics as compared to 2% of the adoptive relatives and control).

Reference: Puri BK, Hall A, Ho R (2014). *Revision Notes in Psychiatry*. London: CRC Press, p. 440.

Question 35 Answer: b, Anosmia
Explanation: Tumour of frontal lobe is a known cause of anosmia (loss of olfactory function). Other common causes include injury to olfactory nerve, Alzheimer's disease and Parkinson's disease. Amusia is caused by lesions in the superior temporal lobe. Anterograde amnesia is caused by lesions in the medial temporal lobe. Apraxia is caused by lesions in the non-dominant parietal lobe. Bitemporal hemianopia is caused by tumours in the pituitary gland.

Reference: Malhi GS, Malhi S (2006). *Examination Notes in Psychiatry: Basic Sciences* (2nd edition). London: Hodder Arnold.

Question 36 Answer: c, Bystander effect
Explanation: This refers to the phenomenon where individuals are less likely to extend help during an emergency in the presence of others.

Reference: Puri BK, Treasaden I (2010). *Psychiatry: An Evidence-Based Text*. London: Hodder Arnold, p. 290.

Question 37 Answer: a, Cenesthesia
Explanation: Cenesthesia refers a change in the normal quality of feeling tone in a part of the body.

Reference: Sadock BJ, Sadock VA. (2008). *Kaplan and Sadock's Concise Textbook of Psychiatry* (3rd edition). Philadelphia, PA: Lippincott, Williams & Wilkins, p. 23.

Question 38 Answer: c, Delusional misidentification
Explanation: This condition is known as morbid jealousy (or pathological jealousy or Othello syndrome), which is the delusional belief of infidelity of the spouse or sexual partner. Patients with morbid jealousy go to excessive lengths to test their partner's fidelity and make accusations based on insignificant evidence. The condition is more common in men. Some aetiological factors include psychoactive substance use disorders, paranoid schizophrenia, depression, neurosis or personality disorders and organic disorders such as dementia.

Reference and Further Reading: Puri BK, Hall AD (2002). *Revision Notes in Psychiatry*. London: Arnold, p. 381.

Question 39 Answer: e, Insight
Explanation: Attention, retention, reproduction and motivation are all involved in the modelling process. Successful observational learning is more likely when there

is optimal arousal, the presence of an attractive, prestigious, colourful and dramatic model. Reproduction also helps to ensure what has been remembered have been translated into behaviour. It is important to note that unsuccessful observational learning is more likely to occur in association with the following factors including low arousal, over-arousal and in the presence of distracting stimuli.

Reference: Puri BK, Hall A, Ho R (2014). *Revision Notes in Psychiatry*. London: CRC Press, p. 27.

Question 40 Answer: b, Conditioning theory
Explanation: All of the aforementioned are theories that explain interpersonal attraction. Reciprocal reinforcement of the attraction occurs with rewards in both directions. Based on the social exchange theory, people tend to prefer relationships that appear to offer an optimum cost–benefit ratio. Equity theory states that the preferred relationships are those in which each feels that the cost–benefit ratio of the relationship for each person is approximately equal. Proxemics relates to interpersonal space and body buffer zone.

Reference: Puri BK, Hall A, Ho R (2014). *Revision Notes in Psychiatry*. London: CRC Press, p. 59.

Question 41 Answer: a, Automatic obedience
Explanation: Automatic obedience refers to a condition in which the person follows the examiner's instructions blindly without judgement and resistance.

Reference and Further Reading: Puri BK, Treasaden I (eds) (2010). *Psychiatry: An Evidence-Based Text*. London: Hodder Arnold, pp. 294–295.

Question 42 Answer: b, Post-natal psychosis
Explanation: She is likely to be having post-natal psychosis. Post-natal psychosis usually has an abrupt onset, usually within the first 2 weeks after childbirth. In addition, it is characterized by marked restlessness, fear and insomnia. There might be delusions, hallucinations and disturbed behaviour, which develop rapidly. There might be marked perplexity, but with no detectable cognitive impairment. Usually, there is noted to be rapid fluctuations in the mental state, sometimes from hour to hour.

Reference: Puri BK, Hall A, Ho R (2014). *Revision Notes in Psychiatry*. London: CRC Press p. 568.

Question 43 Answer: b, Foot in the door technique
Explanation: This is an example of the foot in the door technique. Foot in the door technique involves asking for a small commitment, followed by a bigger commitment after gaining initial compliance.

Reference: Puri BK, Tresaden I (2010). *Psychiatry: An Evidence-Based Text*. London: Hodder Arnold, pp. 290–291.

Question 44 Answer: b, Gegenhalten

Explanation: Gegenhalten is a form of paratonia consisting of uneven resistance of the limbs to passive movement.

Reference and Further Reading: Campbell RJ (1996). *Psychiatric Dictionary*. Oxford, UK: Oxford University Press.

Question 45 Answer: c, Fourth cranial nerve

Explanation: The fourth cranial nerve is likely to be affected, as it supplies the superior oblique muscle of the eye, which has been affected in this clinical example.

Reference: Puri BK, Hall A, Ho R (2014). *Revision Notes in Psychiatry*. London: CRC Press, p. 159.

Question 46 Answer: e, Emotional arousal might or might not increase aggression.

Explanation: Emotional arousal would potentially increase aggression. In addition, the frustration–aggression hypothesis proposes that preventing a person from reaching their goal will induce an aggressive drive resulting in a behaviour intended to harm the one causing the frustration. Expressing this aggression will reduce the aggressive drive.

Reference: Puri BK, Hall A, Ho R (2014). *Revision Notes in Psychiatry*. London: CRC Press, p. 60.

Question 47 Answer: b, Cataplexy

Explanation: Cataplexy refers to the temporary paralysis and loss of antigravity muscle tone without loss of consciousness. Cataplexy is often precipitated by emotional excitement and associated with narcolepsy.

Reference and Further Reading: Campbell RJ (1996). *Psychiatric Dictionary*. Oxford, UK: Oxford University Press.

Question 48 Answer: b, Mannerism

Explanation: Mannerisms are repeated involuntary movements that are goal directed. An example would be 'A person repeatedly moving his hand when he talks and tries to convey his message to the examiner'.

Reference and Further Reading: Rajagopal S (2007). Catatonia. *Advances in Psychiatric Treatment*, 13: 51–59.

Question 49 Answer: e, Chlorpromazine increases the serum concentration of valproate.

Explanation: Chlorpromazine inhibits the metabolism of valproate and decreases its clearance. Hence, chlorpromazine increases the serum level of valproate. Option A is incorrect. A significant increase in the serum chlorpromazine concentration was observed when administered with amitriptyline.

Reference and Further Reading: Rasheed A, Javed MA, Nazir S, Khawaja O (1994). Interaction of chlorpromazine with tricyclic anti-depressants in schizophrenic patients. *J Pak Med Assoc*, 44: 233–234; Puri BK, Treasaden I (eds) (2010). *Psychiatry: An Evidence-Based Text*. London: Hodder Arnold, pp. 12, 893, 901–902, 903.

Question 50 Answer: a, Cognitive behaviour therapy

Explanation: Generally for outpatients, cognitive analytical therapy, cognitive behaviour therapy, interpersonal therapy and focal dynamic therapy would help. The main aims of psychotherapy would be to reduce the risk, enhance patient's motivation, encourage healthy eating and reduce other symptoms related to AN. In particular, CBT is able to target specific cognitive distortions and also behaviours that are related to weight, body image and eating. The minimum duration for outpatient psychological treatment is 6 months. It should be noted that psychotherapy is difficult for patients with severe emaciation. It has been advised that psychotherapy should wait until the weight has increased.

Reference: Puri BK, Hall A, Ho R (2014). *Revision Notes in Psychiatry*. London: CRC Press, p. 580.

Question 51 Answer: d, Jargon aphasia

Explanation: In jargon aphasia, the patient utters incoherent meaningless neologistic speech. There are two forms of intermediate aphasia: In central aphasia, in which there is difficulty in arranging words in the proper sequence; and nominal aphasia, in which there is difficulty with naming objects. In expressive aphasia, this refers to the difficulty in expressing thoughts in words whilst comprehension remains. In global aphasia, both receptive aphasia and expressive aphasia are present at the same time. Semantic aphasia refers to the errors in using the target words due to deficits in semantic memory.

Reference: Puri BK, Hall A, Ho R (2014). *Revision Notes in Psychiatry*. London: CRC Press, p. 10.

Question 52 Answer: d, Schemas tend to persist even after evidence for the schema has been discredited.

Explanation: Schemas have been known to persist after evidence for the schema has been discredited because the old schema has been activated more times than the new, modified schema and will be reactivated when there are little cognitive resources or time to activate the new schemas.

Reference: Aronson E, Wilson TD, Akert RM (2007). *Social Psychology*. Upper Saddle River, NJ: Prentice Hall, pp. 58–72.

Question 53 Answer: e, Schnauzkrampf

Explanation: Schnauzkrampf is a feature of catatonia and described as a protrusion of the lips such that they resemble a snout.

Reference and Further Reading: Roper P, Grad B (1968). A sign of schizophrenia: Clinical response of possible significance observed during electroconvulsive therapy. *Can Med Assoc J*, 99: 798–804.

Question 54 Answer: b, Conversion disorder

Explanation: The clinical diagnosis is likely to be that of conversion disorder. In conversion disorders, there is no evidence of physical disorder that may explain the symptoms. Instead, there is evidence for psychological causation, and usually there is a clear association in time with related stressful events. There might be calm acceptance known as la belle indifference. Conversion disorders are presumed to be psychogenic in origin. They are associated with traumatic events, insoluble problems or disturbed relationships.

Reference: Puri BK, Hall A, Ho R (2014). *Revision Notes in Psychiatry*. London: CRC Press, p. 433.

Question 55 Answer: c, Hypothermia

Explanation: All of the aforementioned are features of Wernicke's encephalopathy, with the exception of hypothermia. It is usually caused by the deficiency of thiamine, which is due to prolonged alcohol abuse in the Western countries. There are also other medical causes that need to be excluded as well. An estimated 10% of patients with the condition have the classical triad. Peripheral neuropathy may also be present in some individuals.

Reference: Puri BK, Hall A, Ho R (2014). *Revision Notes in Psychiatry*. London: CRC Press, p. 517.

Question 56 Answer: e, Attributing others' mistakes to their personal dispositions

Explanation: Fundamental attribution error is the tendency to overestimate the extent to which a person's behaviour is due to internal, dispositional factors and to underestimate the role of external, situational factors.

Reference and Further Reading: Aronson E, Wilson TD, Akert RM (2007). *Social Psychology*. Upper Saddle River, NJ: Prentice Hall, p. 109.

Question 57 Answer: b, Extinction

Explanation: Extinction is the gradual disappearance of the conditioned response (i.e. nausea) following repeated presentations of the conditioned stimulus (i.e. hospital) without the unconditioned stimulus (i.e. chemotherapy).

Reference and Further Reading: Puri BK, Treasaden I (eds) (2010). *Psychiatry: An Evidence-Based Text*. London: Hodder Arnold, p. 199.

Question 58 Answer: a, Conditioned response

Explanation: In this scenario, the unconditioned stimulus is chemotherapy and the conditioned stimulus is hospital building. The nausea feeling associated with the hospital building is a conditioned response.

Reference and Further Reading: Puri BK, Treasaden I (eds) (2010). *Psychiatry: An Evidence-Based Text*. London: Hodder Arnold, pp. 197–200.

Question 59 Answer: c, Generalization
Explanation: Stimulus generalization refers to a stimulus (i.e. alarm from the alarm clock) that is similar to a conditioned stimulus (i.e. mobile phone alarm) spontaneously causing a conditioned response (i.e. nausea).

Reference and Further Reading: Puri BK, Treasaden I (eds) (2010). *Psychiatry: An Evidence-Based Text*. London: Hodder Arnold, p. 199.

Question 60 Answer: c, Delusion of persecution
Explanation: Schneiderian first-rank symptoms include auditory hallucinations (audible thoughts, voices heard arguing and voices giving a running commentary), delusion of passivity (thought insertion, withdrawal and broadcasting; made feelings, actions and impulses), somatic passivity and delusional perception. Other delusions such as delusion of persecution, hallucinations and emotional blunting are second-rank symptoms.

Reference and Further Reading: Puri BK, Hall AD (2002). *Revision Notes in Psychiatry*. London: Arnold, p. 368.

Question 61 Answer: a, Levator palpebrae muscle paralysis
Explanation: Levator palpebrae muscle paralysis, Horner's syndrome and III nerve palsy are common causes of unilateral ptosis. Options (b) to (e) are common causes of bilateral ptosis.

Reference and Further Reading: Ward N, Frith P, Lipsedge M (2001). *Medical Masterclass Neurology, Ophthalmology and Psychiatry*. London: Royal College of Physicians; Puri BK, Treasaden I (eds) (2010). *Psychiatry: An Evidence-Based Text*. London: Hodder Arnold, pp. 336–338, 351, 525–527.

Question 62 Answer: d, Bias towards attributing a behaviour to situational causes
Explanation: The fundamental attribution error is best viewed as a bias towards attributing an actor's behaviour to dispositional causes rather than as an attribution error towards situational causes. It has been found that people in individualistic, Western cultures prefer dispositional attributions compared to those in collectivistic cultures, who take situational factors into account when making attributions.

Reference and Further Reading: Aronson E, Wilson TD, Akert RM (2007). *Social Psychology*. Upper Saddle River, NJ: Prentice Hall, pp. 109–110

Question 63 Answer: a, Low positive predictive value, low negative predictive value, low sensitivity and low specificity
Explanation: APOE screening is not recommended as a result of low positive predictive value, low negative predictive value, low sensitivity and low specificity.

Reference: Puri BK, Treasaden I (eds) (2010). *Psychiatry: An Evidence-Based Text.* London: Hodder Arnold, p. 473.

Question 64 Answer: e, Presence of altered consciousness
Explanation: Delirium is commonly defined as a state of fluctuating global disturbance of the cerebral function, which is abrupt in onset and of short duration, usually arising as a consequence of physical illnesses. Awareness is always impaired. Alertness tends to change and can be either increased or decreased. Orientation is always impaired, particularly for time. Recent and immediate memory is impaired with poor learning and lack of recall for events occurring during the delirious period. However, the knowledge base remains intact.

Reference: Puri BK, Hall A, Ho R (2014). *Revision Notes in Psychiatry.* London: CRC Press, p. 707.

Question 65 Answer: e, Treat systolic hypertension (>160 mm Hg) in older people (age >60 years).
Explanation: Option (e) is based on good evidence. Option (a) is recommended in first-degree relatives of Alzheimer's disease but not for the general population. There is insufficient evidence to support options (b), (c), and (d). High-dose vitamin E is associated with excess mortality and should not be recommended.

Reference: Puri BK, Treasaden I (eds) (2010). *Psychiatry: An Evidence-Based Text.* London: Hodder Arnold, pp. 511–513, 1100–1108.

Question 66 Answer: b, Thought block
Explanation: The classical first-rank symptoms include auditory hallucinations (thought echo, in third person, in the form of a running commentary), delusions of passivity (thought insertion, withdrawal and broadcasting and made feelings, impulses and actions) and somatic passivity and delusional perception. Second-rank symptoms include perplexity, emotional blunting, hallucination and other delusions. First-rank symptoms could occur in other psychosis and, although highly suggestive of schizophrenia, are not pathognomonic.

Reference: Puri BK, Hall A, Ho R (2014). *Revision Notes in Psychiatry.* London: CRC Press, p. 351.

Question 67 Answer: b, Perceived lack of social support during the trauma
Explanation: The following are psychosocial factors that are responsible for the development of PTSD: female gender, low intelligence quotient at the age of five, previous trauma history, previous psychiatric history, hyperactivity, anti-social behaviour, severity of trauma, perceived life threat, peri-traumatic dissociation, impaired social support and low socioeconomic status.

Reference: Puri BK, Hall A, Ho R (2014). *Revision Notes in Psychiatry.* London: CRC Press, p. 427.

Question 68 Answer: a, The scientific study of the way in which people's thoughts, feelings and behaviours are influenced by the real, imagined or implied presence of other people.
Explanation: Social psychology is the scientific study of the way in which people's thoughts, feelings and behaviours are influenced by the real, imagined or implied presence of other people. Option (d) defines psychology.

Reference and Further Reading: Puri BK, Treasaden I (eds) (2010). *Psychiatry: An Evidence-Based Text*. London: Hodder Arnold, p. 131.

Question 69 Answer: d, Ekbom's syndrome
Explanation: This woman suffers from delusions of parasitosis or Ekbom's syndrome, which is the belief that one is infested with parasites that live on or under the skin. The primary symptom is a cutaneous pruritus. This itch causes continuous picking of the skin to extract the suspected parasites. Patients often present with foreign objects or debris from their skin in small containers. This is called the 'matchbox sign'.

The syndrome is associated with bipolar disorder, paranoia, schizophrenia, depression as well as abuse of drugs, such as cocaine, ritalin and amphetamines. Risperidone or olanzapine are the current treatments of choice.

Reference and Further Reading: Edlich RF, Cross CL, Wack CA, Long WB 3rd (2009). Delusions of parasitosis. *American Journal of Emergency Medicine*, 8: 997–999.

Question 70 Answer: a, Discrimination
Explanation: Stimulus discrimination refers to the tendency to stop responding to the stimulus similar to the conditioned stimulus, as the similar stimulus is not paired with the unconditioned stimulus. The man learns to differentiate or discriminate between the two alarm sounds and learns to respond differently to each alarm.

Reference and Further Reading: Puri BK, Treasaden I (eds) (2010). *Psychiatry: An Evidence-Based Text*. London: Hodder Arnold, p. 199.

Question 71 Answer: e, Recovery
Explanation: Spontaneous recovery is the recurrence of a conditioned response after extinction. Extinction is the weakening of the conditioned response after the removal of the unconditioned stimulus (i.e. Drug A).

Reference and Further Reading: Puri BK, Treasaden I (eds) (2010). *Psychiatry: An Evidence-Based Text*. London: Hodder Arnold, pp. 199, 208.

Question 72 Answer: a, Dyslexia without agraphia
Explanation: Dyslexia without agraphia refers to word blindness with writing impairments and is caused by lesions in the left occipital lobe. Homonymous hemianopia occurs in optic tract, radiation and cortex lesions. Papilloedema and loss of pupillary reflex are caused by optic nerve lesions. Quadrantopia is caused by optic radiation lesions.

Reference: Malhi GS, Malhi S (2006). *Examination Notes in Psychiatry: Basic Sciences* (2nd edition). London: Hodder Arnold.

Question 73 Answer: c, Daniel M'Naghten trial
Explanation: Daniel M'Naghten suffered from delusions of persecution for years and stalked Prime Minister Sir Robert Peel. He mistook Edward Drummond, Peel's secretary, for Peel and shot him. Drummond 'languished' for 4 months and then died while M'Naghten was found not criminally responsible in 2 minutes. The M'Naghten trail led to public outrage, and Queen Victoria requested clarification of the 'not criminally responsible' standard. M'Naghten rule tests criminality of murder committed by a person who is deemed to be mentally insane. For option (a), bifurcated trial means that the person must be proven guilty of each offence first and the 'not criminally responsible' issue is the second part of the trial. For option (b), the first right versus wrong test is associated with the Bellingham trial in 1812. For option (e), the wild beast test is associated with the trial Rex versus Arnold in 1724.

Reference and Further Reading: Puri BK, Treasaden I (eds) (2010). *Psychiatry: An Evidence-Based Text*. London: Hodder Arnold, pp. 1162, 1163, 1168.

Question 74 Answer: c, Moderate
Explanation: Based on the ICD-10 diagnostic classification system, he is likely to be suffering from moderate degree of depression. Duration of 2 weeks of symptoms is required for the diagnosis. This applies to the first episode only. Severity is classified into mild depressive disorder, moderate depressive disorder, severe depressive episode without psychotic symptoms and severe depressive episode with psychotic symptoms.

Reference: Puri BK, Hall A, Ho R (2014). *Revision Notes in Psychiatry*. London: CRC Press, p. 378.

Question 75 Answer: b, 10%
Explanation: His son has 10% risk of developing schizophrenia.

Reference and Further Reading: Puri BK, Treasaden I (eds) (2010). *Psychiatry: An Evidence-Based Text*. London: Hodder Arnold, pp. 474–475, 597, 599.

Question 76 Answer: d, Four times increased risk
Explanation: Cannabis would cause an estimated fourfold increment in the risk of psychosis.

Reference: Puri BK, Hall A, Ho R (2014). *Revision Notes in Psychiatry*. London: CRC Press, p. 361.

Question 77 Answer: e, There has been found to be an association, but there is no strong evidence to support the estimated increment in risk.
Explanation: Previous research has found that patients with Down's syndrome are at a higher risk to develop Alzheimer's disease. Other psychiatric co-morbidities include

obsessive-compulsive disorder, depression, autism, bipolar disorder and psychosis. There has not been strong evidence to support the estimated increment in risk.

Reference: Puri BK, Hall A, Ho R (2014). *Revision Notes in Psychiatry*. London: CRC Press, p. 665.

Question 78 Answer: e, Trace conditioning
Explanation: This phenomenon is known as trace conditioning. In trace conditioning, the conditioned stimulus is removed before the onset of the unconditioned stimulus. In this example, the conditioned stimulus is the doctor's white coat. As the girl has to wait for her turn before she receives her injection (i.e. the unconditioned stimulus), there is an interval between the conditioned stimulus and the unconditioned stimulus, which is why this phenomenon is trace conditioning and not delayed conditioning. The conditioned response in trace conditioning is usually weaker than that in delayed conditioning. Trace conditioning becomes less effective as the delay between the two stimuli increases.

Reference and Further Reading: Puri BK, Treasaden I (eds) (2010). *Psychiatry: An Evidence-Based Text*. London: Hodder Arnold, p. 198.

Question 79 Answer: c, 1930s
Explanation: The term schizoaffective psychosis was introduced by Kasanin in 1933 in order to describe a condition with both affective and schizophrenic symptoms, usually with sudden acute onset after good premorbid functioning and with almost complete recovery.

Reference: Puri BK, Hall A, Ho R (2014). *Revision Notes in Psychiatry*. London: CRC Press, p. 373.

Question 80 Answer: d, 6 months
Explanation: Based on the advice given by the DVLA to doctors, it has been stated that patients with bipolar disorder requiring admission should be placed off the road for 6–12 months.

Reference: Puri BK, Hall A, Ho R (2014). *Revision Notes in Psychiatry*. London: CRC Press, p. 150.

Question 81 Answer: c, 35%–40%
Explanation: Research has found that people with Down syndrome are at a higher risk of developing Alzheimer's disease. For those who are between the ages of 50 and 59 years, the increased incidence has been estimated to be around 36%–40%. For those between the ages of 60 and 69 years, the increased incidence has been found to be around 55%. Research has shown that as age advances, there is a higher incidence of neurofibrillary tangle and plaques being deposited.

Reference: Puri BK, Hall A, Ho R (2014). *Revision Notes in Psychiatry*. London: CRC Press, p. 665.

Question 82 Answer: b, People with mental illnesses are not at a higher risk of offending compared to general population.

Explanation: Since the peak of deinstitutionalization in the 1970s, the proportion of inmates in prisons with serious mental illnesses has increased significantly. People with mental illnesses are at a higher risk of offending compared to the general population, and the rates of mental illness among prisoners have increased steadily since deinstitutionalization.

Reference and Further Reading: Puri BK, Treasaden I (eds) (2010). *Psychiatry: An Evidence-Based Text*. London: Hodder Arnold, pp. 3–15.

Question 83 Answer: c, Simultaneous conditioning

Explanation: In simultaneous conditioning, the onset and termination of the conditioned and unconditioned stimuli occur at the same time. In this example, the spider (i.e. unconditioned stimulus) and the ringing sound (i.e. conditioned stimulus) are presented at the same time, and this elicits fear (conditioned response) in the girl.

Reference and Further Reading: Puri BK, Treasaden I (eds) (2010). *Psychiatry: An Evidence-Based Text*. London: Hodder Arnold, p. 198.

Question 84 Answer: a, Bleuler

Explanation: It was in 1911 that Bleuler introduced the term schizophrenia and applied it.

Reference: Puri BK, Hall A, Ho R (2014). *Revision Notes in Psychiatry*. London: CRC Press, p. 349.

Question 85 Answer: d, Kasanin

Explanation: The term 'schizoaffective psychosis' was introduced by Kasanin in 1933 to describe a condition with both affective and schizophrenic symptoms, with sudden onset after good premorbid functioning and usually with complete recovery.

Reference: Puri BK, Hall A, Ho R (2014). *Revision Notes in Psychiatry*. London: CRC Press, p. 373.

Question 86 Answer: e, Under the consequentialist approach, confidentiality is an absolute condition in psychiatric practice.

Explanation: Confidentiality is recognized as a *prima facie* obligation. An action is morally right only if it promotes the best consequences for the greatest number of people.

Reference: Green SA (1998). The ethics of managed mental health care, in Bloch S, Chodoff P, Green SA (eds) *Psychiatric Ethics* (3rd edition). Oxford, UK: Oxford University Press.

Question 87 Answer: b, MSE provides important information in establishing a psychiatric diagnosis.
Explanation: The Mini Mental State Examination (MMSE) is a cognitive assessment and is not a shorter version of the Mental State Examination. The MSE should be conducted as soon as the interview begins, and the mental state of the patient is observed throughout the process of history taking. Physical examination is required in psychiatric assessment, and the MSE cannot replace physical examination. Information obtained from history taking is affected by the patient's subjective views and defence mechanisms. Observations during the MSE are more objective and reliable.

Reference and Further Reading: Puri BK, Treasaden I (eds) (2010). *Psychiatry: An Evidence-Based Text*. London: Hodder Arnold, pp. 92, 515, 786, 1101.

Question 88 Answer: c, Emotional liability
Explanation: The presence of emotional labiality suggests the diagnosis of bipolar disorder.

Reference and Further Reading: Puri BK, Treasaden I (eds) (2010). *Psychiatry: An Evidence-Based Text*. London: Hodder Arnold, pp. 593–609.

Question 89 Answer: d, Neologism
Explanation: The person exhibits neologism while condensing words such as 'syringe' and 'risperidone'. It is defined as a new word that is constructed by the person or an everyday word is being used in a special way by the person.

Reference and Further Reading: Puri BK, Hall AD (2002). *Revision Notes in Psychiatry*. London: Arnold, p. 4.

Question 90 Answer: c, 3 months
Explanation: According to the ICD-10, a delusional disorder is an ill-defined condition, manifesting as a single delusion or a set of related delusions, being persistent, sometimes life-long and not having an identifiable organic basis. Delusions are the most obvious or are the only symptoms that are present for at least 3 months. For the diagnosis to be made, there must be no evidence of schizophrenia symptoms or brain diseases.

Reference: Puri BK, Hall A, Ho R (2014). *Revision Notes in Psychiatry*. London: CRC Press, p. 370.

Question 91 Answer: d, The ratio for MZ to DZ concordance is around 56:5.
Explanation: The ratio of MZ to DZ concordance has been found to be 56:5 (Holland et al.). Twin studies have found higher concordance rates for monozygotic twins than for dizygotic twins. Five per cent of the first-degree relatives are usually affected. The heritability of AN has been estimated to be around 80%. Linkage genes controlling serotonin function on chromosome 1 and AN have been found.

Reference: Puri BK, Hall A, Ho R (2014). *Revision Notes in Psychiatry*. London: CRC Press, p. 575.

Question 92 Answer: a, Checking

Explanation: Checking is the most common compulsion, followed by washing and counting. Symmetry and doubting are associated obsessions. Compulsions are defined as repetitive behaviours or mental acts in response to an obsession. The behaviours or mental acts are aimed at preventing or reducing anxiety or distress. Obsession is defined as recurrent and intrusive thoughts, urges or images that cause marked anxiety or distress. Thus, an individual would resort to attempts to suppress such thoughts, urges or images or attempt to neutralize them using compulsive behaviour.

Reference: Puri BK, Hall A, Ho R (2014). *Revision Notes in Psychiatry*. London: CRC Press, p. 418.

Question 93 Answer: d, Benzodiazepine withdrawal syndrome

Explanation: She is likely to be experiencing benzodiazepine withdrawal syndrome. This would include withdrawal symptoms such as autonomic hyperactivity, malaise and weakness, tinnitus and grand mal convulsions. There are cognitive effects with impaired memory and concentration. There are also perceptual effects with hypersensitivity to sound, light and touch; depersonalization and derealization. Delirium may develop within a week of cessation, associated with visual, auditory and tactile hallucinations and delusions. Affective effects such as irritability, anxiety and phobic symptoms may also occur.

Reference: Puri BK, Hall A, Ho R (2014). *Revision Notes in Psychiatry*. London: CRC Press, p. 548.

Question 94 Answer: b, Drawing the face of a clock, indicating 10 past 11

Explanation: Folstein's MMSE does not include drawing a clock face, which requires intact frontal lobe and parietal lobe function.

Reference and Further Reading: Puri BK, Treasaden I (eds) (2010). *Psychiatry: An Evidence-Based Text*. London: Hodder Arnold, pp. 92, 515, 786, 1101.

Question 95 Answer: c, Pibloktoq

Explanation: Pibloktoq is characterized by prodromal fatigue, depression or confusion followed by a 'seizure' including stripping off clothes, frenzied running, rolling in snow, glossolalia or echolalia, echopraxia, property destruction and coprophagia.

Reference and Further Reading: Puri BK, Treasaden I (eds) (2010). *Psychiatry: An Evidence-Based Text*. London: Hodder Arnold, pp. 309–318; World Health Organisation (1994) *ICD-10 Classification of Mental and Behavioural Disorders*. Edinburgh, UK: Churchill Livingstone.

Question 96 Answer: e, Duty to warn

Explanation: There were two court hearings of Tarasoff's case. After the first hearing in 1974, the California court held that the mental health professionals bear a duty to use reasonable care to give threatened persons such warnings because warnings are essential to avert foreseeable danger arising from a patient's condition.

Reference and Further Reading: Puri BK, Treasaden I (eds) (2010). *Psychiatry: An Evidence-Based Text*. London: Hodder Arnold, pp. 1228–1229.

Question 97 Answer: b, Duty to protect

Explanation: There were two court hearings of Tarasoff's case. After the second hearing in 1976, the California court held that the mental health professionals have a duty to protect potential victims by reasonable means if their patients have plans to harm the others. The protective privilege ends where the public peril begins.

Reference and Further Reading: Puri BK, Treasaden I (eds) (2010). *Psychiatry: An Evidence-Based Text*. London: Hodder Arnold, pp. 1228–1229.

Question 98 Answer: d, Uqamairineq

Explanation: Uqamairineq is characterized by sudden paralysis associated with borderline sleep states. It is accompanied by anxiety, agitation or hallucinations.

Reference and Further Reading: Puri BK, Treasaden I (eds) (2010). *Psychiatry: An Evidence-Based Text*. London: Hodder Arnold, pp. 309–318; World Health Organisation (1994) *ICD-10 Classification of Mental and Behavioural Disorders*. Edinburgh, UK: Churchill Livingstone.

Question 99 Answer: a, Backward conditioning

Explanation: In backward conditioning, the conditioned stimulus is presented after the unconditioned stimulus has been terminated. In this example, the ringing sound is the conditioned stimulus (i.e. ringing sound) and it is presented after the unconditioned stimulus (i.e. the snake).

Reference and Further Reading: Puri BK, Treasaden I (eds) (2010). *Psychiatry: An Evidence-Based Text*. London: Hodder Arnold, p. 198.

Question 100 Answer: c, Normal jaw jerk

Explanation: Candidates are advised to be familiar with the differences between bulbar and pseudobulbar palsies. The differences are summarized as follows:

	Bulbar palsy	Pseudobulbar palsy
Lesions	Lower motor neuron	Upper motor neuron
Causes	Motor neuron diseases, Guillain–Barré syndrome, polio, syringobulbia, brainstem tumours and central pontine myelinolysis in people with alcohol misuse	Bilateral lesions above the mid-pons, for example, in the corticobulbar tracts in multiple sclerosis, motor neuron disease and stroke. It is more common than bulbar palsy
Tongue	Flaccid and fasciculating	Spastic
Jaw jerk	Normal	Increased
Speech	Quiet, hoarse and nasal	Donald Duck speech Inappropriate laughter or emotional incontinence

Reference and Further Reading: Longmore M, Wilkinson I, Turmezei T, Cheung CK (2007). *Oxford Handbook of Clinical Medicine* (7th edition). Oxford, UK: Oxford University Press; Puri BK, Treasaden I (eds) (2010). *Psychiatry: An Evidence-Based Text*. London: Hodder Arnold, pp. 544, 554.

Question 101 Answer: e, Visuospatial abilities are assessed using a clock-drawing task and a three-dimensional cube copy.

Explanation: MoCA was designed as a rapid screening instrument for mild cognitive dysfunction. Hence, option (b) is incorrect. Option (a) is incorrect because a score of 26 or above is considered normal. The total possible score is 30 points. MoCA assesses different cognitive domains: attention and concentration, executive functions, memory, language, visuoconstructional skills, conceptual thinking, calculations and orientation. Time to administer the whole MoCA is approximately 10 minutes. Hence, option (d) is incorrect.

The short-term memory recall task involves two learning trials of five nouns and delayed recall after approximately 5 minutes.

Reference: http://www.mocatest.org/pdf_files/MoCA-Instructions-English_2010.pdf.

Question 102 Answer: b, Brain fag

Explanation: Brain fag refers to brain fatigue from too much thinking demanded of students. Brain fag is a culture-bound syndrome in West Africa.

Reference and Further Reading: Campbell RJ (1996). *Psychiatric Dictionary*. Oxford, UK: Oxford University Press; Puri BK, Treasaden I (eds) (2010). *Psychiatry: An Evidence-Based Text*. London: Hodder Arnold, pp. 309–318.

Question 103 Answer: b, Projection

Explanation: A person with paranoid personality disorder often projects the tendency to harm other people and believes that others are trying to harm him or her. This results in suspicion and lack of trust. Other common defence mechanisms include projective identification and splitting.

Reference and Further Reading: Puri BK, Hall AD (2002). *Revision Notes in Psychiatry*. London: Arnold, pp. 168–169.

Question 104 Answer: c, Confidentiality

Explanation: This case occurred in the 1960s. Prosenjit Poddar was a university student and he fell in love with a female student called Tatiana Tarasoff. Poddar told the university psychologist that he wanted to kill Tarasoff in a psychotherapy session. Without any precedent, the psychologist decided to maintain the confidentiality of Poddar's homicidal plan. Poddar eventually murdered Tarasoff. The Tarasoff family sued the psychologist from the University of California for not informing Tatiana Tarasoff and the police about Poddar's homicidal plan. In 1976, the California Supreme Court concluded that the mental health professionals have to breach confidentiality in such situations.

Reference and Further Reading: Puri BK, Treasaden I (eds) (2010). *Psychiatry: An Evidence-Based Text*. London: Hodder Arnold, pp. 1228–1229.

Question 105 Answer: d, Koro
Explanation: Koro refers to acute panic or anxiety reaction involving fear of genital retraction.

Reference and Further Reading: World Health Organisation (1994) *ICD-10 Classification of Mental and Behavioural Disorders*. Edinburgh, UK: Churchill Livingstone; Puri BK, Treasaden I (eds) (2010). *Psychiatry: An Evidence-Based Text*. London: Hodder Arnold, pp. 309–318.

Question 106 Answer: b, Bipolar disorder type II
Explanation: The clinical diagnosis should be bipolar disorder type II. This disorder lasts for a minimum of 4 days. There is at least one major depressive episode and at least one hypomanic episode. Individuals usually have no impairments in terms of their functioning. It is important to note that the number of symptoms required to diagnose hypomania is similar to that of a manic episode.

Reference: Puri BK, Hall A, Ho R (2014). *Revision Notes in Psychiatry*. London: CRC Press, p. 378.

Question 107 Answer: c, The cut-off score gives rise to high sensitivity and 100% specificity for diagnosing dementia.
Explanation: The cut-off score of 82 gives rise to high sensitivity (84%) and 100% specificity for diagnosing dementia. The ACE-R incorporates MMSE and frontal lobe assessment. The Addenbrooke's Cognitive Examination Revised (ACE-R) is available in Mandarin for people in Mainland China but not in Cantonese for Chinese people in Hong Kong. It is used to screen for dementia but not delirium.

Reference: Mioshi E, Dawson K, Mitchell J, Arnold R, Hodges R (2006). The Addenbrooke's Cognitive Examination Revised (ACE-R): A brief cognitive test battery for dementia screening. *Int J Geriatr Psychiatry*, 21: 1078–1085.

Question 108 Answer: e, Suppression
Explanation: This person suffers from narcissistic personality disorder. Options A to D are common narcissistic defence mechanisms.

Reference: Gabbard GO, Beck JS, Holmes J (2005). *Oxford Textbook of Psychotherapy*. Oxford, UK: Oxford University Press.

Question 109 Answer: e, Second-order conditioning
Explanation: In this scenario, the white coat is new conditioned stimulus. This new conditioned stimulus is learnt through the original conditioned

stimulus (i.e. the hospital building or hospital environment) but not the original unconditioned stimulus (i.e. the chemotherapy). The nausea feeling associated with white coat is known as second-order conditioning.

Reference and Further Reading: Puri BK, Treasaden I (eds) (2010). *Psychiatry: An Evidence-Based Text*. London: Hodder Arnold, pp. 198–199.

Question 110 Answer: b, 82
Explanation: The two cut-offs were defined in ACE-R (score 88: sensitivity = 0.94, specificity = 0.89; score 82: sensitivity = 0.84, specificity = 1.0). Hence, the cut-off at 82 is the most specific.

Reference: Mioshi E, Dawson K, Mitchell J, Arnold R, Hodges R (2006). The Addenbrooke's Cognitive Examination Revised (ACE-R): A brief cognitive test battery for dementia screening. *Int J Geriatr Psychiatry*, 21: 1078–1085.

Question 111 Answer: c, Displacement
Explanation: Displacement is the redirecting of feelings from a threatening target to a less threatening one. Projection involves placing one's unacceptable or threatening thoughts onto others. Sublimation is the turning of unacceptable impulses into socially acceptable behaviour.

Reference and Further Reading: Puri BK, Hall AD (2002). *Revision Notes in Psychiatry*. London: Arnold, pp. 168–169.

Question 112 Answer: d, 33 hours per week
Explanation: Schizophrenic patients are more likely to relapse if they have been discharged back to their families in which their relatives displayed highly critical comments and over-involvement. Changes in physiological arousal might account for this. This is especially so for families with highly expressed emotions for more than 33 hours per week. Previously, it was also found that schizophrenics had experienced more independent life events in the 3 weeks prior to the onset of a relapse as compared to controls.

Reference: Puri BK, Hall A, Ho R (2014). *Revision Notes in Psychiatry*. London: CRC Press, p. 360.

Question 113 Answer: e, Short-term memory
Explanation: With regards to short-term memory, the anatomical correlate of auditory verbal short-term memory is in the left (dominant) parietal lobe, while that of the visual verbal short-term memory is possibly in the left temporo-occipital area. The anatomical correlate of non-verbal short-term memory is possibly in the right (non-dominant) temporal lobe.

Reference: Puri BK, Hall A, Ho R (2014). *Revision Notes in Psychiatry*. London: CRC Press, p. 103.

Question 114 Answer: e, Sublimation

Explanation: The son has transformed the unacceptable and destructive impulse into acceptable and constructive form. This defence mechanism is known as sublimation.

Reference and Further Reading: Puri BK, Hall AD (2002). *Revision Notes in Psychiatry*. London: Arnold, pp. 168–169.

Question 115 Answer: b, Reaction formation

Explanation: This girl behaves in an opposite manner to hide her underling fear of the monkey and she exhibits reaction formation.

Reference and Further Reading: Puri BK, Hall AD (2002). *Revision Notes in Psychiatry*. London: Arnold, pp. 168–169.

Question 116 Answer: d, Motor neuron disease

Explanation: Depression does not cause progressive worsening dysphagia and her history is supported by her partner. The attending psychiatrist must rule out underlying neurological conditions because progressive dysphagia may indicate a worsening mechanical lesion. Motor neuron disease is associated with progressive dysphagia. Myasthenia gravis is associated with fluctuating dysphagia, and cerebrovascular accident is associated with static dysphagia.

Reference and Further Reading: Ward N, Frith P, Lipsedge M (2001). *Medical Masterclass Neurology, Ophthalmology and Psychiatry*. London: Royal College of Physicians; Puri BK, Treasaden I (eds) (2010). *Psychiatry: An Evidence-Based Text*. London: Hodder Arnold, pp. 441, 527, 543–544, 441.

Question 117 Answer: d, Dependent personality disorder

Explanation: The most appropriate diagnosis would be dependent personality disorder. Individuals with dependent personality disorder usually have tremendous fear of being left alone, and their expression of disagreement is limited. They tend to avoid decision making and taking on responsibilities. Their relationship is sought urgently with other relationships' end. For individuals with dependent personality disorder, they tend to lack self-confidence as well.

Reference: Puri BK, Hall A, Ho R (2014). *Revision Notes in Psychiatry*. London: CRC Press, p. 453.

Question 118 Answer: e, De-personalization

Explanation: The clinical features of catatonia include all of the following: ambitendency, automatic obedience, mitegehen, mitmachen, mannerism, negativism, echolalia, echopraxia, logorrhea and stereotypy. The common etiological causes for catatonia include schizophrenia, depression of manic (more common than schizophrenia), organic disorders, epilepsy, medications, recreational drugs and psychogenic catatonia.

Reference: Puri BK, Hall A, Ho R (2014). *Revision Notes in Psychiatry*. London: CRC Press, p. 369.

Extended matching items (EMIs)

Theme: Cognitive testing

Question 119 Answer: f, Vineland Social Maturity Scale
Explanation: This is a scale that consists of 117 items that assess different aspects of social maturity and social ability. It can be used for the assessment of dementia, childhood development and learning disability.

Question 120 Answer: e, Clifton Assessment Schedule
Explanation: Both the Clifton Assessment Schedule and the Stockton Geriatric Rating Scale are scales that are used by nurses for assessment.

Question 121 Answer: c, Blessed Dementia Scale
Explanation: This is a questionnaire that is usually administered to a relative or friend who is asked to answer the questions on the basis of performance over the previous 6 months. The first set of questions deals with activities of daily living, the second set deals with further activities of daily living and the third set deals with changes in personality, interest and drive.

Question 122 Answer: d, Geriatric Mental State Schedule
Explanation: The Geriatric Mental State Schedule is a semi-structured interview which assesses the subject's mental state.

Question 123 Answer: b, Cambridge Neuropsychological Test Automated Battery
Explanation: This is an automated computerized task that offers sensitive and specific cognitive assessment, using a touch screen. It consists of 13 computerized tasks.

Question 124 Answer: a, Mini Mental State Examination
Explanation: The answer is Mini Mental State Examination. It in itself has a clear advantage over a combination of cognitive testing and informant questionnaire.

Reference: Puri BK, Hall A, Ho R (2014). *Revision Notes in Psychiatry*. London: CRC Press, p. 98.

Theme: Executive function tests

Question 125 Answer: e, Cognitive Estimates Test
Explanation: In the absence of a reduction of intelligence quotient (IQ), some frontal lobe damaged patients may give outrageous incorrect cognitive estimates of commonly known phenomena. For example, when asked to estimate the length of an adult elephant, they might reply 100 yards.

Question 126 Answer: f, Six elements test

Explanation: In this test, the subject is asked to carry out six different tasks (in two groups of three) during a quarter of an hour. In order to maximize their score, the subject needs adequately to plan and schedule these tasks while also monitoring the time that has elapsed.

Question 127 Answer: h, Trail making test

Explanation: The aforementioned test evaluates all of the above-mentioned abilities. Difficulties with cognitive flexibility or complex conceptual thinking may manifest as much longer times being required for Trail B than would be expected from the Trail A time score.

Question 128 Answer: d, Wisconsin Card Sorting Test

Explanation: This helps to pick up perseverative errors (such as continuing too long to sort the cards by number, well after the indexing rule has changed to colour) and non-perseverative errors. Poor performance on this task is particularly associated with dysfunction of the left dorsolateral prefrontal cortex.

Question 129 Answer: c, Tower of London Test

Explanation: The Tower of London Test is based on the Tower of Hanoi game and test planning. The subject is asked to move coloured discs of varying sizes between three columns, either using a model or via a computer program, in order to achieve a given result. Left frontal lobe lesions are associated with poor performance on this test.

Question 130 Answer: b, Verbal fluency test

Explanation: A typical verbal fluency test involves asking the subject to articulate as many words as possible, during a 2-minute interval, starting with the letters F, A, S and in turn. Proper nouns and derivatives such as plurals and different verb endings are not allowed to count together with the root words. Verbal fluency is impaired in left (dominant) frontal lobe lesions.

Question 131 Answer: a, Stroop Test

Explanation: The aforementioned is true with regards to the description of this test. Inference may occur between reading words and naming colours. Left dominant frontal lobe lesions are associated with poor performance on the Stroop test.

Reference: Puri BK, Hall A, Ho R (2014). *Revision Notes in Psychiatry*. London: CRC Press, p. 96.

Theme: Clinical interview

Question 132 Answer: l

Explanation: This is an example of humour.

Question 133 Answer: o
Explanation: This example demonstrates labile affect.

Reference and Further Reading: Puri BK, Hall AD. (2002). *Revision Notes in Psychiatry*. London: Arnold, p. 150.

Question 134 Answer: d
Explanation: This illustrates disinhibition. If such scenario occurs in the CASC examination, a male candidate should inform the examiner to call in a chaperon.

Reference and Further Reading: Puri BK, Treasaden I (eds) (2010). *Psychiatry: An Evidence-Based Text*. London: Hodder Arnold, p. 510.

Theme: Basic psychology
Question 135 Answer: j
Explanation: The patient has storage failure and cannot recall.

Question 136 Answer: i
Explanation: The cue of the anxiety provoked by the gunshot in the park helps him to remember things he forgot in the past.

Question 137 Answer: f
Explanation: In proactive interference, old learning affects new learning.

Reference and Further Reading: Puri BK, Treasaden I (eds) (2010). *Psychiatry: An Evidence-Based Text*. London: Hodder Arnold, pp. 256–262.

Theme: Classification systems
Question 138 Answer: c, DSM-I
Explanation: DSM-I was written and produced in 1952 and was essentially based on the mental disorders section of the ICD-6.

Question 139 Answer: e, DSM-III
Explanation: The DSM-III, launched in 1980, was essentially an innovative classification system that tried not to appear favourably disposed to competing aetiological theories and introduced the operational diagnostic criteria as well as a multi-axial classification system.

Question 140 Answer: f, DSM-III-R
Explanation: The DSM-III was revised, corrected and published as the DSM-III-TR in 1987.

Reference: Puri BK, Hall A, Ho R (2014). *Revision Notes in Psychiatry*. London: CRC Press, p. 18.

Theme: Learning theories and behavioural change

Question 141 Answer: b, Negative reinforcer
Explanation: It refers to an aversive stimulus, whose removal would increase the probability of occurrence of the operant behaviour. Escape conditioning is an example of this, as the response learnt provides complete escape from the aversive stimulus.

Question 142 Answer: c, Punishment
Explanation: Punishment is the situation that occurs if an aversive stimulus is presented whenever a given behaviour occurs, thereby reducing the probability of occurrence of this response. The removal of the aversive stimulus then allows it to act as a negative reinforcer rather than a punisher.

Question 143 Answer: d, Primary reinforcement
Explanation: This is the reinforcement that occurs through reduction of needs deriving from basic drives such as food and drink.

Question 144 Answer: e, Secondary reinforcement
Explanation: This is reinforcement derived from association with primary reinforcers such as money and stress.

Question 145 Answer: g, Fixed interval schedule
Explanation: This form of reinforcement has been known to be particularly poor at maintaining the conditioned response; the maximum response rate typically occurs only when the reinforcement is expected.

Question 146 Answer: h, Variable interval schedule
Explanation: In a variable interval schedule, reinforcement occurs after variable intervals. It is considered to be very good at maintaining the CR.

Question 147 Answer: i, Fixed ratio schedule
Explanation: In a fixed ratio schedule, reinforcement occurs after a fixed number of responses. It is good at maintaining a high response rate.

Reference: Puri BK, Hall A, Ho R (2014). *Revision Notes in Psychiatry*. London: CRC Press, p. 28.

Theme: Attachment abnormalities

Question 148 Answer: a, Insecure attachment
Explanation: In insecure attachment, there is chronic clinginess and ambivalence towards the mother. Clinically, this may be relevant as it is a precursor towards childhood emotional disorders (including school refusal) and disorders (such as agoraphobia) starting in adolescence and adulthood.

Question 149 Answer: b, Avoidant attachment

Explanation: In avoidant attachment, a distance is typically kept from the mother, who may sometimes be ignored. Clinically, avoidant attachment caused by rejection by the mother may be relevant as it may be a precursor to poor social functioning in later life (including aggression).

Question 150 Answer: c, Separation anxiety

Explanation: Separation anxiety refers to the fear an infant shows of being separated from his or her caregiver. Holding a comfort object or a transitional object would help to deal with these feelings. The rate of disappearance of separation anxiety varies with the child's experiences of previous separations, handling by mother, perception of whether the mother will die or depart and temperament.

Question 151 Answer: f, Maternal separation

Explanation: Following a failure to form adequate attachments, for example due to prolonged maternal separation or rejecting parents, can lead to the development of language delay, indiscriminate affection seeking, shallow relationships, lack of empathy, aggression and social disinhibition.

Reference: Puri BK, Hall A, Ho R (2014). *Revision Notes in Psychiatry*. London: CRC Press, p. 63–65.

Theme: Clinical assessment and neuropsychological processes
Question 152 Answer: a, Lexical dysgraphia
Explanation: This is caused by lesion in the left temporo-parietal region. The person breaks down the word's spelling and has difficulty in writing irregular words.

Question 153 Answer: b, Deep dysgraphia
Explanation: This is caused by extensive left hemisphere lesion and a breakdown of the sound-based route for spelling.

Question 154 Answer: c, Neglect dysgraphia
Explanation: Neglect dysgraphia is caused by right hemispheric lesions and leads to misspelling of the initial part of the word.

Question 155 Answer: e, Alexia without agraphia
Explanation: This is due to the occlusion of the left posterior cerebral artery that leads to infarction of the media; aspect of the left occipital lobe and the splenium of the corpus callosum. The explanation for the clinical presentation is as follows: after the stroke, the patient starts off with right hemianopia and he cannot read in the right visual field. Then, the words have to be seen on the left side, which are projected to the right hemisphere. There is a lesion in the splenium that prevents the transfer of visual information from the right to the left side. The primary language area is

disconnected from incoming visual information. As a result, he cannot comprehend any written material, although he can write. As times goes by, he develops a strategy of identifying the individual letters in the right hemisphere. Saying each letter aloud enables him to access the pronunciation of word in the left hemisphere.

Reference: Puri BK, Hall A, Ho R (2014). *Revision Notes in Psychiatry.* London: CRC Press, p. 107.

Question 156 Answer: j, Shaping
Explanation: In shaping, successively closer approximations to the desired behaviour are reinforced in order to achieve the latter. It finds application clinically in the management of behavioural disturbances in people with learning difficulties and in the therapy of patients suffering from psychoactive substance use disorder.

Reference and Further Reading: Puri BK, Hall A, Ho R (2014). *Revision Notes in Psychiatry.* London: CRC Press, p. 29; Puri B, Treasaden I (eds) 2010: *Psychiatry: An Evidence-Based Text.* London: Hodder Arnold, p. 204.

Question 157 Answer: i, Reciprocal inhibition
Explanation: Reciprocal inhibition is a concept developed by Joseph Wolpe. Opposing emotions cannot exist simultaneously. It can be used in treating conditions associated with anticipatory anxiety.

Reference and Further Reading: Puri B, Treasaden I (eds) (2010). *Psychiatry: An Evidence-Based Text.* London: Hodder Arnold, pp. 655, 990; Puri BK, Hall A, Ho R (2014). *Revision Notes in Psychiatry.* London: CRC Press, p. 28.

Question 158 Answer: k, Systematic desensitization
Explanation: Systemic desensitization was developed by Wolpe.
   During this process, the patient is successfully exposed (in reality or in imagination) to these stimuli in the hierarchy, beginning with the least anxiety-evoking one, each exposure being paired with relaxation.

Reference and Further Reading: Puri B, Treasaden I (eds) (2010). *Psychiatry: An Evidence-Based Text.* London: Hodder Arnold, p. 990; Puri BK, Hall A, Ho R (2014). *Revision Notes in Psychiatry.* London: CRC Press, p. 28.

Question 159 Answer: c, Flooding
Explanation: Flooding involves exposure to the top stimulus in the hierarchy *in vivo*, while implosion involves exposing to the top stimulus by imagination.

Further Reading: Puri B, Treasaden I (eds) (2010). *Psychiatry: An Evidence-Based Text.* London: Hodder Arnold, pp. 665, 991.

Question 160 Answer: h, Premack's principle
Explanation: Premack's principle uses high-frequency behaviour in this case (e.g. playing piano) to reinforce the low-frequency behaviour (e.g. doing homework).

Premack's principle is useful when it is difficult to identify reinforcers. The high-frequency behaviour does not need to be pleasurable.

Question 161 Answer: l, Token economy
Explanation: Token economy or behavioural therapy has been used to reinforce behaviours.

Reference: Puri BK, Hall A, Ho R (2014). *Revision Notes in Psychiatry*. London: CRC Press, p. 501.

Question 162 Answer: a, Aversive conditioning
Explanation: This type of aversive conditioning is known as convert sensitization as the prisoners imagine the adverse outcomes.

Reference: Puri BK, Hall A, Ho R (2014). *Revision Notes in Psychiatry*. London: CRC Press, p. 25.

Question 163 Answer: f, Latent learning
Explanation: Latent learning shows that learning can take place in the absence of reinforcement.

Further Reading: Puri B, Treasaden I (eds) (2010). *Psychiatry: An Evidence-Based Text*. London: Hodder Arnold, pp. 207, 222.

Question 164 Answer: b, Chaining
Explanation: In chaining, the components of a more complex desired behaviour are first taught and then connected in order to teach the latter. Chaining may be conceptualized in the following two different ways: responses that function as discriminative stimuli for subsequent responses or responses that produce stimuli that function as discriminative stimuli for subsequent responses.

Reference: Puri BK, Hall A, Ho R (2014). *Revision Notes in Psychiatry*. London: CRC Press, p. 29.

Question 165 Answer: g, Penalty
Explanation: Penalty refers to the removal of pleasant stimulus following undesirable behaviour. It is different from punishment which gives an unpleasant outcome, for example canning.

Further Reading: Puri B, Treasaden I (eds) (2010). *Psychiatry: An Evidence-Based Text*. London: Hodder Arnold, p. 949.

Question 166 Answer: a, Aversive conditioning
Explanation: This example demonstrates escape conditioning, an example of aversive conditioning.

Further Reading: Puri B, Treasaden I (eds) (2010). *Psychiatry: An Evidence-Based Text*. London: Hodder Arnold, p. 949.

Question 167 Answer: d, Habituation
Explanation: Sensitization is opposite to habituation. In sensitization, the strength of response is increased as the subject is told that the stimulus is significant.

Further Reading: Puri B, Treasaden I (eds) (2010). *Psychiatry: An Evidence-Based Text*. London: Hodder Arnold, p. 990, 949.

Question 168 Answer: e, Insight learning
Explanation: Insight learning involves a spontaneous and sudden gaining of insight and solution to the problems.

Further Reading: Puri B, Treasaden I (eds) (2010). *Psychiatry: An Evidence-Based Text*. London: Hodder Arnold, p. 949.

Question 169 Answer: b, Kahlbaum
Explanation: In 1882, Karl Kahlbaum, who was a German psychiatrist, coined the terminology cyclothymia.

Question 170 Answer: f, Leonard
Explanation: In this condition, the psychotic symptoms appear suddenly a few days before menstruation, resolve with the onset of menstrual bleeding and reappear with the next cycle. Between psychotic episodes, the woman appears largely asymptomatic. Most cases do not show familial psychiatric comorbidity. The first psychotic episode usually occurs at a young age. The psychiatric picture is nonspecific and changes with every menstruation. Some common features include psychomotor retardation, anxiety, perplexity, disorientation and amnestic features.

Reference: Puri BK, Hall A, Ho R (2014). *Revision Notes in Psychiatry*. London: CRC Press, p.559.

Question 171 Answer: d, Kraepelin
Explanation: In 1896, Emil Kraepelin grouped together catatonia, hebephrenia and the deteriorating paranoid psychosis under the name of dementia praecox.

Further Reading: Puri B, Treasaden I (eds) (2010). *Psychiatry: An Evidence-Based Text*. London: Hodder Arnold, pp. 11, 593, 614, 624.

Question 172 Answer: g, Hecker
In 1871, this was described by Hecker.

Question 173 Answer: a, Bleuler
Explanation: In 1911, Bleuler introduced the term schizophrenia, applied it to Kraepelin's cases of dementia praecox and expanded the concept to include what today may be considered to be schizophrenia spectrum disorders.

Further Reading: Puri B, Treasaden I (eds) (2010). *Psychiatry: An Evidence-Based Text*. London: Hodder Arnold, p. 593.

Question 174 Answer: c, Kasanin
Explanation: Oneiroid state consists of a strange, dream-like, psychotic experience with narrowing of consciousness. It can occur in catatonia.

Reference: Puri BK, Hall A, Ho R (2014). *Revision Notes in Psychiatry*. London: CRC Press, p. 351.

Question 175 Answer: h (36%–50%)

Question 176 Answer: c (13%)

Question 177 Answer: e (23%)

Question 178 Answer: a (4%)

Question 179 Answer: a (2.4%)
Explanation: The concordance rate for monozygotic twins is approximately 45%, and for dizygotic twins, it is approximately 10%. The approximate lifetime risks for the development of schizophrenia in the relatives of patients with schizophrenia are as follows:
 a. Parents: 6%
 b. All siblings: 10%
 c. Siblings (when one parent has schizophrenia): 17%
 d. Children: 13%
 e. Children (when both parents have schizophrenia): 46%
 f. Grandchildren: 4%
 g. Uncles, aunts, nephew and nieces: 3%

Reference and Further Reading: Puri B, Treasaden I (eds) (2010). *Psychiatry: An Evidence-Based Text*. London: Hodder Arnold, pp. 474–475, 597, 599; Puri BK, Hall A, Ho R (2014). *Revision Notes in Psychiatry*. London: CRC Press, p. 358.

Question 180 Answer: b

Question 181 Answer: d (12–24 months)

Question 182 Answer: j
Explanation: The following facts should be remembered:

5%–25% of schizophrenics remain unresponsive to conventional neuroleptics.
40%–60% of patients are known to be noncompliant with medications. The possible reasons include having limited insight into the disease, limited beneficial effect, unpleasant side effects, pressure from family and friends and poor communication with the medical team. Depot would help to increase compliance and reduce the relapse rates.
Of patients who have stopped medications, 60%–70% of them would relapse within 1 year and 85% of them within 2 years. This is in comparison to 10%–30% of those who are continued on treatment.

Reference: Puri BK, Hall A, Ho R (2014). *Revision Notes in Psychiatry*. London: CRC Press, p. 365.

EMI on aetiology

Question 183 Answer: k

Explanation: This patient suffers from paediatric autoimmune neuropsychiatric disorders associated with streptococcal infections (PANDAS).

Reference and Further Reading: Puri BK, Treasaden I (eds) (2010). *Psychiatry: An Evidence-Based Text*. London: Hodder Arnold, p. 551.

Question 184 Answer: d, Childhood sexual abuse

Explanation: This patient suffers from borderline personality disorder, and childhood sexual abuse is an important aetiological factor.

Reference and Further Reading: Puri BK, Treasaden I (eds) (2010). *Psychiatry: An Evidence-Based Text*. London: Hodder Arnold, pp. 707, 709.

Question 185 Answer: g, Dysbindin gene, h, Migration, i, Neuregulin gene

Explanation: This patient suffers from schizophrenia, and *dysbindin*, *neuregulin* and migration may be aetiological factors.

Reference and Further Reading: Puri BK, Treasaden I (eds) (2010). *Psychiatry: An Evidence-Based Text*. London: Hodder Arnold, pp. 593–609.

This question has been modified from the 2008–2010 examination.

GET THROUGH MRCPSYCH PAPER A1: MOCK EXAMINATION

Total number of questions: 194 (119 MCQs, 75 EMIs)
Total time provided: 180 minutes

Question 1
Which of the following statements about delusion is false?
 a. It is a false belief based usually on incorrect inference about external reality.
 b. It is firmly sustained despite what almost everyone else believes.
 c. It is firmly sustained despite what constitutes as obvious proof or evidence to the contrary.
 d. It is usually not preceded by a delusional mood.
 e. The belief is not accepted by other members of the person's culture or subculture.

Question 2
A man with a phobia of open spaces is made to draw up a hierarchy of situations, from the least anxiety provoking to the most anxiety provoking. He is then taught relaxation techniques and gradually exposed to the hierarchy of situations that he has previously drawn up. This is known as
 a. Classical conditioning
 b. Operant conditioning
 c. Systematic desensitization
 d. Punishment
 e. Flooding

Question 3
In order to determine whether a client is suitable for intensive psychotherapy, which one of the following needs to be assessed?
 a. Analysis of transference
 b. Analysis of countertransference
 c. Analysis of personality and intelligence
 d. Assessment of client's family
 e. Assessment of dreams

Question 4

An electrocardiogram (ECG) tracing was done as part of the annual assessment for a schizophrenia patient who is on follow-up with the outpatient service. The corrected QTC was noted to be 750 ms. Which of the following medications is most likely to be responsible for this?

a. Risperidone
b. Olanzapine
c. Quetiapine
d. Abilify
e. Clozapine

Question 5

A 22-year-old male has been feeling increasingly troubled by his neighbours, as he believes that they are spying on him consistently. He does not report any other perceptual abnormalities and there has not been any decline in terms of his functioning. The most likely clinical diagnosis would be

a. Paranoid schizophrenia
b. Hebephrenic schizophrenia
c. Delusional disorder
d. Simple schizophrenia
e. Paranoid personality disorder

Question 6

A core trainee has been asked to obtain collaborative history from the family members of a patient who has just been admitted. According to the family members, the patient has been having behavioural changes for the past 6 months. At times, he would be laughing to himself, and he has shown a general decline in his personal functioning. He does have delusional beliefs and auditory hallucinations. Which subtype of schizophrenia would this be?

a. Paranoid schizophrenia
b. Hebephrenic schizophrenia
c. Undifferentiated schizophrenia
d. Residual schizophrenia
e. Post schizophrenia depression

Question 7

An elderly old man looks into the mirror and is shocked that he is unable to see himself in the mirror. What form of psychopathology is this?

a. Autoscopy
b. Negative autoscopy
c. Extracampine hallucination
d. Functional hallucination
e. Reflex hallucination

Question 8

A 25-year-old man, John, has just been discharged from the ward following treatment for first-episode psychosis. He is followed up closely by his community psychiatric nurse. She is concerned that when John is at home, he is being subjected to critical and harsh remarks from his father. She is asking the multi-disciplinary team to consider other interventions that might be appropriate for John. Which of these interventions would be the most appropriate?

a. Interpersonal therapy
b. Cognitive behavioural therapy
c. Psychodynamic therapy
d. Cognitive analytical therapy
e. Family therapy

Question 9

A 20-year-old male has been recently diagnosed with first-episode psychosis. He started on an antipsychotic risperidone around 4 weeks ago. The community psychiatric nurse reports that there has not been any improvement in his symptoms. As a core trainee, what would you want to consider?

a. Increasing the dose of the medications
b. Switching to another antipsychotic
c. Augmentation with another medication
d. Switching to clozapine
e. Exploring potential non-concordance to medications

Question 10

With regards to the treatment of Wernicke's encephalopathy, which of the following should be administered first?

a. Intravenous saline
b. Intravenous glucose
c. Intravenous thiamine and vitamin B
d. Intravenous potassium
e. Intravenous phosphate

Question 11

Based on the *International Classification of Diseases* (ICD)-10 and *Diagnostic and Statistical Manual of Mental Disorders* (DSM)-5 classification system, which of the following psychiatric disorder is believed to be part of a continuum between schizophrenia and mood symptoms?

a. Depression with psychotic features
b. Bipolar affective disorder type I
c. Bipolar affective disorder type II
d. Schizoaffective disorder
e. Post-schizophrenia depression

Question 12

Which of the following statements about persuasion is incorrect?
a. Audience identification with the communicator plays a key role in persuasion.
b. Views of reference groups usually do not play a role if the communicator is credible and has expertise.
c. High self-esteem and intelligence of the recipient increase the likelihood that complex communications will be persuasive.
d. Simple message repetition can be a persuasive influence leading to attitude change.
e. A low anxiety recipient is more influenced by a high fear message and vice versa.

Question 13

A 30-year-old Malaysian man is referred by police for psychiatric assessment. Few days ago, he was arrested by police for shoplifting in the supermarket. Then, he became mildly depressed because he 'lost face' after the incident. This morning, he took a knife and tried to kill pedestrians who walked across his path. He is amnesic for the episode. This man suffers from which of the following culture-bound syndromes?
a. Amok
b. Brain fag
c. Dhat
d. Koro
e. Latah

Question 14

All of the following are considered to be part of the normal stage of grief with the exception of
a. Denial
b. Anger
c. Bargaining
d. Depression
e. Agitation

Question 15

A 22-year-old male has been diagnosed with paranoid schizophrenia and sectioned for treatment in the mental health service three times since the onset of his schizophrenia. He has had an adequate trial of haloperidol and olanzapine, which did not help with his symptoms. It is now decided that he start on a trial of clozapine. Which one of the following investigations should be considered before starting him on clozapine?
a. Full blood count
b. Renal panel
c. Liver function test
d. Thyroid function test
e. Metabolic markers

Question 16

A patient presents with catatonia to the outpatient clinic and a joint decision was made for inpatient admission for further treatment. The trainee should expect to find the following signs of catatonia, with the exception of

a. Neologism
b. Ambitendency
c. Mitgehen
d. Negativism
e. Mannerism

Question 17

A 22-year-old male came for his routine outpatient clinic follow-up and he reported that he had been troubled by voices recently. He shared that he was worried about the voices, as the voices seemed to be commenting on what he is doing. The psychopathology being described would be

a. Command hallucination
b. Running commentary
c. Pseudohallucination
d. Functional hallucination
e. Hallucinosis

Question 18

A 40-year-old man suffers from alcohol dependence. His general practitioner (GP) asked him to take disulfiram but no clear instruction was given. Every time he drinks alcohol, he takes disulfiram. He develops flushing of the face, headache, vomiting, chest pain and sweating when he drinks alcohol. He attributes the unpleasant experiences to alcohol and he has decided not to drink alcohol in his life. This phenomenon is known as

a. Aversive conditioning
b. Backward conditioning
c. Classical conditioning
d. Forward conditioning
e. Systematic desensitization

Question 19

A 21-year old male has a history of bipolar disorder and he has been previously admitted thrice for manic episodes and just recently for a depressive episode. During his routine outpatient review, the core trainee noted that the patient has pervasively low mood with reduced interest and fulfils the criteria for bipolar, depressive episode. Which of the following medications would be most suitable for him?

a. Doxepin
b. Fluoxetine
c. Sertraline
d. Mirtazapine
e. Lamotrigine

Question 20

This is a particular subtype of schizophrenia in which there might be marked psychomotor disturbances that might alternate between extremes. In addition, the patient might also report experiencing a dream-like state with vivid scenic hallucination.

a. Paranoid schizophrenia
b. Simple schizophrenia
c. Residual schizophrenia
d. Post-schizophrenia depression
e. Catatonic schizophrenia

Question 21

A 75-year-old woman has suffered from a recent cerebrovascular accident (CVA). After the CVA, her family members note that she has global dementia and associated frontal lobe personality changes. Which of the following might be implicated?

a. Infarction of the anterior cerebral arteries
b. Infarction of the middle cerebral arteries
c. Infarction of the posterior cerebral artery
d. Subarachnoid bleed
e. Subdural bleed

Question 22

A medical student being attached to the addiction specialty wonders how long an individual needs to have symptoms of alcohol dependence in order for a diagnosis to be made. The correct answer, based on the ICD-10 classification system, would be

a. 1 month
b. 2 months
c. 6 months
d. 1 year
e. 2 years

Question 23

There are five types of social powers that have been proposed. Which of the following types of social power best describes someone who is often being looked up to as a role model, is well liked by many and has the ability to make people around them feel good?

a. Authority
b. Reward
c. Coercive
d. Referent
e. Expert

Question 24

The following defence mechanism is commonly used in borderline personality disorder:

a. Splitting
b. Reaction formation
c. Rationalization
d. Humour
e. Sublimation

Question 25

A patient with obsessive-compulsive disorder (OCD) tends to make use of this particular defence mechanism:

a. Projection
b. Acting out
c. Splitting
d. Reaction formation
e. Projective identification

Question 26

Which of the following medications would be the most helpful for patients diagnosed with catatonia?

a. Benzodiazepines
b. Nonsteroidal anti-inflammatory drugs (NSAIDs)
c. Antipsychotics
d. Antidepressants
e. Mood stabilizers

Question 27

A welfare organization decides to hire a man with schizophrenia for vocational training. This man will be paid £400 at the end of each month if he can make 100 key chains per month. This phenomenon is known as

a. Classical conditioning
b. Fixed interval schedule
c. Fixed ratio schedule
d. Variable interval schedule
e. Variable ratio schedule

Question 28

The following best describe auditory hallucinations that psychotic patients experience, with the exception of

a. Command voices
b. Demeaning voices
c. Voices doing a running commentary
d. Voices telling them that they are useless
e. Voices arguing amongst each other

Question 29

Which of the following factors account for the lower incidence of alcoholism in Orientals?

a. Presence of isoenzyme aldehyde dehydrogenase
b. Absence of isoenzyme aldehyde dehydrogenase
c. Presence of isoenzymes alcohol dehydrogenase
d. Absence of isoenzyme alcohol dehydrogenase
e. Presence of ultra-rapid metabolizing CYP 450 enzymes

Question 30

Which of the following personality disorders might be present in someone who presents with the psychiatric diagnosis of malingering?

a. Schizoid personality disorder
b. Schizotypal personality disorder
c. Antisocial personality disorder
d. Borderline personality disorder
e. Dependent personality disorder

Question 31

On examination of a patient's visual field, the examiner would ask the patient to cover one eye and fixate on the examiner's opposite eye. Mapping of the visual field is then carried out by the examiner. The objective of this examination is to check for

a. Weakness of the extraocular muscles
b. Checking for presence of organic disorders (myasthenia gravis or thyroid eye disease)
c. Lens dislocation
d. Assessment for lesions involving the central visual pathway
e. Myopia

Question 32

A 20-year-old university student presents with delusions, hallucinations, disorganized speech and grossly disorganized behaviour for 3 weeks. He failed an examination 3 weeks ago. Which of the following statements is correct?

a. This patient does not fulfil both DSM-IV-TR and ICD-10 diagnostic criteria for brief and acute psychotic disorders respectively.
b. This patient fulfils the DSM-IV-TR diagnostic criteria for brief psychotic disorder.
c. This patient fulfils the ICD-10 diagnostic criteria for acute and transient psychotic disorder.
d. This patient fulfils both DSM-IV-TR and ICD-10 diagnostic criteria for brief and acute psychotic disorders respectively.
e. DSM-IV-TR diagnostic criteria for brief psychotic disorder do not consider the person's culture.

Question 33

Colon cancer patients have a tendency to compare themselves with other patients who are deemed to be more ill than them. Which of the following terminology best describes this phenomenon?
  a. Downward social comparison
  b. Upward social comparison
  c. Normative social comparison
  d. Relative social comparison
  e. Absolute social comparison

Question 34

Attitudes are made up of which of the following components?
  a. Motivational only
  b. Motivational and emotional only
  c. Motivational, emotional and perceptual
  d. Motivational, emotional, perceptual and cognitive
  e. Motivational, emotional and cognitive

Question 35

A 30-year-old female has been too afraid recently to step out of her house. She feels that other people around her can know what she is thinking just by looking at her. This form of psychopathology is known as
  a. Thought insertion
  b. Thought withdrawal
  c. Thought broadcast
  d. Thought interference
  e. Delusion of reference

Question 36

A talented child believes that he will get the highest marks in class if he wears a red watch on the day of examination. When he does not have an examination, he usually wears a blue watch. The interval for him to get the highest mark varies. Nevertheless, his habit of wearing a red watch during examination remains stable over the years. He tends to wear the red watch more often if he has not obtained the highest marks in class for a long time. This phenomenon is known as
  a. Classical conditioning
  b. Fixed interval schedule
  c. Fixed ratio schedule
  d. Variable interval schedule
  e. Variable ratio schedule

Question 37

A 30-year-old man suffering from schizophrenia used to take chlorpromazine 100 mg orally per day. He wants to change antipsychotics and requests a list of

drugs. Which of the following lists indicate the correct dosage which is equivalent to oral chlorpromazine 100 mg per day?
   a. 0.5 mg/day for haloperidol, 0.5 mg/day for risperidone, 2.5 mg/day for olanzapine, 37.5 mg/day for quetiapine, 15 mg/day for ziprasidone and 3.75 mg/day for aripiprazole
   b. 1 mg/day for haloperidol, 1 mg/day for risperidone, 2.5 mg/day for olanzapine, 37.5 mg/day for quetiapine, 30 mg/day for ziprasidone and 3.75 mg/day for aripiprazole
   c. 1.5 mg/day for haloperidol, 1.5 mg/day for risperidone, 2.5 mg/day for olanzapine, 37.5 mg/day for quetiapine, 30 mg/day for ziprasidone and 3.75 mg/day for aripiprazole
   d. 2 mg/day for haloperidol, 2 mg/day for risperidone, 5 mg/day for olanzapine, 75 mg/day for quetiapine, 60 mg/day for ziprasidone and 7.5 mg/day for aripiprazole
   e. 4 mg/day for haloperidol, 4 mg/day for risperidone, 10 mg/day for olanzapine, 150 mg/day for quetiapine, 120 mg/day for ziprasidone and 15 mg/day for aripiprazole.

Question 38
Which of the following is considered to be a poor prognostic factor for patients with schizophrenia?
   a. Being male
   b. Being married
   c. No ventricular enlargement on computed tomography (CT) imaging
   d. Affective component to the illness
   e. Good initial response to treatment

Question 39
A 60-year-old male sustained head injuries, after being involved in a major road traffic accident about one year ago. Recently, his wife has noticed marked changes in his behaviour. She is concerned especially about him making inappropriate, rude sexual remarks when he is out. The symptoms that he is currently experiencing suggest an injury to which part of his brain?
   a. Frontal lobe
   b. Temporal lobe
   c. Parietal lobe
   d. Cerebellum
   e. Hippocampus

Question 40
A 25-year-old woman develops brief psychosis following childbirth. In order for her to fulfil the diagnostic criteria for postpartum psychosis, which of the following statements is incorrect?
   a. The DSM-IV-TR specifies the onset of her psychotic episode has to be within 4 weeks postpartum.
   b. The ICD-10 states that her psychotic episode should commence within 6 weeks of delivery.

c. The DSM-IV-TR provides postpartum onset specifier associated with brief psychotic disorder.
d. In the ICD-10, her condition is classified under schizophrenia.
e. There is no specific diagnostic criterion for postpartum psychosis in the DSM-IV-TR and the ICD-10.

Question 41
A 28-year-old specialist registrar was at the annual Royal College of Psychiatrist academic conference. There were a lot of participants and she was having a discussion with Professor Brown regarding her latest research. She was able to identify Professor Wilson, who called out for her. Which form of attention process was Jane using?
a. Selective/focused attention
b. Divided attention
c. Sustained attention
d. Non-sustained attention
e. Differentiated attention

Question 42
A 30-year-old motorcyclist suffers from head injuries after a road traffic accident. His partner comments that his memory has become very poor. Which of the following is not a standardized test to assess his memory?
a. Auditory–Verbal Learning Test (AVLT)
b. California Verbal Learning Test (CVLT)
c. Recognition Memory Test (RMT)
d. Wechsler Memory Test (WMT)
e. Weigl Colour–Form Sorting Test (WCFST)

Question 43
A 35-year-old male has a diagnosis of narcissistic personality disorder. He is rejected from further admission to the ward because he has made the nurses very upset by making unreasonable complaints. The nurses are begging the consultant not to admit him, although he is highly suicidal. This is an example of
a. Acting out
b. Countertransference
c. Displacement
d. Irresponsibility
e. Narcissistic injury

Question 44
All of the following are immature defence mechanisms except
a. Denial
b. Humour
c. Hypochrondriasis
d. Repression
e. Somatization

Question 45

A 60-year-old man is admitted to the gastroenterology ward because of abdominal pain. He has been complaining for the past 6 months that his intestines have stopped working, and said to the gastroenterologist, 'My intestines are rotten and you can smell it.' He has also told the doctor that he could hear his neighbours saying bad things about him. What is the most likely ICD-10 diagnosis?

a. Acute and transient psychosis
b. Late onset schizophrenia
c. Persistent delusional disorder
d. Schizophrenia
e. Severe depressive episode with psychotic features

Question 46

Which of the following statements with regards to the respective delusions is incorrect?

a. Delusional jealousy – Othello syndrome
b. Delusion of doubles – i'illusions de sosies
c. Delusion of infestation – Ekbom's syndrome
d. Doppelganger – Cotard's syndrome
e. Delusion of pregnancy – Couvade syndrome

Question 47

A gambler thinks that the more often he gambles, the more often he will win. He is not certain about the number of times gambling resulted in winning. The time interval between two episodes of winning is also unpredictable. His wife complains that he often has emotional outbursts when he pursues to win. This phenomenon is known as

a. Classical conditioning
b. Fixed interval schedule
c. Fixed ratio schedule
d. Variable interval schedule
e. Variable ratio schedule

Question 48

The following are findings from the Clinical Antipsychotic Trials of Intervention Effectiveness (CATIE) study, except

a. More patients taking second-generation antipsychotics continue the antipsychotic treatment compared with patients taking conventional antipsychotics.
b. Olanzapine was the most effective in terms of the rates of discontinuation.
c. The efficacy of the conventional antipsychotic agent perphenazine appeared similar to that of quetiapine, risperidone and ziprasidone.
d. Olanzapine was associated with greater weight gain and increases in measures of glucose and lipid metabolism.
e. Perphenazine was associated with more discontinuation for extrapyramidal effects.

Question 49

A medical student reading up on the history of psychiatry found out that lactate infusion was given in the late 1960s. From his reading, the intravenous infusion of lactate caused patients to have several symptoms, which included sudden onset of palpitations, chest pain, choking sensations, dizziness, depersonalization and also a significant fear of losing control and dying. What is the psychiatric condition that has resulted from intravenous lactate infusion?
  a. Specific phobia
  b. Generalized anxiety disorder
  c. Panic disorder
  d. Post-traumatic stress disorder
  e. Lactic acidosis

Question 50

A trainee wants to start a research about attitudes. He has only basic understanding that attitudes are usually based on pre-existing beliefs. Which one of the following statements associated with the measurement scale is incorrect?
  a. Thurstone Scale – Dichotomous scale indicating agreement or disagreement
  b. Thurstone Scale – Ranking is unbiased
  c. Likert Scale – More sensitive in comparison to the dichotomous Thurstone Scale
  d. Semantic Differential Scale – Easy to use and has good test-retest reliability
  e. Semantic Differential Scale – Positional response bias might occur

Question 51

A 50-year-old woman has received six sessions of electroconvulsive therapy (ECT). She complains of significant recent memory loss while remote memories remain intact. This phenomenon is known as
  a. Gestalt's law
  b. Marr's law
  c. Ribot's law
  d. Tarasoff's law
  e. Weber–Fechner law

Question 52

This particular ethical principle emphasizes minimization of the risks and maximizing the benefits for the greatest number of individuals. This ethical principle is referred to as
  a. Utilitarian
  b. Deontology
  c. Virtue
  d. Paternalism
  e. Beneficence

Question 53

Based on your understanding of the basic ethical principles in psychiatry, deontology refers to

a. Providing a duty-based approach.

b. Acting in the patient's best interest.

c. Ensuring that the action performed is considered to be morally right if it would lead to the greatest human pleasure, happiness and satisfaction.

d. Ensuring that all individuals receive equal and impartial consideration.

e. A doctor's native motive is to provide morally correct care to his or her patients and focus solely on the rightness and wrongness of the actions themselves, and not on the consequences of the actions.

Question 54

The following are ICD-10 diagnostic criteria for delusional disorder, except

a. There is a set of related delusions (e.g. persecutory, grandiose, hypochondriacal, jealous or erotic delusions).

b. The minimum duration of delusions is 6 months.

c. There must be no persistent hallucination.

d. The general criteria for schizophrenia and depressive disorder should not be fulfilled.

e. There must be no evidence of primary or secondary organic mental disorders.

Question 55

A 40-year-old man wants to transfer from another NHS trust to your trust. He is admitted to the psychiatric ward because of low mood. He complains to the ward manager that the inpatient service is not up to standard. After discharge, he has written 15 letters to the chief executive about the delay in psychologist appointment. Which of the following personality disorders is the most likely diagnosis?

a. Anankastic

b. Anxious (avoidant)

c. Antisocial

d. Borderline

e. Narcissistic

Question 56

A patient was called into the interview room. Throughout the interview process, he was noted to be moving his hand repeatedly whenever he talks. This form of psychopathology is known as

a. Automatic obedience

b. Catalepsy

c. Cataplexy

d. Mannerism

e. Echopraxia

Question 57

A 35-year-old patient with schizophrenia previously on olanzapine was diagnosed by his GP to suffer from diabetes mellitus. Her GP has written a letter to consult you on the most suitable antipsychotics to prescribe in this case. Which of the following antipsychotics would you recommend in this case?

a. Amisulpride
b. Chlorpromazine
c. Clozapine
d. Risperidone
e. Quetiapine

Question 58
Individuals usually tend to feel uneasy when cognitive dissonance occurs and this might lead to increased anxiety. There is always a motivation to achieve internal cognitive consistency. All of the following help with the reduction of anxiety associated with cognitive dissonance, except

a. Changing one or more of the thought processes involved in the dissonant relationship
b. Changing the behaviour that is considered inconsistent with the cognition
c. Addition of new thoughts that are consistent with pre-existing thought processes
d. Altering attitude
e. Challenging negative automatic thoughts

Question 59
During routine outpatient review, a patient with a diagnosis of schizophrenia, who has been concordant to his medications and has not had a relapse in the last decade, informs the psychiatrist that he wishes to stop medical treatment. The psychiatrist is concerned and cautioned him about the risk of relapse as well as the advantage and benefits of staying on the medications. The patient has mental capacity to understand and formulate a decision. However, his decision in this case would not be the best option. The psychiatrist feels compelled to go along with the wishes of the patient. This is an example of the ethical principle of

a. Utilitarianism
b. Deontology
c. Nonmaleficence
d. Autonomy
e. Beneficence

Question 60
A 40-year-old female teacher suffering from depression has been on sick leave for the past 6 months. She has asked the core trainee to continue giving her sick leave. The core trainee is concerned and consults you. Which of the following is an indicator for not issuing a medical certificate to this patient?

a. She is willing to continue the antidepressant as suggested by the core trainee.
b. She is keen to see a psychologist for psychotherapy as suggested by the core trainee.

c. She wants to be in a depressive state because her husband gives her more support when she is sick.

d. She is very depressed and cannot focus on teaching. She needs to be exempted from her normal social role.

e. She is very depressed and worries that the school will blame her for being responsible for causing her own depression.

Question 61

A concerned sister brought her 50-year-old brother to see you. She feels that he suffers from obsessive-compulsive personality disorder based on the information available on the Internet. Which of the following clinical features highly suggest that he indeed suffers from anankastic personality disorder?

a. He was asked to leave a church because he said obscene things to fellow church members.

b. He was fined by the traffic police for illegal parking because he tends to park anywhere on the street.

c. He was penalized by the HM Revenue & Customs for delay in filling up income tax form because he could not make up his mind what to report and feared making mistakes.

d. He was sued by his ex-wife for refusing to pay maintenance fee because he believes that she can support herself.

e. He was suspended from school when he was young because he vandalized school properties.

Question 62

Which of the following statements correctly defines what is meant by delusional perception?

a. It means that an abnormal perception has taken on delusional significance.

b. It refers to a delusional mood with delusional significance.

c. It means that a normal perception has taken on a delusional significance.

d. It means that a normal perception has been misinterpreted.

e. It arises due to the recall of an abnormal memory.

Question 63

A 3-year-old boy was playing with his toy car when it rolled under the sofa. He attempted reaching for the toy car with his hands but it was too far in. After several tries at using his hands, he picked up an umbrella and succeeded at using the hook of the umbrella to reach for his toy car. Which of the following learning theories best describes the aforementioned phenomenon?

a. Cognitive learning

b. Mowrer's two-factor theory

c. Psychological imprinting

d. Observational learning

e. Operant conditioning

Question 64
Which of the following phenomenon is the most common extrapyramidal side effect associated with the first generation antipsychotics?
a. Akathisia
b. Acute dystonia
c. Galactorrhoea
d. Pseudo-parkinsonism
e. Tardive dyskinesia

Question 65
A 45-year-old doctor wakes up at 6.00 AM every day and goes to the hospital to ensure that the parking lot closest to the hospital main entrance is not occupied. She is easily upset with other doctors who occupy this parking lot. She could only buy fish and chips from the same store in the last 10 years and she usually declines to try other foods during lunch. She is a very clean person and likes to document in great details. Her colleagues consult you about her personality. Your answer is
a. Anankastic personality
b. Anxious avoidance personality
c. Normal personality
d. Schizoid personality
e. Schizotypal personality

Question 66
A 14-year-old teenager is experiencing and undergoing which stage, based on Erikson's stage of development?
a. Initiative
b. Accomplishment and duty
c. Identity
d. Intimacy
e. Generativity

Question 67
In an experiment, it was found that when there were more people around during an emergency, the participants were less likely to help. Which of the following best describes the aforementioned phenomenon?
a. Propinquity effect
b. Overjustification effect
c. Bystander effect
d. Social dilemma
e. Moral dilemma

Question 68
A psychotherapist, on knowing the difficulties that his patient has had experienced recently (being dismissed from work and working through the grief associated

with the loss of his loved ones), mentioned to his client that 'You have indeed coped extremely well despite the circumstances that you have been in'. This is an example of

a. Summarizing
b. Reflective listening
c. Affirmation
d. Normalization
e. Empathetic statement

Question 69

A medical student was shown a list of symptoms during his psychiatry examinations and he was asked which one of the following would be helpful towards arriving at a psychiatric diagnosis for schizophrenia. What would the correct answer be?

a. Diminished interest
b. Short-term memory difficulties
c. Long-term memory difficulties
d. Attention and concentration difficulties
e. Thought withdrawal

Question 70

A 35-year-old man suffering from treatment-resistant schizophrenia is treated with clozapine. He wants to know the most common side effect. Your answer is

a. Agranulocytosis
b. Hypersalivation
c. Sedation
d. Seizure
e. Weight gain

Question 71

A 30-year-old woman with a history of depression complains of 1-week history of worsening diplopia. During physical examination, her left eye is medially deviated giving a diplopia best prevented by closing her left eye. On attempted left lateral gaze, her right eye achieves full adduction but her left eye remains static, producing a widely separated image horizontally. Which of the following conditions is the most likely?

a. IV nerve palsy
b. Left VI nerve palsy
c. Left III nerve palsy
d. Right VI nerve palsy
e. Right III nerve palsy

Question 72

A neurosurgeon was concerned about the cognitive deficits after he operated on a 23-year-old driver who had recently been involved in a traumatic road traffic accident. He referred him to the psychiatrist for further evaluation. It was found

that the driver had impaired parietal lobe functioning. Which one of the following is NOT a test of parietal lobe functioning?
a. Left and right orientation
b. Acalculia
c. Dysgraphia
d. Cognitive estimates
e. Ideomotor apraxia

Question 73
You are performing a risk assessment on a 20-year-old man suffering from paranoid schizophrenia. Which of the following factors is least likely to be associated with violence?
a. The person has well-planned violence.
b. The person has access to weapons.
c. The person retains the ability to plan.
d. The person is staying in the community.
e. The person is totally losing touch with reality.

Question 74
You are performing a risk assessment on a 22-year-old man suffering from acute psychosis. Which of the following conditions is least likely to be associated with violence?
a. He experiences hallucinations causing positive emotions.
b. He feels dominated by forces beyond his control.
c. He feels that there are people wanting to harm him.
d. He feels that his thoughts are being put into his head.
e. He reacts in despair by striking out against others.

Question 75
A 40-year-old man is referred by his GP because he needs to drink one bottle of beer first thing in the morning, two bottles of beer during lunch time and at least few glasses of hard liquor in the evening. He needs to drink to calm his nerves as he finds his job is very stressful. According to his wife, he was previously diagnosed with personality disorder. Which of the following personality disorders is most likely?
a. Antisocial personality disorder
b. Anxious avoidant personality
c. Borderline personality disorder
d. Dependent personality disorder
e. Narcissistic personality disorder

Question 76
Which of the following is not considered to be a formal thought disorder?
a. Asyndesis
b. Condensation

c. Derailment
d. Fusion
e. Perseveration

Question 77

A 23-year-old female has just been recently diagnosed with an anxiety condition known as agoraphobia. The consultant has recommended that she be started on a course of medication (antidepressants) and also a course of psychological therapy. She has been concordant thus far and has improved such that she is now able to leave home independently. Which of the following psychological interventions has helped her?
a. Classical conditioning
b. Operant conditioning
c. Habit reversal
d. Exposure and response prevention
e. Extinction

Question 78

A 24-year-old female patient comes for review to your outpatient clinic. The inpatient consultant prescribed olanzapine and she has taken this medication for 3 months since discharge. She complains of a weight gain of 10 kg and increased appetite. She has a family history of diabetes. She requests a change in antipsychotic. Which of the following medications would you recommend?
a. Aripiprazole
b. Paliperidone
c. Quetiapine
d. Risperidone
e. Ziprasidone

Question 79

A medical student new to her posting wonders at roughly what age newborns will acquire skills of accommodation and colour vision. Which of the following would be correct?
a. Immediately at birth
b. 2 months
c. 4 months
d. 6 months
e. 1 year

Question 80

Psychiatry is the only specialty whose diagnoses are not confirmed by investigations but rests upon history taking. Which of the following statements regarding history taking is the most incorrect?

a. Assessment proforma such as admission sheets which could be found in the case notes of long-stay patients in large mental hospitals is not a good example of psychiatric history taking.
b. Clinical errors often occur because the clinical history itself is inadequate.
c. Continuing history taking is sometimes neglected because the patient is 'well-known' to a psychiatrist.
d. History taking should not be a passive process of information collection.
e. The standard schema of psychiatric history taking is a good guide to the structure of the psychiatric interview.

Question 81
A core trainee-1 resident was interviewing an elderly man in his clinic. He decided to perform a bedside Mini Mental State Examination on the patient in view of his recent difficulties with his memory. He asked the man to copy intersecting polygons. This is a test of which part of the brain functions?
  a. Frontal lobes
  b. Parietal lobes
  c. Temporal lobes
  d. Corpus callosum
  e. Hippocampus

Question 82
A 30-year-old woman with a history of depression complains of 1-week history of worsening diplopia. When her right eyelid is lifted, her right eye is looking down and out and the pupil is fixed and dilated. When she is asked to gaze to the left, her right eye remains in position while her left eye achieves full abduction. Which of the following conditions is most likely?
  a. IV nerve palsy
  b. Left VI nerve palsy
  c. Left III nerve palsy
  d. Right VI nerve palsy
  e. Right III nerve palsy

Question 83
A 40-year-old man needs to drink alcohol immediately after he wakes up in the morning, again a few pints of beer during lunch time and again at least 8 units of alcohol in the evening. He annoys his family members who always ask him to cut down his alcohol intake. He claims that he is not an alcoholic and he needs to drink to keep himself calm. Based on the clinical information, which of the following is your diagnosis?
  a. Anankastic personality disorder
  b. Antisocial personality disorder
  c. Alcohol-dependent syndrome
  d. Generalized anxiety disorder
  e. OCD

Question 84

Which of the following statements with regards to delusional perception is incorrect?

a. Delusional perception is a primary delusion.
b. Delusional perception is a secondary delusion.
c. It might be preceded by a period of delusional mood in which the person might be aware that something strange and threatening might be happening.
d. It is considered to be one of the first-rank symptoms.
e. It usually arises fully formed without any discernible connections with prior events.

Question 85

A 20-year-old man agreed to participate in a research project. He was first given Drug A, which caused tachycardia. Five minutes later, he was given Drug B, which was supposed to cause bradycardia. Drug B was not strong enough to overcome the tachycardia associated with Drug A. The subject still had tachycardia after administration of Drug B. The administration of Drug A and Drug B was repeated 12 times over the 3 days. On the fourth day, the investigator only gave the subject Drug B and was surprised to find that he developed tachycardia. The tachycardia associated with administration of Drug B on the fourth day is known as

a. Conditioned response
b. Conditioned stimulus
c. Unconditioned response
d. Unconditioned stimulus
e. Second-order conditioning

Question 86

A 30-year-old man suffers from treatment-resistant schizophrenia and he is on clozapine. He also suffers from post-schizophrenia depression. Augmentation with which of the following antidepressants is the safest option in view of the potential risk of epilepsy?

a. Amitriptyline
b. Bupropion
c. Clomipramine
d. Fluoxetine
e. Venlafaxine

Question 87

Who was responsible for discovering the use of lithium?

a. John Cade
b. Maxwell Jones
c. Viktor Frankl
d. Carl Rogers
e. Joseph Wolpe

Question 88
The individual who was responsible for the development of existential therapy was
a. Maxwell Jones
b. Viktor Frankl
c. Jacob Kasanin
d. Cerletti
e. John Bowlby

Question 89
Which of the following terms best describes 'the presence of clearly demarcated total memory loss, with no recovery of this lost memory over time', for individuals who have experienced alcoholic blackouts?
a. State-dependent memory
b. Fragmentary blackouts
c. En bloc blackouts
d. Episodic memory impairments
e. Declarative memory impairments

Question 90
A 30-year-old woman with a history of depression complains of 1-week history of worsening diplopia. She describes difficulty looking down, often notable when reading or walking down stairs. Which of the following conditions is most likely?
a. II nerve palsy
b. III nerve palsy
c. IV nerve palsy
d. VI nerve palsy
e. VII nerve palsy

Question 91
A 55-year-old male who has a history of alcohol dependence was admitted just 2 days ago for an emergency hip operation following a fall. He now reports that he is troubled by visions of multiple small spiders running around the room. Which of the following correctly describes his experience?
a. Lilliputian hallucination
b. Functional hallucination
c. Reflex hallucination
d. Macropsia
e. Micropsia

Question 92
A 39-year-old man with a history of cocaine dependence continues taking the drug to avoid experiencing withdrawal symptoms. This phenomenon is known as
a. Aversion
b. Negative reinforcement
c. Partial reinforcement

d. Positive reinforcement

e. Punishment

Question 93

A medical student wants to know the most common sign of neuroleptic malignant syndrome. Your answer is

a. Altered mental state

b. Hyperhidrosis

c. Incontinence

d. Labile blood pressure

e. Rigidity

Question 94

Based on Piaget's theory, which stage would a child be in if he is able to recognize that containers, even though they are of different shapes, contain similar amounts of water?

a. Sensorimotor

b. Preoperational

c. Operational

d. Concrete operational

e. Formal operational

Question 95

A 30-year-old woman with a history of depression complains of a 3-month history of worsening diplopia and ptosis in the evenings. Which of the following conditions is the most likely?

a. Cavernous sinus thrombosis

b. Guillain–Barre syndrome

c. Mitochondrial diseases

d. Myasthenia gravis

e. Multiple sclerosis

Question 96

A 60-year-old retired naval officer with depression believes that he is in danger of imminent arrest and life imprisonment for stealing a uniform from the Royal Navy 30 years ago. The psychopathology being described is

a. Delusional mood

b. Delusional perception

c. Delusion of guilt

d. Delusion of reference

e. Nihilistic delusion

Question 97
A 25-year-old woman with a history of methamphetamine abuse reports that she continues smoking the drug because of 'euphoria' she experiences. This phenomenon is known as
a. Aversion
b. Negative reinforcement
c. Partial reinforcement
d. Positive reinforcement
e. Punishment

Question 98
There are reported differences in the development of boys versus girls. In particular, the average age of onset of puberty of boys is much later. Which of the following is the average age of puberty for boys?
a. 10 years old
b. 11 years old
c. 12 years old
d. 13 years old
e. 14 years old

Question 99
There are several theories that explain interpersonal attraction. Which of the following is not a theory of interpersonal attraction?
a. Proxemics
b. Social exchange theory
c. Equity theory
d. Reinforcement theory
e. Mutual attraction

Question 100
Please choose the most appropriate statements with regards to schizophrenia:
a. Afro-Caribbean immigrants to the United Kingdom have a much lower risk of developing schizophrenia.
b. The winter excess of births in schizophrenics is due to a seasonal prevalence of a viral infection or other perinatal hazard.
c. Males have generally a later onset of schizophrenia as compared to females.
d. It has been found that there is a reduction in the relapse rates of schizophrenia in those who have lived with families in which the relatives displayed high EE.
e. Obstetric complications are less likely in individuals with schizophrenia.

Question 101

A mother worries that her daughter will develop depression because of the family history of depressive disorder. Which of the following genes is associated with increased risk?

a. APO E4 gene on chromosome 21
b. Catechol-O-methyltransferase (COMT) gene on chromosome 21
c. Presenilin-2 gene on chromosome 1
d. Presenilin-1 gene on chromosome 14
e. Serotonin transporter gene

Question 102

During a clinical examination, a core trainee was asked what terminology would best describe 'memories for events occurring while intoxicated are lost when sober, but returns when next intoxicated'. Which of the following would the most appropriate terminology?

a. State-dependent memory
b. Fragmentary blackouts
c. En bloc blackouts
d. Episodic memory impairments
e. Declarative memory impairments

Question 103

A 22-year-old male, Jack, is usually not an aggressive person. However, in 2011, while participating in a large-scale riot in London that turned violent, Jack found himself engaged in violence as well. Which of the following best explains Jack's behaviour?

a. Social loafing
b. Social facilitation
c. Social norms
d. Deindividuation
e. Social tuning

Question 104

At what age does a British child start to have early comprehension of English grammar?

a. 1–2 years
b. 2–3 years
c. 3–6 years
d. 6–9 years
e. 9–12 years

Question 105

A 65-year-old man presents with unequal pupils, right-sided ptosis and anhidrosis of the right half of the face and body. The patient is most likely suffering from?

a. Argyll Robertson pupils
b. Diabetic neuropathy

c. Holmes–Adie syndrome

d. Horner's syndrome

e. Pupillary defect

Question 106

A 23-year-old man meets the diagnostic criteria for schizophrenia and exhibits passivity phenomena. Passivity phenomena include the following, except

a. Made feelings

b. Made impulses

c. Thought blocking

d. Thought broadcasting

e. Somatic passivity

Question 107

A 14-year-old girl was disallowed to meet her friends over the weekend as she was caught lying to her parents. This phenomenon is known as

a. Aversion

b. Negative reinforcement

c. Partial reinforcement

d. Positive reinforcement

e. Punishment

Question 108

A 40-year-old man has been prescribed with lithium, haloperidol and fluoxetine. A trainee consults you because the patient has developed a tremor. Which of the following features suggest that the tremor is caused by haloperidol?

a. Coarse tremor

b. Dysdiadochokinesis

c. Fine tremor

d. Parkinsonism

e. Wide-based gait

Question 109

Attention refers to an intensive process in which information selection takes place. Which one of the following statements is true?

a. Dichotic listening studies test for selective attention.

b. With divided attention, performance is enhanced.

c. Attention is the equivalent of working memory.

d. Attention involves information retrieval from the short-term memory storage.

e. Attention involves information retrieval from the long-term memory storage.

Question 110

You are the trainee psychiatrist in the child and adolescent mental health service (CAMHS). An anxious mother brings her 2-year-old daughter for developmental assessment. She is concerned about her daughter's language and speech development. Which of the following developmental milestones is expected of her daughter?

a. Cooing
b. Repetitive babbling
c. Grammatical morphemes
d. Vocabulary of five words
e. Telegraphic speech

Question 111

Autochthonous delusions are

a. ego-dystonic
b. ego-syntonic
c. secondary to hallucinations
d. shared with a partner
e. starting with an idea

Question 112

The case of Phineas Gage describes which of the following syndrome?

a. Frontal lobe syndrome
b. Temporal lobe syndrome
c. Parietal lobe syndrome
d. Vascular dementia
e. Alzheimer's dementia

Question 113

Which of the following will predispose the child to emotional problems later in life?

a. Thumb-sucking at age 4
b. Transitional object for more than 6 months in the first year of life
c. Nocturnal enuresis
d. Upbringing in an authoritarian family setting
e. Adoption after 2 months

Question 114

A core trainee presents a list of symptoms for neuroleptic malignant syndrome (NMS). The following are symptoms of NMS, except?

a. NMS presents within 48 hours after the initiation of a new antipsychotic
b. Dysphagia
c. Labile blood pressure
d. Leucocytosis
e. Mutism

Question 115

A drug company wants to promote its new antidepressants. Patients will get one box of antidepressants free of charge if they purchase three boxes of antidepressants at one time. This phenomenon is known as

a. Classical conditioning
b. Fixed interval schedule

c. Fixed ratio schedule
d. Variable interval schedule
e. Variable ratio schedule

Question 116
Morbid jealousy is not
a. a misidentification phenomenon
b. associated with erectile dysfunction
c. associated with violence
d. encapsulated
e. more common in men than in women

Question 117
A 60-year-old man has had a stroke recently. He is concerned about developing dementia and wants to find out which medication could prevent vascular dementia. The correct answer is
a. Low-dose aspirin
b. High dose of statins
c. Low dose of hypoglycaemic agents
d. Thiamine
e. Vitamin E

Question 118
Previous research has found which of the following to be an important protective factor for Alzheimer's dementia?
a. High level of education
b. Occasional physical activities
c. Early retirement
d. Smoking
e. Previous history of depression

Question 119
Which of the following is not a primary prevention strategy in children and adolescents?
a. Easing the impact of traumatic milestones and transitional events in school and family
b. Preventing vulnerable population from succumbing to psychiatric disorder
c. Preventing the onset of carefully defined psychiatric disorder
d. Promoting and enhancing adaptability and healthy functioning
e. Measuring intelligence at regular intervals from children to adolescence

Extended matching items (EMIs)

Theme: Attention
Options:
a. Selective/focused attention
b. Divided attention

c. Sustained attention
d. Controlled attention
e. Automatic attention
f. Stroop effect

Lead in: Select the most appropriate answer for each of the following. Each option may be used once, more than once or not at all.

Question 120
In this particular type of attention, at least two sources of information are attended to simultaneously and the performance is inefficient.

Question 121
This particular type of attention is commonly described as the cocktail party effect.

Question 122
In this particular type of attention, the environment is monitored over a long period of time.

Question 123
In this particular type of attention, the subject becomes so skilled with the task that little conscious effort is now required.

Theme: Memory tests
Options:
  a. Benton Visual Retention Test
  b. Rey–Osterrieth Test
  c. Paired Associate Learning Test
  d. California Verbal Learning Test
  e. Rivermead Behavioural Memory Test
  f. National Adult Reading Test
  g. Raven Progressive Matrices

Lead in: Select the most appropriate answer for each of the following. Each option may be used once, more than once or not at all.

Question 124
This is a memory test that could be utilized in clinical settings to estimate the premorbid intelligence quotient.

Question 125
This is a test that tests for the perception of relations between abstract items.

Question 126
This is a memory test battery that has an emphasis on tests related to skills required in daily living.

Question 127
This particular test is effective in testing for brain damage as well as early cognitive decline.

Question 128
Non-dominant temporal lobe damage can lead potentially to impaired performance on this test, whereas dominant temporal lobe damage tends not to.

Theme: Social sciences and stigma

Options:
a. Stereotype
b. Enacted stigma
c. Felt stigma
d. Prejudice
e. Discrimination

Lead in: Select the most appropriate answer for each of the following. Each option may be used once, more than once or not at all.

Question 129
This is the dogmatic belief that one race is superior to another one and that there exist identifiable racial characteristics which influence cognition, achievement and behaviour.

Question 130
This terminology refers to the enactment of prejudice.

Question 131
This terminology refers to the experience of discrimination of an individual who bears a stigma.

Question 132
This terminology refers to the fear of discrimination of an individual who bears a stigma.

Theme: Dynamic psychopathology and theories

Options:
a. Unconscious
b. Preconscious
c. Conscious
d. Primary process
e. Secondary process
f. Pleasure principle
g. Id
h. Ego
i. Superego

Lead in: Select the most appropriate answer for each of the following. Each option may be used once, more than once or not at all.

Question 133
This is the operating system of the preconscious and the conscious.

Question 134
This is deemed to be the operating system of the unconscious.

Question 135
This contains memories, ideas and affects that are typically repressed.

Question 136
This is the part of the mind that develops during childhood and serves to maintain repression and censorship.

Question 137
Based on the structural model of the mind, this is considered to be unconscious. It contains primordial energy reserves derived from instinctual drives.

Question 138
Based on the structural model of the mind, this helps to fulfil the task of self-preservation.

Theme: Clinical psychiatry – old age psychiatry
Options:
   a. Alzheimer's dementia
   b. Vascular dementia
   c. Binswanger's disease
   d. Fronto-temporal dementia
   e. Dementia with Lewy bodies
   f. Parkinson's disease dementia

Lead in: Select the most appropriate answer for each of the following. Each option may be used once, more than once or not at all.

Question 139
Antipsychotics are usually not indicated for mild-to-moderate non-cognitive symptoms because of the risk of severe adverse events.

Question 140
Patients with this form of dementia tend to have a younger age of onset, with more severe apathy, disinhibition, reduction in speech output, loss of insight and coarsening of social behaviour.

Question 141
This form of dementia is characterized by a stepwise deteriorating course with a patchy distribution of neurological and neuropsychological deficits.

Question 142
In this form of dementia, on CT scan, there is noted to be progressive subcortical vascular encephalopathy with CT scan revealing markedly enlarged ventricles secondary to infarction in hemispheric white matter.

Question 143
This is a form of dementia that is more common in males.

Theme: Clinical psychiatry – somatoform and dissociative disorder

Options:
a. Somatization disorder
b. Somatoform autonomic dysfunction
c. Persistent somatoform pain disorder
d. Hypochondriacal disorder
e. Conversion disorder
f. Factitious disorder
g. Malingering

Lead in: Select the most appropriate answer for each of the following. Each option may be used once, more than once or not at all.

Question 144
This is a condition in which the patient intentionally produces physical or psychological symptoms and the patient is fully aware of his or her underlying motives.

Question 145
In this condition, the patient intentionally produces physical and psychological symptoms but the patient is unconscious about his or her underlying motives.

Question 146
Patients with this condition usually presents with persistent, severe, distressing pain, which cannot be explained by physical disorder.

Theme: Clinical psychiatry – women's mental health

Options:
a. Premenstrual syndrome
b. Cyclic psychosis
c. Depressive disorder in pregnancy
d. Bipolar disorder in pregnancy
e. Puerperal psychosis
f. Postnatal blues
g. Postnatal depression

Lead in: Select the most appropriate answer for each of the following. Each option may be used once, more than once or not at all.

Question 147
This occurs usually on the third to the fifth day after pregnancy and occurs in about 50% of women.

Question 148
Poor social adjustment, marital relationship and fear of labour are predisposing factors leading to the development of this condition.

Question 149
This condition has an abrupt onset, usually within the first 2 weeks after childbirth, and there might be rapid changes in mental state, sometimes from hour to hour.

Question 150
This condition occurs in 10%–15% of postpartum women usually within 3 months of childbirth.

Question 151
This is a condition that a higher prevalence in those around the age of 30 years, and the prevalence increases with increasing parity.

Theme: History of psychiatry
Options:
  a. Phineas Gage
  b. Wilhelm Griesinger
  c. Benedict Morel
  d. Jacob Mendes Da Costa
  e. Paul Broca
  f. Carl Wernicke
  g. Emil Kraepelin
  h. Sigmund Freud
  i. Carl Jung
  j. Henry Maudsley

Lead in: Select the most appropriate answer for each of the following. Each option may be used once, more than once or not at all.

Question 152
This is one of the best-known psychiatrists during the Victorian era. He was the first person to propose the abolishment of physical restraints in England.

Question 153
He was first to develop the technique of psychoanalysis.

Question 154
This led to the formation of the terminology 'Soldier's heart' during the American Civil War.

Question 155
Broca's aphasia was coined by which one of the aforementioned individuals?

Question 156
This individual proposed the degeneration theory that states that mental illness affecting one generation can be passed on to the next generation in ever-worsening degrees.

Theme: Ethics and psychiatric research
Options:
  a. Nuremberg code
  b. Declaration of Helsinki
  c. Belmont report

Lead in: Select the most appropriate answer for each of the following. Each option may be used once, more than once or not at all.

Question 157
This code emphasizes that all experiments should avoid suffering and injury.

Question 158
This code emphasizes that seeking consent from research subjects is absolutely necessary.

Question 159
This code states the importance of formulation in research protocol and informs the subjects of the protocol details.

Question 160
This code emphasizes on the importance of justice.
Answer: (c) Belmont report

Theme: Clinical psychiatry – personality disorder
Options:
  a. Paranoid personality disorder
  b. Schizoid personality disorder
  c. Schizotypal personality disorder
  d. Antisocial personality disorder
  e. Histrionic personality disorder
  f. Narcissistic personality disorder
  g. Avoidant personality disorder
  h. Obsessive-compulsive personality disorder
  i. Borderline personality disorder

Lead in: Select the most appropriate answer for each of the following. Each option may be used once, more than once or not at all.

Question 161
These patients tend to have marked emotional coldness and have little interest in activities that provide pleasure or in relationships.

Question 162
These patients tend to have unusual perceptions, are friendless and have odd beliefs and speech. They might also have ideas of reference.

Question 163
These are individuals who bear grudges without justification and are excessively sensitive to attacks.

Question 164
The age of onset of this disorder is usually from adolescence or early adulthood. This disorder is associated with a suicide rate of 9%.

Question 165
Patients with this disorder usually have very low tolerance to frustration and a low threshold for discharge of aggression, including violence.

Theme: Clinical psychiatry – substance misuse disorders
Options:
  a. Alcoholic blackouts
  b. Withdrawal fits
  c. Wernicke's encephalopathy
  d. Korsakoff's syndrome
  e. Alcoholic dementia
  f. Alcoholic hallucinosis
  g. Pathological jealousy

Lead in: Select the most appropriate answer for each of the following. Each option may be used once, more than once or not at all.

Question 166
Individuals with this condition usually present with the following clinical symptoms: ophthalmoplegia, nystagmus, ataxia and clouding of consciousness.

Question 167
Approximately 10% of patients with this condition have the classical triad, but for others, peripheral neuropathy might also be present.

Question 168
This is commonly described as an abnormal state in which memory and learning are affected, out of proportion to other cognitive functions in an otherwise alert and responsive patient.

Question 169
This usually occurs within 48 hours of stopping drinking.

Question 170
Intoxication of alcohol usually leads to episodes of short-term amnesia and blackouts.

Theme: Basic psychopharmacology
Options:
  a. Carbamazepine
  b. Diazepam
  c. Electroconvulsive therapy
  d. Haloperidol
  e. Lamotrigine
  f. Lithium
  g. Olanzapine
  h. Quetiapine
  i. Sodium valproate
  j. Sertraline

k. St John's wort

l. Topiramate

Lead in: Choose the appropriate physical treatments for the following clinical scenarios. Each option might be used more than once or not at all.

Question 171
A 45-year-old man suffers from bipolar disorder. He has had five episodes of depression and one episode of hypomania over the past 5 years. He had hypothyroidism 20 years ago. He prefers to take medications. (Choose one option.)

Question 172
A Foundation Year 2 doctor consults you regarding which anticonvulsant is not recommended for routine use in the prophylaxis in bipolar disorder. (Choose one option.)

Question 173
A 40-year-old man suffers from bipolar disorder. He has had two episodes of depression and three episodes of mania over the past 1 year. He has not responded well to the monotherapy with lithium. You suggest augmentation therapy with another medication. (Choose one option.)

Question 174
A 35-year-old man who suffered from bipolar disorder was treated by the psychiatrist in a tropical country. He was referred by the urologist to review his psychotropic medication as he has developed renal calculi after coming back to the UK. Which medication is associated with the development of renal calculi? (Choose one option.)

Question 175
A 45-year-old man suffers from bipolar disorder and hypertension. His GP prescribes angiotensin-converting enzyme (ACE) inhibitor to treat his hypertension. The ACE inhibitor increases the serum level of one medication. (Choose one option.)

Theme: Basic psychopharmacology
Options:
  a. Carbamazepine
  b. Diazepam
  c. Electroconvulsive therapy
  d. Haloperidol
  e. Lamotrigine
  f. Lithium
  g. Olanzapine
  h. Quetiapine
  i. Sodium valproate
  j. Fluoxetine
  k. St John's wort
  l. Topiramate

Lead in: Choose the appropriate physical treatments for the following clinical scenarios based on the NICE guidelines. Each option might be used more than once or not at all.

Question 176

A 35-year old woman with rapid cycling bipolar disorder was admitted to the hospital due to severe depressive symptoms. She takes Lithium CR 800 mg nocte and has been adherent to lithium. Which medication would you consider to add onto the lithium? (Choose one option.)

Question 177

A 35-year old woman with rapid cycling bipolar disorder is being managed in the community. She does not respond to monotherapy. The GP consults you on the long-term management. Combination of which two medications is recommended? (Choose two options.)

Theme: Cultural psychiatry

Options:
  a. Amok
  b. Brain fag
  c. Dhat
  d. Koro
  e. Latah
  f. Pibloktoq
  g. Susto
  h. Taijin Kyofusho
  i. Windigo

Lead in: Identify which of the aforementioned resembles the following clinical scenarios.

Question 178

A 20-year-old African university student preparing for pharmacology examination presents with burning headache, blurring eye sight and difficulty in understanding the meaning of the textbook, and cannot remember the drugs he studied. (Choose one option.)

Question 179

A 20-year-old Chinese national serviceman in Singapore was referred by the army doctor. He complains that his penis is getting shorter and it will go into his abdomen. He measures his penis every day and he cannot concentrate on his work. (Choose one option.)

Question 180

A 25-year-old Malaysian woman becomes dissociative after a road traffic accident, followed by echopraxia, echolalia, command obedience and utterance of obscene words. (Choose one option.)

Question 181
A 30-year-old indigenous Indian staying near Yellowknife, Canada, complains that he is possessed by a spirit to eat human flesh of the tribe leader after long-term conflict with him. (Choose one option.)

Theme: Psychopathology

Options:
- a. Acting-out
- b. Ambivalence
- c. Anger
- d. Disinhibition
- e. Dysphoric mood
- f. Euphoric mood
- g. Failure of empathy
- h. Fatuousness
- i. Flat affect
- j. Good rapport
- k. Guardedness
- l. Humour
- m. Humiliation
- n. Incongruous affect
- o. Labile affect
- p. Resistance
- q. Restricted affective range

Lead in: A 58-year-old woman is admitted to the psychiatric ward for the treatment of depression. The consultant psychiatrist worries that she does not simply suffer from depression because she walks with short shuffling steps and exhibits bradykinesia. During the interview, the consultant psychiatrist observes the following clinical features. Identify which of the aforementioned terminology resembles her clinical features. Each option might be used once, more than once or not at all.

Question 182
She has a mask-like face and shows no feelings at all. (Choose one option.)

Question 183
She stands perplexed at the door, putting one hand forward and then taking it back. (Choose one option.)

Question 184
She shouts and damages the door after she knows that she cannot go for home leave this weekend. (Choose one option.)

Theme: Basic psychology

Options:
- a. Bandura, Albert
- b. Pavlov, Ivan

c. Seligman, Martin
   d. Skinner, Burrhus Frederic
   e. Thorndike, Edward
   f. Watson, John

Lead in: Which of the aforementioned researchers is most strongly associated with the following experiments? Each option may be used once, more than once or not at all.

Question 185
In this experiment, an 11-month infant was allowed to play with a white rat. At this point, the infant showed no fear of the rat. The investigator made a loud sound whenever the infant touched the rat. Two weeks later, the infant showed fear of the rat and rabbit eventhough there was no loud sound. (Choose one option.)

Question 186
In this experiment, a hungry cat was confined in a puzzle box with food visible on the outside. The cat could manipulate some devices to open the gate of the puzzle box. Foods were placed outside the box, and the food served as an incentive for the cat to open the gate. Initially, the cat first behaved aimlessly as if doing things by trial and error. The presence of food made the opening of gate more likely to occur and the cat took lesser time to get the food after repeated trials. (Choose one option.)

Question 187
In this experiment, a dog was placed in a two-compartment box where there was no escape. After repeated failures to escape, the dog realized that there was an absence of contingency, became withdrawn and stopped jumping from one compartment to another. (Choose one option.)

Theme: Basic psychology
Options:
   a. Bandura, Albert
   b. Pavlov, Ivan
   c. Seligman, Martin
   d. Skinner, Burrhus Frederic
   e. Thorndike, Edward
   f. Watson, John

Lead in: Which of the aforementioned researchers is most strongly associated with the following experiments? Each option may be used once, more than once or not at all.

Question 188
The investigator designed a box that had one or more levers. When a starved rat pressed the lever, a small pellet of food was dropped onto a tray. The rat soon learned that when he pressed the lever he would receive some food. (Choose one option.)

Question 189
In this experiment, a child witnessed the different levels of aggression from an adult towards a doll. The child paid attention to the relevant aspects of aggression and created a visual image of the model in her mind. By repeated observations, the child remembered the aggressive behaviour. The child rehearsed the aggressive behaviour and anticipated similar consequences between herself and the adult. (Choose one option.)

Question 190
In this experiment, the investigator performed a minor operation on a dog to relocate its salivary duct to the outside of its cheek. This allowed easy measurement of saliva. Periodically, a bell was rang, followed shortly thereafter by meat being placed in the dog's mouth. (Choose one option.)

Theme: Basic psychology

Options:
  a. Bandura, Albert
  b. Kohler, Wolfgang
  c. Premack, David
  d. Skinner, Burrhus Frederic
  e. Tolman, Edward
  f. Watson, John

Lead in: Which of the aforementioned researchers is most strongly associated with the following experiments? Each option might be used once, more than once or not at all.

Question 191
This investigator constructed a variety of problems involving obtaining food that was not directly accessible for the chimpanzees. The investigator used chimpanzees because chimpanzees have higher intelligence than cats and dogs. Initially, the chimpanzees spent most of their time unproductively rather than slowly working towards a solution. All of a sudden, they would find a way to obtain the food. (Choose one option.)

Question 192
This investigator designed complex maze running experiments and investigated the role of reinforcement in learning. The rats developed and learned the cognitive map of a maze even when there was no reward. These experiments eventually led to a theory of latent learning, which states that learning can occur in the absence of a reward. (Choose one option.)

Question 193
This investigator conducted experiments using monkeys and found that more probable behaviours would reinforce less probable behaviours. (Choose one option.)

MRCPSYCH PAPER AI MOCK EXAMINATION 3: ANSWERS

GET THROUGH MRCPSYCH PAPER AI: MOCK EXAMINATION

Question 1 Answer: d, It is usually not preceded by a delusional mood.
Explanation: A primary delusion is a delusion that arises full formed without any connection with previous events. It could be preceded by a delusional mood in which the person is aware of something strange and threatening happening.

Reference: Puri BK, Hall A, Ho R (2014). *Revision Notes in Psychiatry*. London: CRC Press, p. 6.

Question 2 Answer: c, Systematic desensitization
Explanation: Systematic desensitization is based on the behavioural concept of reciprocal inhibition. This holds that relaxation inhibits anxiety so that the two are considered to be mutually exclusive. During this treatment, patients are successfully exposed (either in reality or in imagination) to stimuli in the hierarchy, beginning with the least anxiety-provoking event and then to the most anxiety-provoking event, with each exposure being paired with relaxation.

Reference: Puri BK, Hall A, Ho R (2014). *Revision Notes in Psychiatry*. London: CRC Press, p. 28.

Question 3 Answer: c, Analysis of personality and intelligence
Explanation: An assessment and analysis of personality and intelligence is essential to determine whether the client is suitable for psychotherapy.

Reference: Puri BK, Hall A, Ho R (2014). *Revision Notes in Psychiatry*. London: CRC Press, p. 331.

Question 4 Answer: c, Quetiapine
Explanation: The cardiac QT interval is a useful, but imprecise, indicator of risk of torsades de pointes and increased cardiac mortality. Quetiapine has been shown to have a moderate effect on the QTC interval (meaning that it has been observed to prolong the QTC by more than 10 ms on average when given at a normal clinical dose). Clozapine, risperidone and olanzapine have a low effect. Other risk factors

for QTC prolongation include: cardiac history, previous long QT syndrome, bradycardia, ischemic heart disease, myocarditis, myocardial infarction, electrolytes abnormalities and female gender.

Reference: Taylor D, Paton C, Kapur S (2009). *The Maudsley Prescribing Guidelines* (10th edition). London: Informa Healthcare, p. 119.

Question 5 Answer: c, Delusional disorder

Explanation: The answer is a delusional disorder. Based on the ICD-10 classification system, a delusional disorder is largely an ill-defined condition, manifesting as either a single delusion or a set of delusions, being persistent and at times lifelong, and not having an identifiable organic basis. There are occasional or transitory auditory hallucinations, particularly in the elderly. Delusions are the most conspicuous or the only symptoms and are present for at least 3 months. For the diagnosis to be made, there must not be any evidence of schizophrenic symptoms or brain disease.

Reference: Puri BK, Hall A, Ho R (2014). *Revision Notes in Psychiatry*. London: CRC Press, p. 372.

Question 6 Answer: b, Hebephrenic schizophrenia

Explanation: The diagnosis is likely to be hebephrenic schizophrenia. The mean age of onset is usually between 15 and 25 years. It is usually associated with a poor prognosis. Affective changes are usually quite prominent. Fleeting and fragmentary delusions and hallucinations, disorganized thoughts, rambling speech and mannerisms are also common. Negative symptoms such as flattening of affect might also be observed.

Reference: Puri BK, Hall A, Ho R (2014). *Revision Notes in Psychiatry*. London: CRC Press, p. 354.

Question 7 Answer: b, Negative autoscopy

Explanation: In autoscopy, the person sees himself or herself and knows that it is him or her. Negative autoscopy occurs when the person looks into the mirror and cannot see one's image.

Reference: Puri BK, Hall A, Ho R (2014). *Revision Notes in Psychiatry*. London: CRC Press, p. 8.

Question 8 Answer: e, Family therapy

Explanation: Family therapy would be recommended in this case. External indicators for family therapy include the fact that John has just been recently diagnosed with an illness that has caused a significant change in his role within the family; internal indicators for family therapy include the fact that there are communication problems and triangulation within his existing family network. Family therapy, by introducing humour, demonstration of warmth and empathy and through role-playing, would help to modify both verbal and non-verbal communication.

Reference: Puri BK, Hall A, Ho R (2014). *Revision Notes in Psychiatry*. London: CRC Press, p. 343.

Question 9 Answer: e, Considering exploring potential nonconcordance to medications

Explanation: Patients with first-episode psychosis need to be treated with antipsychotics for a minimum duration of at least 6 months. One of the commonest reasons why antipsychotic treatment does not seem effective would be underlying nonconcordance. It would be beneficial to explore potential nonconcordance to medications prior to titrating the dose of the medications. Factors that could help to optimize patient compliance include education, setting reasonable expectations and using alternative medications if there are troublesome side effects.

Reference: Puri BK, Hall A, Ho R (2014). *Revision Notes in Psychiatry*. London: CRC Press, p. 240.

Question 10 Answer: c, Intravenous thiamine and vitamin B

Explanation: It is considered to be a medical emergency, and intravenous thiamine and vitamin B should be given. It should be treated early as 80% of untreated individuals would convert to Korsakov's psychosis if untreated.

Reference: Puri BK, Hall A, Ho R (2014). *Revision Notes in Psychiatry*. London: CRC Press, p. 517.

Question 11 Answer: d, Schizoaffective disorder

Explanation: Schizoaffective disorder is believed to be representative of this continuum. The ICD-10 describes these disorders in which both the affective and schizophrenia symptoms are prominent with the same episode of the illness, either simultaneously or within a few days of each other.

Reference: Puri BK, Hall A, Ho R (2014). *Revision Notes in Psychiatry*. London: CRC Press, p. 373.

Question 12 Answer: b, Views of reference groups usually do not play a role if the communicator is credible and has expertise.

Explanation: This is incorrect. Views of the reference groups are important for persuasive communication. In addition, it is important to note that mere repetition of a message in itself could have a persuasive influence leading to a change in the attitude. Also explicit messages are more persuasive, especially so for less intelligent recipient. Interactive personal discussions and one-sided communications tend to be more persuasive.

Reference: Puri BK, Hall A, Ho R (2014). *Revision Notes in Psychiatry*. London: CRC Press, p. 58.

Question 13 Answer: a, Amok

Explanation: Amok stands for battling furiously in Malay. Amok is a culture-specific syndrome of the Malay consisting of an explosive outburst of homicidal fury, vented indiscriminately against anyone who happens to cross his or her path. Once the episode is over, the person is amnesic for the episode and may commit suicide.

Reference and Further Readings: Campbell RJ (1996). *Psychiatric Dictionary*. Oxford, UK: Oxford University Press; Puri BK, Treasaden I (eds) (2010). *Psychiatry: An Evidence-Based Text*, London: Hodder Arnold, pp. 309–318.

Question 14 Answer: e, Agitation
Explanation: The normal stages of grief include denial, anger, bargaining, depression and acceptance. Other theories with regards to grief proposed that it has three core phases. The stunned phase usually last for a few hours to a few weeks. This would then give way to the mourning phase, with intense yearning and autonomic symptoms. After several weeks, the phase of acceptance and adjustments takes over. Grief usually lasts for about 6 months.

Reference: Puri BK, Hall A, Ho R (2014). *Revision Notes in Psychiatry*. London: CRC Press, p. 382.

Question 15 Answer: a, Full blood count
Explanation: Given that clozapine is started, it would be important to do a baseline full blood count (FBC) prior to the commencement of treatment. Based on the guidelines of the Clozapine Patient Management System, it is necessary for the patient to be registered and an initial FBC needs to be obtained. Clozapine needs to be started at 12.5 mg once a green blood result is issued by the CPMS.

Reference: Puri BK, Hall A, Ho R (2014). *Revision Notes in Psychiatry*. London: CRC Press, p. 368.

Question 16 Answer: a, Neologism
Explanation: Catatonic typically involves the presence of the aforementioned clinical features: ambitendency, automatic obedience, mitgehen, mannerism, negativism, echolalia, echopraxia, logorrhea, stereotypy, waxy flexibility and verbigeration. Neologism refers to how a new word is being constructed by the person or an everyday word being used in a special way.

Reference: Puri BK, Hall A, Ho R (2014). *Revision Notes in Psychiatry*. London: CRC Press, p. 371.

Question 17 Answer: b, Running commentary
Explanation: This is an example of a mood incongruent complex auditory hallucination. The voices might discuss the person in third place, perform a running commentary on a person's behaviour or even cause an individual to feel that his thoughts are spoken out loud.

Reference: Puri BK, Hall A, Ho R (2014). *Revision Notes in Psychiatry*. London: CRC Press, p. 7.

Question 18 Answer: a, Aversive conditioning

Explanation: Aversive conditioning helps decrease undesirable behaviour by making use of exposure to adverse stimuli while the person is engaging in a targeted behaviour. Escape conditioning, avoidance conditioning and punishments are known collectively as aversive conditioning.

Reference and Further Reading: Puri BK, Treasaden I (eds) (2010). *Psychiatry: An Evidence-Based Text*. London: Hodder Arnold, pp. 197–200.

Question 19 Answer: e, Lamotrigine

Explanation: Lamotrigine has been shown to be effective both as a treatment for bipolar depression and for preventing against further episodes. It has no tendency to induce switching or rapid cycling of the mood states. Previous research has shown that it is as effective as citalopram and it also causes less weight gain as compared to lithium. It is important to note that the main side effect is rash, which is usually associated with the speed of dose titration.

Reference: Taylor D, Paton C, Kapur S (2009). *The Maudsley Prescribing Guidelines* (10th edition). London: Informa Healthcare, p. 164.

Question 20 Answer: e, Catatonic schizophrenia

Explanation: The description is characteristic for catatonic schizophrenia. Catatonic schizophrenia, very often, may be associated with a dream-like state, along with vivid scenic hallucination. One or more of the following behaviours may dominate: stupor, excitement, posturing, negativism, rigidity, waxy flexibility, command automatism and perseveration of words or phrases.

Reference: Puri BK, Hall A, Ho R (2014). *Revision Notes in Psychiatry*. London: CRC Press, p. 354.

Question 21 Answer: a, Infarction of the anterior cerebral arteries

Explanation: This is likely to be due to an infarction involving the anterior cerebral artery. Physical examination might reveal distal and proximal weakness of both legs with impaired pin-prick sensation that spares the arms and the face.

Reference: Puri BK, Hall A, Ho R (2014). *Revision Notes in Psychiatry*. London: CRC Press, p. 494.

Question 22 Answer: d, 1 year

Explanation: The ICD-10 classification system states that the diagnosis of alcohol dependence would be made if there are three or more of the classical symptoms that have been present together at some time over the past 1 year.

Reference: Puri BK, Hall A, Ho R (2014). *Revision Notes in Psychiatry*. London: CRC Press, p. 508.

Question 23 Answer: d, Referent

Explanation: Referent social power refers to someone who is charismatic and is liked by others. Authority refers to power derived from the assignment of a role.

Reward refers to power derived from the ability to allocate resources. Coercive refers to having the power to punish. Expert refers to the power that is derived from skill, knowledge and also experience.

Reference: Puri BK, Hall A, Ho R (2014). *Revision Notes in Psychiatry*. London: CRC Press, p. 59.

Question 24 Answer: a, Splitting
Explanation: Splitting is the most common defence mechanism used. This involves dividing good objects, affects and memories from bad ones. It is often seen in patients with borderline personality disorder.

Reference: Puri BK, Hall A, Ho R (2014). *Revision Notes in Psychiatry*. London: CRC Press, p. 137.

Question 25 Answer: d, Reaction formation
Explanation: Patients with obsessive-compulsive disorder tend to make use of reaction formation. Reaction formation is defined as a psychological attitude that is diametrically opposed to an oppressed wish and constituting a reaction against it.

Reference: Puri BK, Hall A, Ho R (2014). *Revision Notes in Psychiatry*. London: CRC Press, p. 136.

Question 26 Answer: a, Benzodiazepines
Explanation: Benzodiazepines would be indicated for treatment. Intramuscular lorazepam up to 4 mg per day can be given to help with the symptoms. The other alternative treatment would be the use of electroconvulsive therapy. The common causes include schizophrenia, depression or manic (more common than schizophrenia), organic disorders, epilepsy, medications (such as ciprofloxacin), recreational drugs (cocaine), psychogenic catatonia and lethal catatonia.

Reference: Puri BK, Hall A, Ho R (2014). *Revision Notes in Psychiatry*. London: CRC Press, p. 371.

Question 27 Answer: b, Fixed interval schedule
Explanation: Fixed interval schedule has the lowest response rate and is poor at maintaining conditioned response. Fixed interval schedule is also associated with quick extinction. Response rate usually speeds up prior to the next reinforcement. There is a pause after each reinforcement which results in a scallop-shaped reinforcement curve.

Reference and Further Reading: Puri BK, Treasaden I (eds) (2010). *Psychiatry: An Evidence-Based Text*. London: Hodder Arnold, pp. 203–204.

Question 28 Answer: d, Voices telling them that they are useless
Explanation: A hallucination is a false sensory perception in the absence of a real external stimulus. A hallucination is perceived as being located in the objective

space and having almost the same realistic qualities as a normal perception. (d) refers to a mood congruent complex auditory hallucinations, which usually occurs in those with depressive disorder or mania.

Reference: Puri BK, Hall A, Ho R (2014). *Revision Notes in Psychiatry*. London: CRC Press, p. 7.

Question 29 Answer: b, Absence of isoenzyme aldehyde dehydrogenase
Explanation: The absence of aldehyde dehydrogenase would account for the differences in responses. Due to the absence, roughly half of Orientals would develop an unpleasant flushing response when alcohol is ingested, and this is related to the accumulation of acetaldehyde in the system. This intolerance of alcohol protects them from developing alcoholism, since it is much less prevalent in those of oriental heritage.

Reference: Puri BK, Hall A, Ho R (2014). *Revision Notes in Psychiatry*. London: CRC Press, p. 520.

Question 30 Answer: c, Antisocial personality disorder
Explanation: In malingering, the individual usually intentionally produces the physical or psychological symptoms and he or she is usually fully conscious of his or her underlying motives for doing so. Very often, there is a great resistance and reluctance to cooperate for further investigations and examination. There has been an association between malingering and antisocial personality disorder.

Reference: Puri BK, Hall A, Ho R (2014). *Revision Notes in Psychiatry*. London: CRC Press, p. 471.

Question 31 Answer: d, Assessment for lesions involving the central visual pathway
Explanation: This is essentially an assessment for lesions involving the central visual pathway. Candidates need to know the common lesions in the central visual pathway. Lesions in the optic nerve usually result in unilateral visual loss. Lesions at the optic chiasma at the base of the brain would result with bitemporal hemianopia. Lesions when the optic nerves decussate would result in incongruent homonymous hemianopia. Lesions in the Meyer's loop would be associated with superior homonymous quadrantanopia. Lesions in the optic rations are associated with inferior homonymous quadrantanopia.

Reference: Puri BK, Hall A, Ho R (2014). *Revision Notes in Psychiatry*. London: CRC Press, p. 159.

Question 32 Answer: b, This patient fulfils the DSM-IV-TR diagnostic criteria for brief psychotic disorder.
Explanation: The DSM-IV-TR criteria specify that the duration of a brief psychotic disorder is at least 1 day but less than 1 month. The ICD-10 criteria specify that the presentation of the fully developed acute and transient psychotic disorder should

not exceed 2 weeks. DSM-IV-TR further specifies that brief psychotic disorder may not include a symptom if it is culturally sanctioned response pattern.

References: American Psychiatric Association (2000). *Diagnostic Criteria from DSM-IV-TR*. Washington, DC: American Psychiatric Association; World Health Organisation (1994). ICD-10 Classification of Mental and Behavioural Disorders. Edinburgh, UK: Churchill Livingstone.

Question 33 Answer: a, Downward social comparison
Explanation: Based on the social comparison theory, people tend to evaluate their attitudes and abilities by comparing themselves with others. Downward social comparison involves comparing oneself to those who perform worse than themselves.

Reference: Aronson E, Wilson TD, Akert RM (2007). *Social Psychology*. Upper Saddle River, NJ: Prentice Hall, pp. 274–275.

Question 34 Answer: d, Motivational, emotional, perceptual and cognitive
Explanation: Attitude is an enduring organization of motivational, emotional, perceptual and cognitive processes with respect to some aspect of the individual world. Attitudes are largely based on beliefs, a tendency to behave in an observable way, and also have affective components that are the most resistant to change. A change in one of these three components leads to changes in the other two. When predicting behaviour, it is important that situational variables be taken into account. Otherwise, measured attitudes are deemed to be very poor predictors of behaviours.

Reference: Puri BK, Hall A, Ho R (2014). *Revision Notes in Psychiatry*. London: CRC Press, p. 57.

Question 35 Answer: e, Delusion of reference
Explanation: Delusion of reference refers to the fact that events, objects or even people in one's environment have a particular and unusual significance. A delusion in itself is a false belief based on incorrect inference about external reality and that is firmly sustained despite what almost everyone else believes and despite what constitutes incontrovertible and obvious proof or evidence to the contrary. The belief is not one ordinarily accepted by other members of the person's culture or subculture. When a false belief involves a value judgement, it is regarded as a delusion only when judgement is so extreme as to defy credibility.

Reference: Puri BK, Hall A, Ho R (2014). *Revision Notes in Psychiatry*. London: CRC Press, p. 6.

Question 36 Answer: d, Variable interval schedule
Explanation: Variable interval schedule is effective in maintaining conditioned response. Extinction occurs slowly and gradually.

Reference and Further Reading: Puri BK, Treasaden I (eds) (2010). *Psychiatry: An Evidence-Based Text*. London: Hodder Arnold, pp. 203–204.

Question 37 Answer: d, 2mg/day for haloperidol, 2 mg/day for risperidone, 5 mg/day for olanzapine, 75 mg/day for quetiapine, 60 mg/day for ziprasidone and 7.5 mg/day for aripiprazole

Explanation: Chlorpromazine 100 mg orally = 2 mg/day for haloperidol, 2 mg/day for risperidone, 5 mg/day for olanzapine, 75 mg/day for quetiapine, 60 mg/day for ziprasidone and 7.5 mg/day for aripiprazole.

Reference: Woods SW (2003). Chlorpromazine equivalent doses for the newer atypical antipsychotics. *J Clin Psychiatry*, 64(6):663–667.

Question 38 Answer: a, Being male

Explanation: All of the following are considered to be good prognostic factors, with the exception of gender. Those who are female are considered to have good prognosis. Other factors associated with good prognosis include having good premorbid social adjustment, having a family history of affective disorder and short duration of illness prior to treatment. Symptoms predictive of good prognosis include having an affective component to the illness, paranoid (as compared with non-paranoid), lack of negative symptoms and lack of cognitive impairments.

Reference: Puri BK, Hall A, Ho R (2014). *Revision Notes in Psychiatry*. London: CRC Press, p. 370.

Question 39 Answer: a, Frontal lobe

Explanation: It is very likely that Mr Smith has suffered an injury to his frontal lobe. Frontal lobe lesions are associated with personality changes, perseveration, utilization behaviour, impairments of attention, concentration and initiation and aphasia. The personality changes include disinhibition, reduced social and ethical control, sexual indiscretions, poor judgment, elevated mood and lack of concerns for the feelings of other people.

Reference: Puri BK, Hall A, Ho R (2014). *Revision Notes in Psychiatry*. London: CRC Press, p. 110.

Question 40 Answer: d, In the ICD-10, her condition is classified under schizophrenia.

Explanation: Based on the ICD-10, postpartum psychosis is classified under F.53 mental and behavioural disorders associated with the puerperium but not F.20 schizophrenia. In DSM-IV-TR, her diagnosis is classified under brief psychotic disorder with postpartum onset. Both DSM-IV-TR and ICD-10 do not have specific diagnostic criteria for postpartum psychosis.

References and Further Readings: American Psychiatric Association (2000). *Diagnostic Criteria from DSM-IV-TR*. Washington, DC: American Psychiatric Association; World Health Organisation (1994). ICD-10 Classification of Mental and Behavioural Disorders. Edinburgh, UK: Churchill Livingstone; Puri BK, Treasaden I (eds) (2010). *Psychiatry: An Evidence-Based Text*. London: Hodder Arnold, pp. 725–726.

Question 41 Answer: a, Selective/Focused attention
Explanation: This is an example of the cocktail party effect. Jane was making use of selective or focused attention. Selective or focused attention implies that one type of information is attended to, while additional distracting information is ignored. Dichotic listening studies have proved that whilst participants are attending to one channel of information, unattended channel is actually still active and being processed and individuals can switch rapidly if needed.

Reference: Puri BK, Hall A, Ho R (2014). *Revision Notes in Psychiatry*. London: CRC Press, p. 35.

Question 42 Answer: e, Weigl Colour–Form Sorting Test (WCFST)
Explanation: WCFST is a test mainly for executive function. AVLT is a 15-item five-trial test, from which recall (immediate and delayed) and recognition memory can be assessed. CVLT involves a list of 16 words. The list is repeated five times. Then, a second list is given, serving to interfere with the first list, after which recall of the first list is requested. RMT involves recognition of non-verbal material with interference from distracters after the first initial image is presented. The WMT assesses several memory components including concentration and summary indices that can be derived with a mean of 100. Tasks under WMT include assessment of logical memory (subjects are asked to recall the content of two stores read to them with a 30-minute delay); and a verbal paired associates test (learning word pairs, e.g. baby-cries, and to recall the second word when the first word is given).

Reference: Trimble M (2004). *Somatoform Disorders – A Medico-Legal Guide*. Cambridge, UK: Cambridge University Press.

Question 43 Answer: b, Countertransference
Explanation: The nurses exhibit countertransference because of previous unreasonable complaints.

Reference and Further Reading: Puri BK, Treasaden I (eds) (2010). *Psychiatry: An Evidence-Based Text*. London: Hodder Arnold, p. 948.

Question 44 Answer: b, Humour
Explanation: Immature defence mechanisms include denial, fantasy, projection, somatization, hypochondriasis, passive aggressive, acting out, idealization, projective identification and repression.

Reference and Further Reading: Puri BK, Treasaden I (eds) (2010). *Psychiatry: An Evidence-Based Text*. London: Hodder Arnold, p. 948.

Question 45 Answer: e, Severe depressive episode with psychotic features
Explanation: This man presents with nihilistic delusions and mood congruent auditory hallucinations. This suggests that he suffers from severe depressive episode with psychotic features.

Reference: World Health Organisation (1994). *ICD-10 Classification of Mental and Behavioural Disorders*. Edinburgh, UK: Churchill Livingstone.

Question 46 Answer: d, Doppelanger–Cotard's syndrome
Explanation: Doppelganger refers to a delusion that a double of a person or place exists somewhere else. Cotard syndrome refers to a delusion of death, disintegration of organs and nonexistence. Delusions of doubles refer to a delusion that a person known to the person has been replaced by a double. Delusion of infestation refers to a delusion that one is infested by parasites. Delusion of pregnancy refers to a delusion that one is pregnant (usually the husband of a pregnant wife).

Reference: Puri BK, Hall A, Ho R (2014). *Revision Notes in Psychiatry*. London: CRC Press, p. 6.

Question 47 Answer: e, Variable ratio schedule
Explanation: Variable ratio schedule has a quick and steep responding curve. This schedule shows the most resistance to extinction among all schedules.

Reference and Further Reading: Puri BK, Treasaden I (eds) (2010). *Psychiatry: An Evidence-Based Text*. London: Hodder Arnold, pp. 203–204.

Question 48 Answer: a, More patients taking second-generation antipsychotics continue the antipsychotic treatment compared with patients taking conventional antipsychotics.
Explanation: The majority of patients in both groups discontinued their assigned treatment owing to inefficacy or intolerable side effects or for other reasons. Quetiapine had the highest rate of discontinuation for any cause (82%) versus 79% for those on ziprasidone, 75% for those on perphenazine, 74% for those on risperidone and 64% for those on olanzapine. Discontinuation of the drug because of lack of efficacy was the highest among patients on quetiapine (28%) and lowest for those on olanzapine (15%); 19% of patients on olanzapine cited intolerability as the reason for stopping the drug, while intolerability caused 10% patients on risperidone to stop the drug. It was reported that 30% of olanzapine-treated patients gained more than 7% of their body weight during the study, which was significantly greater than weight gain with other study drugs. Predictors of an earlier time to drug discontinuation included higher PANSS score, younger age and long duration of antipsychotic use. CATIE involved 1493 patients with schizophrenia. They were randomly assigned to receive olanzapine (7.5–30 mg per day), perphenazine (8–32 mg per day), quetiapine (200–800 mg per day) or risperidone (1.5–6.0 mg per day) for up to 18 months.

Reference: Lieberman JA, Stroup TS, McEvoy JP (2005). Effectiveness of antipsychotic drugs in patients with chronic schizophrenia. *The New England Journal of Medicine*, 353: 1209–1223.

Question 49 Answer: c, Panic disorder

Explanation: Pitts and McClure (1967) provoked panic attacks in patients with anxiety neurosis through the usage of intravenous sodium lactate. However, it was found that there were no biochemical or neuroendocrine findings that explain lactate-induced panic.

Reference: Puri BK, Hall A, Ho R (2014). *Revision Notes in Psychiatry*. London: CRC Press, p. 414.

Question 50 Answer: b, Thurstone Scale – ranking is unbiased

Explanation: Option b is incorrect. The Thurstone Scale is a scale that indicates either agreement or disagreement with what is being presented. The disadvantages associated with this scale are that different response patterns may still result in the same mean score; the set-up is unwieldy, and the ranking may also be biased. The Likert Scale is a scale that indicates the level of agreement with varying options (five levels). The semantic differential scale is a bipolar visual analogue scale.

Reference: Puri BK, Hall A, Ho R (2014). *Revision Notes in Psychiatry*. London: CRC Press, p. 57.

Question 51 Answer: c, Ribot's law

Explanation: Théodule Ribot proposed that the dissolution of memory is inversely related to the recency of the event in 1881. This is known as Ribot's law and applies to the phenomenon when the recent memories are more likely to be lost as compared to the remote memories in retrograde amnesia. We have noted that not all patients suffering from retrograde amnesia follow Ribot's law. Gestalt's law is related to perception. Marr's law is related to visual perception and three-dimensional perception. Tarasoff's law is related to breach of confidentiality, and Weber–Fechner law is related to stimulus in perception.

Reference: Ribot T (1882). *Diseases of the Memory: An Essay in the Positive Psychology*. New York: D. Appleton and Company.

Question 52 Answer: a, Utilitarian

Explanation: Utilitarian theories emphasize on minimizing the risks and maximizing the benefits for the greatest number. There are two types of this approach: act utilitarian and also rule utilitarian. For example, a patient has thoughts of harming his or her family. In act utilitarian, the psychiatrist may consider disclosing confidential information to his or her family or police by providing good or avoiding harm to the greatest number who stay with him or her or near him or her. In rule utilitarian, the rule of confidentiality may act against the rule of protecting others.

Reference: Puri BK, Hall A, Ho R (2014). *Revision Notes in Psychiatry*. London: CRC Press, p. 145.

Question 53 Answer: e, A doctor's native motive to provide morally correct care to his or her patients, and focus solely on the rightness and wrongness of the action themselves, and not on the consequences of the action.

Explanation: The deontological theories emphasize on a doctor's motive to provide morally correct care to his or her patients. They focus solely on the rightness and wrongness of the doctor's actions and not on the consequences of the actions themselves.

Reference: Puri BK, Hall A, Ho R (2014). *Revision Notes in Psychiatry*. London: CRC Press, p. 146.

Question 54 Answer: b, The minimum duration of delusions is 6 months.

Explanation: The minimum duration is 3 months. Bizarre delusions are not associated with delusional disorders but correspond to the first-rank symptoms of schizophrenia.

Reference and Further Readings: World Health Organisation (1992). *ICD-10: The ICD-10 Classification of Mental and Behavioural Disorders: Clinical Descriptions and Diagnostic Guidelines*. Geneva: World Health Organisation; Puri BK, Treasaden I (eds) (2010). *Psychiatry: An Evidence-Based Text*. London: Hodder Arnold, p. 677.

Question 55 Answer: e, Narcissistic

Explanation: This man suffers from narcissistic personality disorder which is characterised by sense of entitlement and importance.

Reference and Further Reading: Puri BK, Treasaden I (eds) 2010. *Psychiatry: An Evidence-Based Text*. London: Hodder Arnold, pp. 690, 705, 706, 839.

Question 56 Answer: d, Mannerism

Explanation: The psychopathology being referred to here is that of mannerism. Mannerism refers to repeated involuntary movements that appear to be goal directed. Automatic obedience refers to a condition where the person follows the examiner's instructions blindly without judgement and resistance. For example, the examiner might ask the person to move his or her arm in different directions and the person is unable to resist even if it is against his or her will.

Reference: Puri BK, Hall A, Ho R (2014). *Revision Notes in Psychiatry*. London: CRC Press, p. 2.

Question 57 Answer: a, Amisulpride

Explanation: Amisulpride appears not to elevate plasma glucose and seems not to be associated with diabetes. Chlorpromazine, clozapine, risperidone and quetiapine have not been associated with impaired glucose tolerance and diabetes.

Reference and Further Readings: Taylor D, Paton C, Kapur S (2009). *The Maudsley Prescribing Guidelines*. London: Informa Healthcare; Puri BK, Treasaden I (eds) (2010). *Psychiatry: An Evidenced-Based Text*. London: Hodder Arnold, pp. 425–427, 603.

Question 58 Answer: e, Challenging negative automatic thoughts
Explanation: All of the aforementioned options are methodologies, except (e), that could help to achieve cognitive consistency when dissonance is experienced. Hence, in summary, when cognitive dissonance occurs, the individual feels uncomfortable, may experience increased arousal, and is motivated to achieve cognitive consistency. This may occur by changing one or more of the cognitions involved in the dissonant relationship, changing the behaviour that is inconsistent with the cognition or adding new cognitions that are consonant with the pre-existing ones. Cognitive consistency can also be achieved when attitude and behaviour are inconsistent by altering attitude.

Reference: Puri BK, Hall A, Ho R (2014). *Revision Notes in Psychiatry*. London: CRC Press, p. 58.

Question 59 Answer: d, Autonomy
Explanation: This is an example of autonomy. Autonomy refers to the obligation of the doctor to respect his or her patients' rights to make their own choices in accordance to their beliefs and wishes. Non-maleficence refers to the obligation of a doctor to avoid harm to his or her patients. Beneficence refers to the commitment of a doctor to provide benefits to patients and balance benefits against risks when making such decisions.

Reference: Puri BK, Hall A, Ho R (2014). *Revision Notes in Psychiatry*. London: CRC Press, p. 146.

Question 60 Answer: c, She wants to be in a depressive state because her husband gives her more support when she is sick.
Explanation: The patient has an obligation to get well. The others are criteria that a person has to fulfil for Parsons' sick role.

Further Reading: Puri BK, Treasaden I (eds) (2010). *Psychiatry: An Evidence-Based Text*. London: Hodder Arnold, p. 299, 682.

Question 61 Answer: c, He was penalized by the HM Revenue & Customs for delay in filling up the income tax form because he could not make up his mind what to report and feared making mistakes.
Explanation: Patients with anankastic personality disorder have difficulty to make day-to-day decisions because they fear making mistakes.

Reference and Further Reading: Puri BK, Treasaden I (eds) (2010). *Psychiatry: An Evidence-Based Text*. London: Hodder Arnold, p. 657.

Question 62 Answer: c, It means that a normal perception has taken on a delusional significance.

Explanation: A delusional perception means that a normal perception has now taken on a delusional significance. A delusion in itself is a false belief based on incorrect inference about external reality and that is firmly sustained despite what almost everyone else believes and despite what constitutes incontrovertible and obvious proof or evidence to the contrary. The belief is not one ordinarily accepted by other members of the person's culture or subculture. When a false belief involves a value judgement, it is regarded as a delusion only when judgement is so extreme as to defy credibility.

Reference: Puri BK, Hall A, Ho R (2014). *Revision Notes in Psychiatry*. London: CRC Press, p. 6.

Question 63 Answer: a, Cognitive learning

Explanation: Cognitive learning is the acquisition of knowledge through the formation of cognitive or mental maps. Cognitive learning can occur via latent learning and insight learning. This form of learning shows that learning can occur in the absence of a reward.

Reference and Further Reading: Puri BK, Treasaden I (eds) (2010). *Psychiatry: An Evidence-Based Text*. London: Hodder Arnold, pp. 207–208.

Question 64 Answer: a, Akathisia

Explanation: Akathisia is the most common (25%), followed by pseudo-parkinsonism (20%), acute dystonia (10%) and tardive dyskinesia (5%). Galactorrhoea is not an extrapyramidal side effect.

Reference and Further Reading: Puri BK, Treasaden I (eds) (2010). *Psychiatry: An Evidence-Based Text*. London: Hodder Arnold, pp. 901, 903.

Question 65 Answer: a, Anankastic personality

Explanation: According to the ICD-10 criteria, anankastic personality disorder is characterized by (a) feelings of excessive doubt and caution, (b) preoccupation with details, rules, order and organization on schedule, (c) perfectionism that interferes with task completion, (d) pleasure and interpersonal relationships, (e) excessive pedantry and adherence to social conversations, (f) rigidity and stubbornness, (g) unreasonable insistence by the patient that others submit to exactly her way of dealing things, or unreasonable reluctance to allow others to do things and (h) intrusion of insistent and unwelcome thoughts or impulses.

Reference and Further Readings: World Health Organisation (1994). *ICD-10 Classification of Mental and Behavioural Disorders*. Edinburgh, UK: Churchill Livingstone; Puri BK, Treasaden I (eds) (2010). *Psychiatry: An Evidence-Based Text*. London: Hodder Arnold, p. 657.

Question 66 Answer: c, Identity
Explanation: The teenager would be negotiating the identity stage based on Erikson's stages of development model. The age and the corresponding stage that an individual is undergoing are listed as follows: 0–1 (trust/security); 1–4 (autonomy); 4–5 (initiative); 5–11 (duty/accomplishment); 11–15 (identity); 15: adult (intimacy), adulthood (generativity), maturity (integrity).

Reference: Puri BK, Hall A, Ho R (2014). *Revision Notes in Psychiatry*. London: CRC Press, p. 48.

Question 67 Answer: c, Bystander effect
Explanation: Bystander effect is the phenomenon where individuals are less likely to extend help during an emergency when in the presence of others. The most classic example is the murder of Kitty Genovese, during which none of her neighbours called the police despite hearing her cries.

Reference and Further Readings: Puri BK, Treasaden I (eds) (2010). *Psychiatry: An Evidence-Based Text*. London: Hodder Arnold, pp. 290–291; Darley JM, Latané B (1968). Bystander intervention in emergencies: Diffusion of responsibility. *Journal of Personality and Social Psychology*, 8: 377–383.

Question 68 Answer: b, Reflective listening
Explanation: This is an example of reflection and reflective listening. Reflective listening entails repeating the patient's own accounts by paraphrasing and using words that add meaning to what the client has just mentioned.

Reference: Puri BK, Hall A, Ho R (2014). *Revision Notes in Psychiatry*. London: CRC Press, p. 332.

Question 69 Answer: e, Thought withdrawal
Explanation: The presence of thought withdrawal would be of tremendous help in arriving at the diagnosis of schizophrenia. It is part of the first-rank symptoms. The following are first-rank symptoms: auditory hallucinations that either repeat the thoughts out loud, in the third person or performing a running commentary; delusions of passivity which include thought insertion, withdrawal and broadcasting; and somatic passivity and delusional perception.

Reference: Puri BK, Hall A, Ho R (2014). *Revision Notes in Psychiatry*. London: CRC Press, p. 351.

Question 70 Answer: c, Sedation
Explanation: Sedation is the most common side effect, and hypersalivation is the second most common side effect.

Reference and Further Reading: Puri BK, Treasaden I (eds) (2010). *Psychiatry: An Evidence-Based Text*. London: Hodder Arnold, pp. 425–427, 603.

Question 71 Answer: b, Left VI nerve palsy
Explanation: This patient presents with left rectus palsy and horizontal diplopia. This indicates left VI nerve palsy.

Reference and Further Readings: Ward N, Frith P, Lipsedge M (2001). *Medical Masterclass Neurology, Ophthalmology and Psychiatry*. London: Royal College of Physicians; Puri BK, Treasaden I (eds) (2010). *Psychiatry: An Evidence-Based Text*. London: Hodder Arnold, pp. 336–338, 351, 525–527.

Question 72 Answer: d, Cognitive estimates
Explanation: Assessment of the dominant parietal lobe involves the following: finger agnosia (inability to recognize the name of the finger), left and right orientation (inability to recognize left and right), acalculia (inability to recognize number and calculation), dysgraphia, asteroagnosia (inability to recognize the size, shape and texture of an object by palpation), dysgraphesthesia (inability to recognize letters or numbers written on the hand), ideomotor apraxia, Wernicke's or Broca's aphasia as well as impairment of two-point discrimination. Assessment of non-dominant parietal lobe involves asomatognosia (lack of awareness of the condition of all or parts of the body) and constructional dyspraxia (inability to copy double interlocking pentagons). Cognitive estimates is not a test of parietal lobe functioning.

Reference: Puri BK, Hall A, Ho R (2014). *Revision Notes in Psychiatry*. London: CRC Press, p. 114.

Question 73 Answer: e, The person is totally losing touch with reality.
Explanation: Most serious violence is associated with retained ability to plan and reality testing. People with paranoid schizophrenia staying in the community pose higher risk of violence compared to those who are more ill and stay in the hospitals.

Reference and Further Reading: Puri BK, Treasaden I (eds) (2010). *Psychiatry: An Evidence-Based Text*. London: Hodder Arnold, pp. 598, 1175, 1241.

Question 74 Answer: a, He experiences hallucinations causing positive emotions.
Explanation: Hallucinations causing negative emotions such as anger, anxiety or sadness generate more violence. Options B, C and D refer to 'threat/control-override' delusions which appear most risky. Option D is correct because depression is associated with violence.

Reference and Further Reading: Puri BK, Treasaden I (eds) (2010). *Psychiatry: An Evidence-Based Text*. London: Hodder Arnold, p. 1175.

Question 75 Answer: b, Anxious avoidant personality
Explanation: This man needs to use alcohol to calm his nerves and he develops alcohol-dependence syndrome. Hence, anxious personality disorder is the most

likely in this case and this personality disorder can be a maintaining factor in the alcohol dependence.

Reference and Further Reading: Puri BK, Treasaden I (eds) (2010). *Psychiatry: An Evidence-Based Text*. London: Hodder Arnold, p. 653.

Question 76 Answer: e, Perseveration
Explanation: All of the aforementioned options are considered to be part of formal thought disorders, with the exception of (e). Asyndesis refers to the juxtaposition of elements without adequate linkage between them. Condensation refers to combining ideas to make the incomprehensible. Derailment refers to how the thought processes are being derailed into a subsidiary thought. Fusion refers to how different elements of the thought are being interwoven with each other. Other features of formal thought disorder include omission and substitution.

Reference: Puri BK, Hall A, Ho R (2014). *Revision Notes in Psychiatry*. London: CRC Press, p. 4.

Question 77 Answer: e, Extinction
Explanation: Extinction refers to the gradual disappearance of a conditioned response (avoidance of going out of the house). This is achieved when the conditioned stimulus (in this case going out of the house) is repeatedly presented without the unconditioned stimulus.

Reference: Puri BK, Hall A, Ho R (2014). *Revision Notes in Psychiatry*. London: CRC Press, p. 25.

Question 78 Answer: a, Aripiprazole
Explanation: The other antipsychotics may produce weight gain.

Further Reading: Puri BK, Treasaden I (eds) (2010). *Psychiatry: An Evidence-Based Text*. London: Hodder Arnold, pp. 425–426, 604, 904.

Question 79 Answer: c, 4 months
Explanation: Accommodation and colour vision take place only at the age of 4 months. At birth, newborns have the ability to distinguish between brightness and also have eye tracking. However, visual acuity is impaired and focusing is typically fixed at 0.2 m. At the age of 2 months, newborns develop depth perception. At the age of 6 months, they would be able to achieve 6:6 visual acuity.

Reference: Puri BK, Hall A, Ho R (2014). *Revision Notes in Psychiatry*. London: CRC Press, p. 33.

Question 80 Answer: e, The standard schema of psychiatric history taking is a good guide to the structure of the psychiatric interview.
Explanation: The standard schema of psychiatric history taking is not a good guide to the structure of the psychiatric interview because it is too rigid. Option A

is correct because assessment proforma signifies the reduction of patient's life to an administrative purpose. Options B and C are correct for obvious reasons. Option D is correct because history taking is an active process which involves understanding and organizing information.

Reference: Poole R, Higgo R (2006). *Psychiatric Interviewing and Assessment.* Cambridge, UK: Cambridge University Press.

Question 81 Answer: b, Parietal lobe
Explanation: This is an assessment of the non-dominant parietal lobe functions. When there is a lesion involving the non-dominant parietal lobe, this would result in constructional dyspraxia, which refers to the inability to copy double interlocking pentagons. Lesions involving the dominant parietal lobe would result in Gerstmann's syndrome, asteroagnosis, dysgraphesthesia, ideomotor apraxia, Wernicke's or Broca's aphasia and impairment in two-point discrimination.

Reference: Puri BK, Hall A, Ho R (2014). *Revision Notes in Psychiatry*. London: CRC Press, p. 114.

Question 82 Answer: e, Right III nerve palsy
Explanation: In right III nerve palsy, there is usually ptosis. The pupil may be dilated and completely nonreactive. The eye is abducted (by the lateral rectus muscle), depressed and looking down and out (by the superior oblique muscle).

References and Further Readings: Malhi GS, Matharu MS, Hale AS (2000) *Neurology for Psychiatrists*. London: Martin Dunitz; Ward N, Frith P, Lipsedge M (2001). *Medical Masterclass Neurology, Ophthalmology and Psychiatry*. London: Royal College of Physicians; Puri BK, Treasaden I (eds) (2010). *Psychiatry: An Evidence-Based Text*. London: Hodder Arnold, pp. 336–338, 351, 525–527.

Question 83 Answer: c, Alcohol-dependent syndrome
Explanation: This is another version of the MCQ which tries to confuse candidates between the concept of alcohol dependence and personality disorders. The man suffers from alcohol dependence syndrome based on the CAGE questionnaire. There is not enough information from this vignette to suggest that he suffers from other psychiatric disorders.

Reference and Further Reading: Puri BK, Treasaden I (eds) (2010). *Psychiatry: An Evidence-Based Text*. London: Hodder Arnold, pp. 782, 1026–1027.

Question 84 Answer: b, Delusional perception is a secondary delusion.
Explanation: Delusional perception is a primary delusion and not a secondary delusion. It is a delusion that arises fully formed, without any discernible connection with previous events. It may be preceded by a delusional mood in which the person is aware of something strange and threatening happening.

Reference: Puri BK, Hall A, Ho R (2014). *Revision Notes in Psychiatry*. London: CRC Press, p. 6.

Question 85 Answer: a, Conditioned response
Explanation: In this experiment, drug A is an unconditioned stimulus and drug B is an unconditioned stimulus. The conditioned response is tachycardia associated with drug B.

Reference and Further Reading: Puri BK, Treasaden I (eds) (2010). *Psychiatry: An Evidence-Based Text*. London: Hodder Arnold, pp. 197–200.

Question 86 Answer: d, Fluoxetine
Explanation: SSRI seems to be the safest option in view of the potential risk of epilepsy.

Reference: Taylor D, Paton C, Kapur S (2009). *The Maudsley Prescribing Guidelines*. London: Informa Healthcare.

Question 87 Answer: a, John Cade
Explanation: John Cade was the one who discovered the properties of lithium. He injected guinea pigs with urine from patients with mania to see if mania was caused by a toxic product. Lithium was used to dissolve the uric acid prior to injection. Guinea pigs injected with lithium were noted to be more stable in mood. Hence, in the late 1940s, Cade decided to inject manic patients with lithium.

Reference: Puri BK, Hall A, Ho R (2014). *Revision Notes in Psychiatry*. London: CRC Press, p. 142.

Question 88 Answer: b, Viktor Frankl
Explanation: Victor Frankl was the one who developed existential therapy.

Reference: Puri BK, Hall A, Ho R (2014). *Revision Notes in Psychiatry*. London: CRC Press, p. 142.

Question 89 Answer: c, En bloc blackouts
Explanation: This is a description of an en bloc blackout. It should be noted that if the memory disturbances carry on for days, it is highly likely that the subject would experience what is deemed as a fugue state, in which he or she may travel some distance before coming around, with no memory of the events occurring during this time.

Reference: Puri BK, Hall A, Ho R (2014). *Revision Notes in Psychiatry*. London: CRC Press, p. 516.

Question 90 Answer: c, IV nerve palsy
Explanation: The common cause of isolated vertical diplopia is superior oblique palsy. This indicates fourth nerve palsy.

Reference and Further Readings: Ward N, Frith P, Lipsedge M (2001). *Medical Masterclass Neurology, Ophthalmology and Psychiatry*. London: Royal College of Physicians; Puri BK, Treasaden I (eds) (2010). *Psychiatry: An Evidence-Based Text*. London: Hodder Arnold, pp. 336–338, 351, 525–527.

Question 91 Answer: a, Lilliputian hallucination

Explanation: Mr Green is experiencing what is commonly termed as lilliputian hallucination. Hallucinated objects tend to appear greatly reduced in size. Reflex hallucination refers to how a stimulus in one sensory field might lead to a stimulus in another sensory field. In contrast, a functional hallucination refers to a stimulus causing the hallucination is being experienced in addition to the hallucination itself.

Reference: Puri BK, Hall A, Ho R (2014). *Revision Notes in Psychiatry*. London: CRC Press, p. 8.

Question 92 Answer: b, Negative reinforcement

Explanation: In negative reinforcement, an unpleasant stimulus (i.e. withdrawal symptoms) is removed, hence resulting in a strengthening of the behaviour (i.e. drug use).

Reference and Further Reading: Puri BK, Treasaden I (eds) (2010). *Psychiatry: An Evidence-Based Text*. London: Hodder Arnold, pp. 200–205.

Question 93 Answer: e, Rigidity

Explanation: Almost all patients would have fever; 90% present with rigidity and 75% present with altered mental state. Hence, rigidity is the most common sign among the options.

Further Reading: Puri BK, Treasaden I (eds) (2010). *Psychiatry: An Evidence-Based Text*. London: Hodder Arnold, pp. 874, 925.

Question 94 Answer: d, Concrete operational

Explanation: Piaget's model of cognitive development has four main stages, which include sensorimotor, preoperational, concrete operational and formal operational. The concrete operational stage is the third stage of development and this usually occurs from the age of 7 to around 12–14 years of age. It is thought that during this particular stage of development, the child would demonstrate logical thought processes and would be able to make more subjective moral judgements. During this stage, there will be an understanding of the laws of conservation of the number and volume and, in the later stages, the concept of weight.

Reference: Puri BK, Hall A, Ho R (2014). *Revision Notes in Psychiatry*. London: CRC Press, p. 68.

Question 95 Answer: d, Myasthenia gravis
Explanation: The severity of symptoms in myasthenia gravis fluctuates during the day, being less severe in the morning and more severe at the day goes on. Myasthenia gravis is associated with other weaknesses such as dysphagia, slurred speech, shortness of breath or limb weakness.

Reference and Further Readings: Ward N, Frith P, Lipsedge M (2001). *Medical Masterclass Neurology, Ophthalmology and Psychiatry*. London: Royal College of Physicians; Puri BK, Treasaden I (eds) (2010). *Psychiatry: An Evidence-Based Text*. London: Hodder Arnold, pp. 533–534.

Question 96 Answer: c, Delusion of guilt
Explanation: Delusion of guilt is the false belief of guilt. Such beliefs may dominate the patient's thoughts and are common in depression. An example of delusion of guilt is the false belief that one committed a crime and needs to be punished. There is usually no logical connection between the situation and the guilt feelings the person perceives.

Reference and Further Reading: Sims A (2003). *Symptoms of the Mind: An Introduction to Descriptive Psychopathology*. London: Saunders, p. 137.

Question 97 Answer: d, Positive reinforcement
Explanation: Positive reinforcement is the strengthening of a response by the addition of a pleasurable stimulus.

Reference and Further Reading: Puri BK, Treasaden I (eds) (2010). *Psychiatry: An Evidence-Based Text*. London: Hodder Arnold, pp. 200–205.

Question 98 Answer: d, 13 years old
Explanation: The onset of puberty in girls would be between 9 and 13 years in 95% of the sample population. The very initial signs include breast formation and also pubic hair growth. The average age of onset in the Western countries has been estimated to be around 13.5 years. For boys, in 95% of them, the onset usually occurs between the ages of 9.5 to 13.5 years. The initial signs include testicular and scrotal enlargement. This is in turn followed by the growth of the penis and also the pubic hair. On average, the mean age of onset is around 13 years.

Reference: Puri BK, Hall A, Ho R (2014). *Revision Notes in Psychiatry*. London: CRC Press, p. 71.

Question 99 Answer: e, Mutual attraction
Explanation: Mutual attraction is a factor that predisposes interpersonal attraction but not a theory. Proxemics relates interpersonal attraction to interpersonal space. Social exchange theory suggests that people prefer relationships that offer optimal cost–benefit ratio. Equity theory states that

preferred relationships are those in which there is equal cost and benefits for both parties. Reinforcement theory states that rewards for both parties reciprocally reinforce interpersonal attraction.

Reference and Further Reading: Puri BK, Hall AD (2002). *Revision Notes in Psychiatry*. London: Arnold, pp. 53–54.

Question 100 Answer: b, The winter excess of births in schizophrenics is due to a seasonal prevalence of a viral infection or other perinatal hazard.

Explanation: Only (b) is correct. Afro-Caribbean immigrants to the United Kingdom would have a higher risk of schizophrenia due to the interaction of multiple factors. Males usually have an earlier onset of schizophrenia as compared to females. Those living in higher EE families tend to have an increased relapse rate of schizophrenia. More obstetric complications are suggested for those with schizophrenia.

Reference: Puri BK, Hall A, Ho R (2014). *Revision Notes in Psychiatry*. London: CRC Press, p. 360.

Question 101 Answer: e, Serotonin transporter gene

Explanation: The serotonin transporter gene is implicated in the aetiology of depressive disorder.

Reference and Further Reading: Puri BK, Treasaden I (eds) (2010). *Psychiatry: An Evidence-Based Text*. London: Hodder Arnold, pp. 476–477, 610–611.

Question 102 Answer: a, State-dependent memory

Explanation: The terminology that would best describe the aforementioned would be state-dependent memory loss. State-dependent memory loss means that memory of events occurring while intoxicated is lost when sober but returns on next intoxication. In fragmentary blackouts, there is no clear demarcation of the memory loss, and islets of memory exist within the gaps. Some recovery occurs with time. In en bloc blackouts, there is a clearly demarcated total memory loss, with no recovery of the lost memory over time.

Reference: Puri BK, Hall A, Ho R (2014). *Revision Notes in Psychiatry*. London: CRC Press, p. 516.

Question 103 Answer: d, Deindividuation

Explanation: Deindividuation is the loosening of social constraints or norms when in a group. This leads to an increase in deviant behaviour, as individuals feel less accountable for their actions when they are carried out as a group. This is because, in a group, it is more difficult to identify and blame an individual. Deindividuation also increases an individual's obedience to group norms. Hence, if an individual is in a group riot where the norm is violence, deindividuation will make the individual act violently.

Social facilitation is the tendency to do better on simple tasks in the presence of other people. Social loafing is the tendency to do worse on a task when working in a group and when performance cannot be evaluated. Social norms are behaviours that are acceptable in a society or group. Social tuning is the process whereby people adopt another person's attitudes.

Reference and Further Reading: Aronson E, Wilson TD, Akert RM (2007). *Social Psychology*. Upper Saddle River, NJ: Prentice Hall, pp. 150–151, 277–286.

Question 104 Answer: c, 3–6 years
Explanation: A child starts to have early comprehension of grammar at the age 6–9 years. Between the ages of 1 and 2 years, the child can master 3 words at 12 months to 40 words at 18 months. Between 2 and 3 years, the child is at two-word stage characterized by telegraphic grammar. Between 6 and 12 years, the speech ability of a child is similar to an adult.

Reference and Further Reading: Puri BK, Hall AD (2002). *Revision Notes in Psychiatry*. London: Arnold, p. 72.

Question 105 Answer: d, Horner's syndrome
Explanation: The triad of Horner's syndrome is classically described as miosis, ipsilateral partial ptosis and sometimes anhidrosis. If anhidrosis affects the entire half of the body and face, the lesion is in the central nervous system. If it affects only the face and neck, the lesion is in the preganglionic fibres. If sweating is unaffected, the lesion is above the carotid artery bifurcation.

Reference and Further Readings: Ward N, Frith P, Lipsedge M (2001). *Medical Masterclass Neurology, Ophthalmology and Psychiatry*. London: Royal College of Physicians; Puri BK, Treasaden I (eds) (2010). *Psychiatry: An Evidence-Based Text*. London: Hodder Arnold, pp. 526, 531.

Question 106 Answer: c, Thought blocking
Explanation: Passivity phenomenon is a delusional belief that one's free will has been removed and the self is being controlled by an outside agency. Examples of passivity phenomena are thought alienation (person believes his or her thoughts are controlled by an external agency: thought insertion, thought withdrawal, thought broadcasting), made feelings (person believes his or her feelings are controlled by an external agency), made impulses, made actions and somatic passivity (the delusional belief that one is passively receiving bodily sensations from an external agency).

Reference and Further Reading: Puri BK, Hall AD (2002). *Revision Notes in Psychiatry*. London: Arnold, p. 153.

Question 107 Answer: e, Punishment
Explanation: This phenomenon is known as punishment, which is any stimulus that is applied after a response and causes a weakening of that behaviour.

Punishment is the opposite of reinforcement (both positive and negative). Reinforcement causes a strengthening of the behaviour, whereas punishment suppresses it.

Reference and Further Reading: Puri BK, Treasaden I (eds) (2010). *Psychiatry: An Evidence-Based Text*. London: Hodder Arnold, p. 205.

Question 108 Answer: d, Parkinsonism
Explanation: Option (c) is a side effect of lithium and option (a) occurs in lithium toxicity. Options (b) and (e) are cerebellar signs.

Further Reading: Puri BK, Treasaden I (eds) (2010). *Psychiatry: An Evidence-Based Text*. London: Hodder Arnold, pp. 541–543.

Question 109 Answer: a, Dichotic listening studies test for selective attention
Explanation: The various types of attention include selective attention, divided attention and sustained attention. For divided attention, performance is impaired. In dichotic listening, studies in which subjects attend to one channel, evidence indicates that the unattended channel is still being processed and the listener can switch rapidly if appropriate.

Reference: Puri BK, Hall A, Ho R (2014). *Revision Notes in Psychiatry*. London: CRC Press, p. 35.

Question 110 Answer: e, Telegraphic speech
Explanation: Telegraphic speech is defined as short two- or three-word sentences using nouns, verbs and adjectives, with some basic form of grammar. An example is 'daddy go', which might represent the child's father going out of the house. This occurs between 19 and 36 months.

Cooing and babbling occur before the age of 1 year. Grammatical morphemes are acquired from 3 to 5 years of age. Morphemes are the smallest units of meaning within a language. Grammatical morphemes or bound morphemes have no meaning in itself but are attached to free morphemes to change its grammatical function. Examples are plurals '-s' and past tense '-ed'. A 2-year-old child should have a vocabulary of around 50–300 words.

Reference and Further Readings: Puri BK, Hall AD (2002). *Revision Notes in Psychiatry*. London: Arnold, p. 72; Puri BK, Treasaden I (eds) (2010). *Psychiatry: An Evidence-Based Text*. London: Hodder Arnold, pp. 115–116.

Question 111 Answer: b, egosyntonic
Explanation: Autochthonous delusions (primary delusions) are egosyntonic and refer to the acceptability of ideas or impulses to the ego, which receives the impulses as constant and compatible with one's own principles. Egodystonic refers to a phenomenon (e.g. obsession) which is unacceptable to the ego and prevented from reaching the ego (e.g. compulsion). Secondary delusions are secondary to

hallucinations. Shared delusions (e.g. folie a deux) are shared with a partner. Primary delusions (e.g. delusional perception and delusional memory) do not start with an idea.

Reference and Further Reading: Campbell RJ (1996). *Psychiatric Dictionary.* Oxford, UK: Oxford University Press.

Question 112 Answer: a, Frontal lobe syndrome
Explanation: This was the earliest case that was described. Phineas Gage suffered from a frontal lobe lesion in 1835, and it was documented that he had changes to his personality, but not his memory or intelligence.

Reference: Puri BK, Hall A, Ho R (2014). *Revision Notes in Psychiatry.* London: CRC Press, p. 109.

Question 113 Answer: d, Upbringing in an authoritarian family setting
Explanation: Parents using authoritarian child-rearing style are high in coercive control and low in warmth, acceptance and autonomy granting. Such parents often criticize, command and threaten to exert control, and use force, punishment or withdrawal of love (psychological control) to ensure compliance to their wishes. These parents make decisions on behalf of their children and their points of view are disregarded. Children brought up in authoritarian family settings are often unhappy and anxious, have low self-esteem and self-reliance, and have a tendency to be hostile when frustrated.

Reference and Further Reading: Berk LE (2006). *Child Development* (7th edition). Boston: Pearson, pp. 564–566.

Question 114 Answer: a, NMS presents within 48 hours after the initiation of a new antipsychotic.
Explanation: NMS can occur at any time during the course of antipsychotic treatment.

Further Reading: Puri BK, Treasaden I (eds) (2010). *Psychiatry: An Evidence-Based Text.* London: Hodder Arnold, pp. 874, 925.

Question 115 Answer: c, Fixed ratio schedule
Explanation: In fixed ratio schedule, there is a pause after each reinforcement. There is a high rate of responding leading to the next reinforcement shortly afterwards. Extinction occurs quickly in fixed ratio schedule.

Reference and Further Reading: Puri BK, Treasaden I (eds) (2010). *Psychiatry: An Evidence-Based Text.* London: Hodder Arnold, pp. 203–204.

Question 116 Answer: a, a misidentification phenomenon
Explanation: Misidentification syndrome refers to Capgras and Fregoli syndrome. Morbid jealousy is a delusional disorder that the marital or sexual partner is

unfaithful, typically accompanied by intense searching for evidence of infidelity and repeated interrogations and direct accusations of the partner that may lead to violent quarrels. Morbid jealousy is more common in men than in women. Morbid jealousy is associated with erectile dysfunction and alcohol misuse.

Reference and Further Reading: Campbell RJ (1996). *Psychiatric Dictionary*. Oxford, UK: Oxford University Press.

Question 117 Answer: a, Low-dose aspirin
Explanation: The NICE guidelines do not recommend the use of anti-dementia drugs in the prevention of cognitive decline. The guidelines recommend that it is worthwhile to try to treat the underlying condition in order to slow or halt the progression of vascular dementia.

Reference: Puri BK, Hall A, Ho R (2014). *Revision Notes in Psychiatry*. London: CRC Press, p. 700.

Question 118 Answer: a, High level of education
Explanation: Protective factors for Alzheimer's dementia include being bilingual, cognitive engagement and late retirement. High level of education of more than 15 years and high level of physical activities are also protective factors.

Reference: Puri BK, Hall A, Ho R (2014). *Revision Notes in Psychiatry*. London: CRC Press, p. 694.

Question 119 Answer: e, Measuring intelligence at regular intervals from children to adolescence
Explanation: Measuring intelligence at regular intervals does not offer primary prevention of any psychiatric illness among children and adolescents. Option (b) works by focusing on children with one or two schizophrenic parents, children of alcohol and drug addicts or those experiencing the death of a parent. Option (c) refers to prevention of poisoning of lead-based plants, neurosyphilis, school phobias in children or addictive behaviour patterns in adolescents.

Reference: Paykel ES, Jenkins R (1994). *Prevention in Psychiatry*. London: Gaskell.

Extended matching items (EMIs)

Theme: Attention
Question 120 Answer: b, Divided attention
Explanation: In divided attention, at least two sources of information are attended to at the same time. Performance is inefficient. The loss of performance is called dual-task interference.

Question 121 Answer: a, Selective/focused attention
Explanation: In selective/focused attention, one type of information is attended to while additional distracting information is ignored.

Question 122 Answer: c, Sustained attention

Explanation: In sustained attention, the environment is monitored over a long period of time. Performance actually deteriorates with time.

Question 123 Answer: e, Automatic attention

Explanation: In automatic attention, the subject becomes skilled at a task and therefore little conscious effort is required.

Reference: Puri BK, Hall A, Ho R (2014). *Revision Notes in Psychiatry*. London: CRC Press, p. 35.

Theme: Memory tests

Question 124 Answer: f, National Adult Reading Test

Explanation: The National Adult Reading Test is a reading test consisting of phonetically irregular words that have to be read aloud by the subject. If a patient suffers deterioration in intellectual abilities, their premorbid vocabulary may remain less affected or unaffected. The NART could thus be used to estimate the premorbid IQ.

Question 125 Answer: g, Raven Progressive Matrices

Explanation: This test of non-verbal intelligence consists of a series of printed designs from each of which a part is missing. The subject is required to correctly choose the missing part for each design from the alternatives offered. The test requires the perception of relations between abstract items.

Question 126 Answer: e, Rivermead Behavioural Memory Test

Explanation: It is actually just another memory test battery. However, it lays emphasis on tests that are related to skills required in daily living. The subtests include orientation, name recall, picture recognition, face recognition, story recall, route memory and prospective memory.

Question 127 Answer: a, Benton Visual Retention Test

Explanation: The subject is serially presented with 10 designs, which he or she has to reproduce from memory. It may be used in subjects aged 8 years and over. It may be used to test for brain damage and early cognitive impairment.

Question 128 Answer: b, Rey–Osterrieth Test

Explanation: In this visual memory test, the subject is present with a complex design. The subject is asked to copy this design, and then, 40 minutes later, without previous notification that this will occur, the subject is then asked to draw the same design again from memory. Non-dominant temporal lobe damage could lead to impaired performance on this test, whereas domain temporal lobe damage tends not to, but that could be associated with verbal memory difficulties.

Reference: Puri BK, Hall A, Ho R (2014). *Revision Notes in Psychiatry*. London: CRC Press, p. 95.

Theme: Social sciences and stigma

Question 129 Answer: d, Prejudice
Explanation: Prejudice is a preconceived set of beliefs held about others who are prejudged on this basis: the negative meaning of the term is the one usually used. It is not amenable to discussion and is resistant to change. Prejudiced individuals may believe in ways that create stereotyped behaviour that sustains their prejudice.

Question 130 Answer: e, Discrimination
Explanation: This refers to the enactment of prejudice. In the case of racism, the enactment is also termed racialism.

Question 131 Answer: b, Enacted stigma
Explanation: This refers to the experience of discrimination of an individual who bears a stigma. Stigma is an attribute of an individual that marks him or her as being unacceptable, inferior or dangerous.

Question 132 Answer: c, Felt stigma
Explanation: This refers to the fear of discrimination of an individual who bears a stigma.

Reference: Puri BK, Hall A, Ho R (2014). *Revision Notes in Psychiatry*. London: CRC Press, p. 125.

Theme: Dynamic psychopathology and theories

Question 133 Answer: e, Secondary process
Explanation: Secondary process is the operating system of the preconscious as well as the conscious.

Question 134 Answer: d, Primary process
Explanation: Primary process is the operating system of the unconscious. It consists of the following: displacement, condensation and symbolization.

Question 135 Answer: a, Unconscious
Explanation: The unconscious contains memories, ideas and affects that are repressed. Characteristic features include it being outside of awareness and that it involves primary process thinking. The motivating principle is the pleasure principle. Access to the repressed contents is difficult and occurs only when the censor gives way, for example, when one is relaxed, fooled, or overpowered.

Question 136 Answer: b, Preconscious
Explanation: The characteristic features of preconscious are that it is outside awareness and the operating system is secondary process thinking. The access can occur through focused attention.

Question 137 Answer: g, Id
Explanation: Most of the Id is unconscious. It contains primordial energy reserves derived from instinctual drives. Its aim is to maximize pleasure by fulfilling these drives.

Question 138 Answer: h, Ego
Explanation: The ego has the task of self-preservation. With regards to external events, it performs the task by becoming aware of the stimuli by storing experiences about them, and by avoiding excessively strong stimuli. With regards to internal events in relation to the id, it performs the task by gaining control over the demands of the instinct, by deciding whether they be allowed satisfaction and by postponing the satisfaction at times.

Reference: Puri BK, Hall A, Ho R (2014). *Revision Notes in Psychiatry*. London: CRC Press, pp. 131–132.

Theme: Clinical psychiatry – old age psychiatry
Question 139 Answer: e, Dementia with Lewy bodies
Explanation: In this condition, there is marked neuroleptic sensitivity for patients. Antipsychotics are not indicated for mild-to-moderate noncognitive symptoms in DLB because of the risk of severe adverse reactions. If it needs to be used, consider 'Quetiapine' and monitor carefully for the extrapyramidal side effects.

Question 140 Answer: d, Fronto-temporal dementia
Explanation: These are the typical symptoms for patients with fronto-temporal dementia. In addition, they might have also primitive reflexes such as grasp, pour and palm mental reflexes.

Question 141 Answer: b, Vascular fementia
Explanation: The aforementioned is true for vascular dementia. In addition, there is usually evidence of vascular diseases on physical examination.

Question 142 Answer: c, Biswanger's disease
Explanation: The aforementioned are characteristic CT scan changes for this disorder. The age of onset is usually 50–65 with a gradual accumulation of neurological signs, dementia and disturbances in motor function.

Question 143 Answer: B, Vascular dementia
Explanation: An excess of vascular dementia has been noted in males, which is likely to be due to the increased prevalence of cardiovascular disease in men.

Reference: Puri BK, Hall A, Ho R (2014). *Revision Notes in Psychiatry*. London: CRC Press, p. 699.

Theme: Clinical psychiatry – somatoform and dissociative disorder

Question 144 Answer: g, Malingering

Explanation: In this disorder, the motivation is usually external gain and the signs and symptoms are usually intentionally produced. There is poor cooperation in evaluation and also treatment.

Question 145 Answer: f, Factitious disorder

Explanation: The primary motivation is to assume the sick role. There is intentional production or feigning the signs or symptoms. Often, these patients provide only a vague and confusing history.

Question 146 Answer: c, Persistent somatoform pain disorder

Explanation: Pain usually occurs in association with emotional conflict and results in increased support and attention.

Reference: Puri BK, Hall A, Ho R (2014). *Revision Notes in Psychiatry*. London: CRC Press, p. 470.

Theme: Clinical psychiatry – women's mental health

Question 147 Answer: f, Postnatal blues

Explanation: Postnatal blues is a brief psychological disturbance, characterized by tearfulness, labile emotions and confusion in mothers occurring in the first few days after childbirth.

Question 148 Answer: f, Postnatal blues

Explanation: Postnatal blues have been associated with poor social adjustment, poor marital relationship, high scores on the Eysench Personality Inventory neuroticism scale, fear of labour and also anxious and depressed mood during pregnancy.

Question 149 Answer: e, Puerperal psychosis

Explanation: It has been shown that the risk of developing a psychotic illness is increased 20-fold in the first postpartum month. Certain distinctive symptoms include abrupt onset, marked perplexity, rapid changes in mental state, marked restlessness fear and insomnia and associated delusions, hallucinations and disturbed behaviour.

Question 150 Answer: g, Postnatal depression

Explanation: Postnatal depression is characterized by low mood; reduced self-esteem; tearfulness; anxiety, particularly about the baby's health; and an inability to cope. Mothers may experience reduced affection for their baby and have difficulty with breast-feeding.

Question 151 Answer: a, Premenstrual syndrome

Explanation: The aforementioned are true with regards to the disorder. There is a higher prevalence in those women who have experienced natural menstrual cycles for longer periods of time.

Reference: Puri BK, Hall A, Ho R (2014). *Revision Notes in Psychiatry*. London: CRC Press, p. 567.

Theme: History of psychiatry

Question 152 Answer: j, Henry Maudsley

Explanation: He was the first person to propose the abolishment of physical restraints in England. He went on to become one of the best known psychiatrists. He believed psychiatric illness to be a physical disorder of the body, much similar to other medical illnesses.

Question 153 Answer: h, Sigmund Freud

Explanation: He initially started studying cases of hysteria using hypnosis. Then he began to develop the technique of psychoanalysis, which was later used to explain the psychological causes of symptoms.

Question 154 Answer: d, Jacob Mendes Da Costa

Explanation: He coined the term Da Costa's syndrome or soldier's heart during the American Civil War. This condition is a functional heart disease and the solders presented with left-sided chest pain, palpitation, breathlessness, sweating and fatigue during exertion.

Question 155 Answer: e, Paul Broca

Explanation: Paul Broca coined the terminology Broca's aphasia, which involves a lesion in the ventro-posterior region of the frontal lobe. This leads to Broca's aphasia that affects speech production but not comprehension.

Question 156 Answer: c, Benedict Morel

Explanation: He proposed the degeneration theory that states that mental illness affecting one generation could be passed on to the next in ever worsening degrees.

Reference: Puri BK, Hall A, Ho R (2014). *Revision Notes in Psychiatry*. London: CRC Press, p. 140.

Theme: Ethics and psychiatric research

Question 157 Answer: a, Nuremberg code

Explanation: The Nuremberg code was developed in wartime tribunal against the Nazi German doctors. The main objective is to protect human rights during experiments and research. An experiment should avoid suffering and injury.

Question 158 Answer: a, Nuremberg code

Explanation: It is stated in the code that proper preparations should be performed to protect research subjects and the experiments should be conducted by qualified personnel. During the experiment, the research subjects have the liberty to withdraw at any time, and the investigators should stop the experiment if continuation results in potential injury or death of research subjects. The design should be based on results obtained from animal experiments and natural history of disease. Seeking consent from research subjects is necessary.

Question 159 Answer: b, Declaration of Helsinki
Explanation: This declaration states the aforementioned. The principal investigator should balance the predictable risks and the foreseeable benefits, respect integrity and privacy, obtain consent with liberty and free from undue influence, and preserve accuracy in publication of results.

Question 160 Answer: c, Belmont report
Explanation: The Belmont report emphasizes on justice. Individual justice requires the researcher to offer beneficial research to all participants independent of his or her preference. Social justice requires an order of preference in selection of subjects.

Reference: Puri BK, Hall A, Ho R (2014). *Revision Notes in Psychiatry*. London: CRC Press, p. 148.

Theme: Clinical psychiatry – personality disorder
Question 161 Answer: b, Schizoid personality disorder
Explanation: Individuals with schizoid personality disorder tend to have solitary lifestyle, are indifferent to praise and criticism, and have no interest in relationships and sexual experiences. They have few friends and are cold and detached.

Question 162 Answer: c, Schizotypal personality disorder
Explanation: Patients with this disorder tend to have unusual perception, are friendless with the exception of first-degree family, have odd beliefs and speech, have ideas of reference and might also have inappropriate or constricted affect.

Question 163 Answer: a, Paranoid personality disorder
Explanation: They tend to bear grudges without justification, are excessively sensitive to setbacks and tend to read benign remarks into threats with hidden meaning. At times, fidelity of spouse is doubted and the trustworthiness of others are doubted without due course.

Question 164 Answer: i, Borderline personality disorder
Explanation: The aforementioned is true with regards to borderline personality disorder. There are associated clinical signs and symptoms such as identity disturbance, unstable relationships, fear of impulsivity, self-harm, emptiness, dissociative symptoms, affective instability, paranoid ideation, anger, idealization and devaluation and negativistic attitudes towards others.

Question 165 Answer: d, Antisocial personality disorder
Explanation: Patients with antisocial personality disorder usually will have conduct disorder before the age of 15, and tend to engage in antisocial activities.

They tend to lie frequently, are aggressive and do not value the safety of others. They tend to fail to plan and there is denial of obligation.

Reference: Puri BK, Hall A, Ho R (2014). *Revision Notes in Psychiatry*. London: CRC Press, p. 445.

Theme: Clinical psychiatry – substance misuse disorders

Question 166 Answer: c, Wernicke's encephalopathy
Explanation: These are the core clinical features of individuals with the aforementioned condition.

Question 167 Answer: c, Wernicke's encephalopathy
Explanation: Approximately 10% of individuals with the condition have the classical triad. Peripheral neuropathy might be present in some individuals.

Question 168 Answer: d, Korsakoff's syndrome
Explanation: This is a clinical condition that is frequently preceded by Wernicke's encephalopathy. Clinical features include retrograde amnesia, anterograde amnesia, with sparing of immediate recall and disorientation in time. There might be inability to recall the temporal sequence of events, associated with confabulation as well.

Question 169 Answer: b, Withdrawal fits
Explanation: Withdrawal fits may take place within 48 hours of stopping drinking.

Question 170 Answer: a, Alcoholic blackouts
Explanation: This may occur after just one bout of heavy drinking and have been estimated to affect 15%–20% of those who drink. There are three types of blackout, including state-dependent memory loss, fragmentary blackouts and en bloc blackouts.

Reference: Puri BK, Hall A, Ho R (2014). *Revision Notes in Psychiatry*. London: CRC Press, p. 516.

Theme: Basic psychopharmacology

Question 171 Answer: e, Lamotrigine
Explanation: If the patient does not have hypothyroidism, lithium monotherapy is also an option.

Further Reading: Puri B, Treasaden I (eds) (2010). *Psychiatry: An Evidence-Based Text*. London: Hodder Arnold, pp. 532, 536, 906, 910.

Question 172 Answer: l, Topiramate
Explanation: Based on the NICE guidelines, this is not a drug which is recommended for use in the prophylaxis of bipolar disorder.

Further Reading: Puri B, Treasaden I (eds) (2010). *Psychiatry: An Evidence-Based Text*. London: Hodder Arnold, pp. 538, 699, 905, 910.

Question 173 Answer: i, Sodium valproate
Explanation: Sodium valproate could be used as an augmentation strategy.

Further Reading: Puri B, Treasaden I (eds) (2010). *Psychiatry: An Evidence-Based Text*. London: Hodder Arnold, pp. 532, 538.

Question 174 Answer: l, Topiramate
Explanation: Topiramate causes renal stones in poor hydration during the hot weather.

Further Reading: Puri B, Treasaden I (eds) (2010). *Psychiatry: An Evidence-Based Text*. London: Hodder Arnold, pp. 538, 699, 905, 910.

Question 175 Answer: f, Lithium
Explanation: Lithium is increased through sodium depletion.

Further Reading: Puri B, Treasaden I (eds) (2010). *Psychiatry: An Evidence-Based Text*. London: Hodder Arnold, pp. 613, 623, 630, 632, 633, 909–910.

Question 176 Answer: e, Lamotrigine
Explanation: For rapid cycling bipolar disorder, the NICE guidelines recommend to increase the dose of antimanic drug or adding lamotrigine.

Further Reading: Puri B, Treasaden I (eds) (2010). *Psychiatry: An Evidence-Based Text*. London: Hodder Arnold, pp. 532, 536, 906, 910.

Question 177 Answer: f, Lithium and i, sodium valproate
Explanation: For long-term management of rapid cycling bipolar disorder, the NICE guidelines recommend a combination of lithium and valproate as first-line treatment. Lithium monotherapy is the second-line treatment. Antidepressants should be avoided and thyroid function test should be performed every 6 months.

Further Reading: Puri B, Treasaden I (eds) (2010). *Psychiatry: An Evidence-Based Text*. London: Hodder Arnold, pp. 532, 613, 623, 630, 632, 633, 905, 909–910.

Theme: Cultural psychiatry
Question 178 Answer: b, Brain fag
Explanation: This syndrome is commonly encountered among students, probably because of the high priority to education in the African society. Of importance it is particularly prominent during examination times.

Question 179 Answer: d, Koro
Explanation: Koro is common in Southeast Asia and China. It may occur in epidemic form. It involves the belief of genital retraction with disappearance into the abdomen, accompanied by intense anxiety and fear of impending death.

Question 180 Answer: e, Latah
Explanation: This is a condition that usually begins after a sudden frightening experience in Malay women. It is characterized by a response to minimal stimuli with exaggerated startles, coprolalia, echolalia, echopraxia and automatic obedience. It has been suggested that this is merely one form of what is known to psychologists as the hyperstartle reaction and is universally found.

Question 181 Answer: i, Windigo
Explanation: This is described in North American Indians and ascribed to depression, schizophrenia, hysteria or anxiety. It is a disorder in which the subject believes he or she has undergone a transformation and become a monster who practises cannibalism.

Further Reading: Puri B, Treasaden I (eds) (2010). *Psychiatry: An Evidence-Based Text*. London: Hodder Arnold, pp. 309–318.

Theme: Psychopathology
Question 182 Answer: i, Flat affect
Explanation: This is an example of flat affect.

Reference and Further Reading: Puri BK, Hall AD (2002). *Revision Notes in Psychiatry*. London: Arnold, p. 150.

Question 183 Answer: b, Ambivalence
Explanation: This is an example of ambivalence.

Question 184 Answer: a, Acting-out
Explanation: This is an example of acting-out.

Reference and Further Reading: Puri BK, Treasaden I (eds) (2010). *Psychiatry: An Evidence-Based Text*. London: Hodder Arnold, pp. 940, 948–949.

Theme: Basic psychology
Question 185 Answer: f, Watson, John
Explanation: Watson conducted the Little Albert experiment, which demonstrated stimulus generalization.

Reference and Further Reading: Puri BK, Treasaden I (eds) (2010). *Psychiatry: An Evidence-Based Text*. London: Hodder Arnold, p. 199.

Question 186 Answer: e, Thorndike, Edward
Explanation: Thorndike investigated learning in animals by using cats and formulated the law of effect.

Reference and Further Reading: Puri BK, Treasaden I (eds) (2010). *Psychiatry: An Evidence-Based Text*. London: Hodder Arnold, pp. 200–201.

Question 187 Answer: c, Seligman, Martin
Explanation: Seligman demonstrated learned helplessness.

Reference and Further Reading: Puri BK, Treasaden I (eds) (2010). *Psychiatry: An Evidence-Based Text*. London: Hodder Arnold, pp. 206, 298, 614.

Theme: Basic psychology
Question 188 Answer: d, Burrhus Frederic
Explanation: Skinner demonstrated positive and negative reinforcement.

Reference and Further Reading: Puri BK, Treasaden I (eds) (2010). *Psychiatry: An Evidence-Based Text*. London: Hodder Arnold, pp. 200–205.

Question 189 Answer: a, Bandura, Albert
Explanation: Bandura conducted the 'doll experiment' to demonstrate observational learning and vicarious conditioning.

Reference and Further Reading: Puri BK, Treasaden I (eds) (2010). *Psychiatry: An Evidence-Based Text*. London: Hodder Arnold, p. 207.

Question 190 Answer: b, Pavlov, Ivan
Explanation: Pavlov conducted this experiment to demonstrate classical conditioning.

Reference and Further Reading: Puri BK, Treasaden I (eds) (2010). *Psychiatry: An Evidence-Based Text*. London: Hodder Arnold, pp. 197–200.

Theme: Basic psychology
Question 191 Answer: b, Kohler, Wolfgang
Explanation: Kohler used chimpanzees to study insight learning. Insight learning occurs when the animals suddenly realizes how to solve a problem. In the experiment, a banana is placed above the reach of chimpanzees. In the room there were several boxes but none of them was high enough to enable the chimpanzees to reach the banana. Initially, the chimpanzees would run around, jump, and get upset about their inability to get the banana. All of a sudden, they would pile the boxes on top of each other, climb up and grab the bananas.

Reference and Further Reading: Puri BK, Hall AD (2002). *Revision Notes in Psychiatry*. London: Arnold, p. 5.

Question 192 Answer: e, Tolman, Edward
Explanation: Tolman developed the maze running experiment to demonstrate latent learning. Latent learning occurs in the absence of an obvious reward.

Reference and Further Reading: Puri BK, Treasaden I (eds) (2010). *Psychiatry: An Evidence-Based Text*. London: Hodder Arnold, pp. 207, 222.

Question 193 Answer: c, Premack, David

Explanation: Premack's principle was derived from a study of monkeys. It stated that more probable behaviours will reinforce less probable behaviours.

Reference and Further Reading: Mitchell WS, Stoffelmayr BE (1973). Application of the Premack principle to the behavioral control of extremely inactive schizophrenics. *Journal of Applied Behaviour Analysis*, 6: 419–423.

MRCPSYCH PAPER A1 MOCK EXAMINATION 4: QUESTIONS

GET THROUGH MRCPSYCH PAPER A1: MOCK EXAMINATION

Total number of questions: 195 (139 MCQs, 56 EMIs)
Total time provided: 180 minutes

Question 1
A 25-year-old male has been taken to the emergency services after hurting himself whilst trying to break the computer in his brother's room. He reports to the doctor that he feels that his thoughts have been controlled and are being taken away by the computer. Which of the following best describes this form of psychopathology?
   a. Thought insertion
   b. Thought withdrawal
   c. Thought broadcasting
   d. Made actions
   e. Somatic passivity

Question 2
Which of the following statements about 'Stereotypy' is correct?
   a. The patient would adopt an inappropriate or bizarre bodily posture continuously for a long term.
   b. The patient would have repeated regular fixed patterns of movement that are not goal directed.
   c. There is a feeling of plastic resistance resembling the bending of a soft wax rod as the examiner moves parts of the patient's body.
   d. The patient would have repeated irregular movements involving a muscle group.
   e. The patient would have resting tremors, cogwheel rigidity and postural and gait abnormalities.

Question 3
General practitioners (GPs), though not trained in psychotherapy, could still help patients through the provision of supportive psychotherapy. Supportive psychotherapy's main goal would be to
   a. Allow the GP to provide patients with a source of emotional support
   b. Allow the patients to have a chance to ventilate their feelings

c. Allow the GP to understand more about the patient's environment and assist in enabling changes
d. Allow the GP to help boost the self-esteem of the patients by agreeing with them
e. Allow the GP to strengthen the patient and help them to stabilize

Question 4
A 21-year-old has been sectioned for admission to the mental health unit as he has been experiencing bizarre delusions as well as auditory hallucinations. The ward team has decided to start him on a low dose of olanzapine for stabilization of his condition. However, it was noted that after the commencement of the medication, he developed a temperature as well as marked rigidity of his limbs. Which one of the following is the most likely clinical diagnosis?
a. Neuroleptic malignant syndrome
b. Serotonin syndrome
c. Lethal catatonia
d. Sepsis
e. Established side effects to olanzapine

Question 5
All of the following statements regarding individuals diagnosed with paranoid personality disorder are true, with the exception of
a. There is a tendency to bear grudges.
b. There is marked suspiciousness.
c. Threats and hidden meanings are read into benign remarks.
d. They confide readily.
e. There is excessive sensitivity to setbacks.

Question 6
Which of the following traits is not seen in individuals with schizoid personality disorder?
a. They tend to lead a solitary lifestyle.
b. They tend to appear indifferent to praise and criticism.
c. They have no interest in relationships.
d. There are times when they desire for the presence of close friends.
e. They usually appear to be cold and detached in their emotions.

Question 7
Based on prior research, it has been established that bulimics are more prone to which of the following psychiatric disorder as compared to anorexics?
a. Substance abuse
b. Personality disorders
c. Dementia
d. Obsessive-compulsive disorder (OCD)
e. Generalized anxiety disorder

Question 8
Which of the following is true regarding higher-order conditioning?
a. The onset of the conditioned stimulus precedes the unconditioned stimulus, and the conditioned stimulus continues until the response occurs.
b. The onset of both stimuli is simultaneous, and the conditioned stimulus continues until the response occurs.
c. The conditioned stimulus ends before the onset of the unconditioned stimulus, and the conditioning becomes less effective as the delay between the two increases.
d. The presentation of the conditioned stimulus occurs only after that of the unconditioned stimulus.
e. The conditioned stimulus is paired with a second conditioned stimulus, which, on presentation, by itself elicits the original conditioned response.

Question 9
An elderly Chinese man complained, 'My guts are rotten and blood stopped flowing to my heart. I am dead.' The psychopathology being described is
a. Acute intestinal obstruction
b. Delirium
c. Delusion of control
d. Nihilistic delusion
e. Hypochondriasis

Question 10
A 24-year-old man covers his head with a helmet because he believes that other people can receive his thoughts. The psychopathology being described is
a. Delusional memory
b. Running commentary
c. Thought broadcasting
d. Thought echo
e. Thought insertion

Question 11
A 10-year-old boy prefers playing computer games to doing his homework. His mother allows him 30 minutes of computer games if he finishes his homework and this motivates him to work on his homework diligently. Which of the following learning theories best describes the aforementioned phenomenon?
a. Backward conditioning
b. Forward conditioning
c. Mowrer's two-factor theory
d. Premack's principle
e. Trace conditioning

Question 12
To which class of antidepressants does duloxetine belong to?
a. Tricyclic antidepressants
b. Selective serotonin reuptake inhibitors

c. Serotonergic and noradrenergic reuptake inhibitors
d. Monoamine oxidase inhibitors
e. Adrenergic type 2 antagonists

Question 13
Which of the following antipsychotics belongs to the class of a substituted benzamide?
a. Amisulpride
b. Haloperidol
c. Clozapine
d. Quetiapine
e. Risperidone

Question 14
A 26-year-old male has a known history of bipolar disorder. He has been concordant with his medications. Recently, he has been experiencing constipation and weight gain, and routine investigation diagnosed him with hypothyroidism. Which one of the following medications might predispose James to have this new clinical condition?
a. Sodium valproate
b. Lithium
c. Carbamazepine
d. Lamotrigine
e. Gabapentin

Question 15
A 35-year-old unemployed woman firmly believes Prince William is in love with her even though she has never met him. Collateral history of her family reveals that she has never contacted him. The condition being described is
a. De Clerambault's syndrome
b. Capgras' syndrome
c. Fregoli syndrome
d. Intermetamorphosis syndrome
e. Othello syndrome

Question 16
A 50-year-old man suffered from prostate cancer 2 years ago. He came to the hospital daily to receive chemotherapy. However, when he received chemotherapy, he threw up because of side effects. From that point forward, whenever he was in the hospital, he felt sick to his stomach. The chemotherapy was stopped 1 year ago, and the nausea associated with hospital environment also disappeared. Which of the following statements regarding the disappearance of nausea associated with hospital environment is correct?
a. This process has no treatment implication.
b. This process only applies to biological responses (e.g. nausea) but not psychological responses.

c. This process was developed in conjunction with both classical conditioning and operant conditioning.
d. The response (i.e. nausea) disappeared suddenly.
e. The response (i.e. nausea associated with hospital environment) would never occur again.

Question 17
A medical student states that a hypomanic episode usually differs from a manic episode in terms of the degree of impairment of baseline functioning and also in terms of the duration of the symptoms. What should be the correct answer with regards to how long the symptoms would need to typically last in a hypomanic episode?
a. 1 day
b. 2 days
c. 3 days
d. 4 days
e. 1 week

Question 18
Theory of mind refers to the ability of an individual to understand and comprehend the thoughts, feelings, beliefs and knowledge about others. In which of the following condition is the development of a theory of mind lacking?
a. Pervasive development disorder
b. Hyperkinetic disorder
c. Depressive disorder in children
d. Anxiety disorder in children
e. Conduct disorder in children

Question 19
Attachment theory is a theory that was proposed by
a. Bowlby
b. Harlow
c. Lorenz
d. Freud
e. Piaget

Question 20
A core trainee has assessed a 70-year-old gentleman to be suffering from depression and is keen to recommend antidepressant treatment. He wonders which one of the following pharmacokinetics parameters would be affected in the elderly. All of the following are likely changes, with the exception of
a. Changes in the serum protein binding of the psychotropic medication
b. Changes in the renal clearance of the medication
c. Changes in the percentage of the total body fat

d. Changes in the gastric pH
e. Increased tubular secretion

Question 21
Which of the following hallucinations typically occurs for patients diagnosed with depression with psychotic features?
a. Somatic
b. Visual
c. Gustatory
d. Auditory
e. Olfactory

Question 22
Which of the following statements regarding eidectic image is false?
a. It typically affects those who are more advanced in age.
b. It is classified as one form of pseudohallucination.
c. It occurs usually in the outer objective space.
d. It is common in depression.
e. It can be considered to be a vivid reproduction of a previous perception.

Question 23
A 20-year-old British soldier was seriously wounded in an attack on troops in a southern Iraqi city in 2004. He returned to the United Kingdom for further treatment. After this episode, he experiences recurrent nightmares and flashbacks. He does not want to return to the army camp in the UK and avoids touching firearms. He does not want to talk about anything related to Iraq. His superior wants to find out from you the underlying reason to explain his avoidance. Which of the following learning theories explains his avoidance?
a. Avoidance conditioning
b. Aversive conditioning
c. Classical conditioning
d. Escape conditioning
e. Operant conditioning

Question 24
A 29-year-old woman undergoes psychotherapy for the treatment of OCD. She has hand-washing compulsions and cannot stand touching any surface that has not been sterilized with antibacterial agents. The psychologist makes her turn the door knob with her bare hands when she enters the room to see the psychologist and she is not allowed to wash her hands throughout the psychotherapy session. Which of the following learning theories best describes the aforementioned phenomenon?'
a. Habituation
b. Simultaneous conditioning
c. Spontaneous recovery

d. Stimulus generalization
e. Stimulus discrimination

Question 25
A man sees a blue car driving past him and he realizes that the terrorists are going to kill him. This is most likely which of the following?
a. Delusion of hypochondriasis
b. Delusion of passivity
c. Delusional perception
d. Delusion of persecution
e. Visual hallucination

Question 26
Which of the following statements about psychological imprinting is correct?
a. An example of this is when a young animal learns the characteristics of its parents.
b. Expression of inheritance is in a parent-of-origin-specific manner.
c. It involves learning that is slow.
d. It involves learning that is dependent on the consequences of behaviour.
e. This concept is studied extensively by Tolman.

Question 27
The latest research findings report that the combination of the first- and second-generation antipsychotics significantly increases the risk of metabolic syndrome amongst people with schizophrenia. Which of the following pharmacodynamic properties of the first-generation antipsychotics is most responsible for the aforementioned research findings?
a. Antiadrenergic
b. Antimuscarinic
c. Antidopaminergic
d. Antihistaminergic
e. Antinicotinic

Question 28
Which of the following statements regarding alcoholic dementia is incorrect?
a. Alcoholics might suffer from mild to moderate degree of cognitive impairment if they have been using alcohol on a chronic basis for some years.
b. Women are more likely to develop cognitive impairment much earlier as compared to men.
c. Brain imaging would show the presence of ventricular enlargement and sulcal widening.
d. Chronic alcoholics might show changes in their personality, likely due to frontal lobe atrophy.
e. The mild or moderate cognitive impairment due to long-term use of alcohol would not improve with abstinence.

Question 29

A 28-year-old female noticed that her friend's 3-year-old son seemed to always keep a distance from his mother, and at times, even ignores his mother. What form of attachment does the child have towards his mother?

a. Secure attachment
b. Insecure attachment
c. Avoidant attachment
d. Anxious attachment
e. Ambivalent attachment

Question 30

The following subtypes of schizophrenia could be found within the 10th revision of *International Classification of Diseases* (ICD-10) diagnostic criteria, with the exception of

a. Catatonic schizophrenia
b. Disorganized schizophrenia
c. Hebephrenic schizophrenia
d. Paranoid schizophrenia
e. Simple schizophrenia

Question 31

Confabulation, pseudologia, and retrospective falsification or false memory all have the following in common:

a. Presence of delusional beliefs
b. Presence of hallucinations
c. Presence of suggestibility
d. Presence of passivity phenomenon
e. Presence of abnormal thought content

Question 32

A medical student is curious about the Folstein's Mini Mental State Examination (MMSE). She wants to know the purpose of the Serial Sevens Test. Your answer is

a. Assess attention
b. Assess mathematical skills
c. Assess memory
d. Assess registration
e. Assess recall

Question 33

A medical student being attached to the addiction specialty wonders how long an individual needs to have symptoms of alcohol dependence in order for a diagnosis to be made. The correct answer, based on the ICD-10 classification system, would be

a. 1 month
b. 2 months

c. 6 months
d. 1 year
e. 2 years

Question 34
A medical student asks the consultant psychiatrist of the addictions service how soon would a chronic alcoholic experience alcoholic withdrawal fits. The correct answer would be
a. 12 hours
b. 24 hours
c. 36 hours
d. 48 hours
e. 72 hours

Question 35
A 50-year-old woman is referred by her GP to you for psychiatric assessment. She sees her son when she looks at various strangers walking down the street. The psychopathology being described is
a. De Clerambault's syndrome
b. Capgras syndrome
c. Fregoli syndrome
d. Munchausen syndrome
e. Othello syndrome

Question 36
A person describes the feeling of familiarity when stored material returns to consciousness. The phenomenon being described is
a. Déjà-vu
b. Jamais vu
c. Recognition
d. Recollection
e. Retrieval

Question 37
A 32-year-old married woman with a history of recurrent depressive episodes takes fluoxetine 40 mg on a daily basis. She wants to conceive in the near future but she is concerned about the safety of fluoxetine during pregnancy. She wants to stop taking fluoxetine but wants to know from the chance of having a relapse of depressive episode. Your answer is
a. 5%
b. 15%
c. 35%
d. 55%
e. 75%

Question 38

A 28-year-old female is seductive and always likes to be the centre of attention. She values her own appearance, and at times, she views certain interpersonal relationships as much closer than what others view. Under which one of the following personality disorders would you classify her?
a. Schizoid personality disorder
b. Borderline personality disorder
c. Paranoid personality disorder
d. Histrionic personality disorder
e. Obsessive-compulsive personality disorder

Question 39

At a certain stage of human development, one is able to process new concepts according to a pre-existing system of understanding. Which of the following concepts from Piaget's theory of cognitive development best describes this phenomenon?
a. Accommodation
b. Animism
c. Assimilation
d. Equilibrium
e. Schema

Question 40

A trainee who is more familiar with DSM-5 wonders where, in ICD-10, neurasthenia is classified. The consultant informs him that neurasthenia is classified under
a. Other mood (affective) disorders F35
b. Other anxiety disorders F41
c. Reaction to stress and adjustment disorders F43
d. Somatoform disorders F45
e. Other Neurotic disorders F48

Question 41

A medical student was asked how best the orientation of an inpatient could be determined. Which one of the following statements is the most accurate?
a. Checking with the patient whether he could remember and recall his own address
b. Checking with the patient whether he could perform serial sevens or spell the word 'World' forwards then backwards
c. Checking whether the patient can name specific objects
d. Checking with the patient whether he is able to tell the occupation or the identity of a doctor or an allied health-care staff
e. Checking with the patient whether he is able to name as many words as possible beginning with the letter 'F' in 1 minute

Question 42
A core trainee-2 is seeing a patient who has an alcohol addiction problem. He wishes to use one of the standardized alcohol assessment questionnaires to help him in his assessment. Please select the questionnaire that is not suitable for him to use.
 a. CAGE
 b. Alcohol Use Disorders Identification Test (AUDIT)
 c. Brief Psychiatric Rating Scale (BPRS)
 d. Michigan Alcohol Screening Test (MAST)
 e. Clinical Institute Withdrawal Assessment for Alcohol Scale (CIWA)

Question 43
Which of the following statements about memory is incorrect?
 a. Both primacy and recency effects are involved in remembering a list of names.
 b. Primary memory has been found to have a duration of approximately 7 seconds.
 c. Working memory and primary memory are synonymous.
 d. Chunking increases the capacity of short-term memory.
 e. Short-term memory has a limited capacity.

Question 44
An 80-year-old man says, 'I have a headache because there is too much blood in my head. I feel my throat being blocked and hence, blood cannot leave my head'. The psychopathology being described is
 a. Hypochondriasis
 b. Nihilistic delusion
 c. Passivity experience
 d. Somatic delusion
 e. Stroke

Question 45
A 32-year-old married woman with a history of recurrent depressive episodes takes fluoxetine 40 mg on a daily basis. She wants to conceive in the near future but she is concerned about the safety of fluoxetine during pregnancy. She wants to know the rate of major malformations in the foetus associated with prenatal exposure to fluoxetine. Your answer is
 a. 0%
 b. 1%–3%
 c. 5%–7%
 d. 9%–11%
 e. 13%–15%

Question 46
Which of the following statements about the Sequenced Treatment Alternatives to Relieve Depression (STAR*D) trial is incorrect?
 a. Approximately one-third of the patients did reach a remission state or has had virtual absence of their symptoms during the initial phase of the study.
 b. The remission rate was 20%.

c. Patients who took T3 complained of lesser side effects than those taking lithium.

d. The discontinuation rate for T3 was 10%, whereas the rate for lithium was 23%.

e. The level 4 findings suggested that venlafaxine or mirtazapine treatment would be a better choice than a monoamine oxidase inhibitor (MAO-I).

Question 47

There are known differences between the ICD-10 and the DSM-IV-TR classification system. Which one of the following personality disorders is included in the DSM-IV-TR classification system, but cannot be found in the ICD-10 classification system?

a. Schizotypal personality disorder

b. Paranoid personality disorder

c. Antisocial personality disorder

d. Avoidant personality disorder

e. None of the above

Question 48

An 80-year-old man has been brought in by his family as they are very concerned about his progressive memory loss. The old-age psychiatrist assessing him decided to perform baseline blood investigations, a computed tomography (CT) scan and also a specialized scan. On the specialized scan, multiple protein-like, intra-cytoplasmic inclusion bodies were found in the basal ganglia (which could be visualized only with a microscope). This finding suggests that the aetiology of dementia might be due to

a. Alzheimer's dementia

b. Vascular dementia

c. Frontotemporal dementia

d. Lewy body dementia

e. Alcoholic dementia

Question 49

Which of the following is not part of koro?

a. Illness, exposure to cold and excess coitus are common precursors.

b. Men become convinced that the penis will suddenly withdraw into the abdomen.

c. Onset is usually gradual and slow.

d. Women become convinced that their breasts, labia or vulva will retract.

e. Sufferers expect fatal consequences.

Question 50

Which of the following diagnosis would be the most appropriate to describe a patient who fears that he or she would offend others through inappropriate behaviour or self-presentation?

a. Amok

b. Latah

c. Koro

d. Frigophobia

e. Taijinkyofusho

Question 51
A 14-year-old boy was diagnosed with depression about 1 year ago. He has been receiving intensive psychological treatment. He returns to see the Child and Adolescent Mental Health Service (CAMHS) psychiatrist. Which of the following scales would be the most helpful in determining the diagnosis and symptoms which have been present over the past year?
a. Beck's Depression Inventory (BDI)
b. Hospital Anxiety and Depression Scale (HADS)
c. Montgomery–Asberg Depression Rating Scale (MADRAS)
d. Kiddie Schedule for Affective Disorder and Schizophrenia (K-SADS)
e. Brief Psychiatric Rating Scale (BPRS)

Question 52
Social psychologist Philip Zimbardo designed the Stanford prison experiment where students were randomly assigned to act as either a guard or a prisoner. The 'guards' became abrasive and verbally harassed and humiliated the 'prisoners', and the 'prisoners' became withdrawn and helpless and some were physically ill. This experiment illustrates
a. Social identity
b. Social categorization
c. Social role
d. Social norm
e. Social influence

Question 53
Induced psychosis is a rare delusional disorder, most common amongst which group of individuals?
a. Elderly patients
b. Teenagers
c. Those in a couple relationship
d. Those with blood relationships
e. Any particular group of men or women

Question 54
In a psychological experiment, the subjects find it difficult to remember the following phone number, 18003377924. Which of the following methods would make the phone number most easy to remember?
a. Convert the phone number into two items: 180033-77924
b. Convert the phone number into six items: 18-00-33-77-92–4
c. Convert the phone number into 10 items: 18-0-0-3-3-7-7-9-2-4
d. Remember the phone number, one by one: 1-8-0-0-3-3-7-7-9-2-4
e. Convert the phone number into reverse order: 4-2-9-7-7-3-3-0-0-8-1

Question 55
Hypnagogic hallucinations
  a. Are usually visual
  b. Occur in slow wave sleep
  c. Occur in stage 1 of non-REM sleep
  d. Occur in transition to wakefulness
  e. Require antipsychotic medication

Question 56
A MRCPsych Paper 1 revision course organizer wants to help the participants accurately retain the information in working memory as long as possible. Which of the following methods is the least useful?
  a. The course organizer should keep the number of pieces of information small enough for participants to study.
  b. The course organizer should keep attention constantly focused on the information under consideration in each topic.
  c. The course organizer should rehearse the information often whilst the student is working on sample MCQs or EMIs.
  d. The course organizer should emphasize the participants to store the information in their brain and advise them to reduce access to the information during the course.
  e. The course organizer should help participants to move the information to long-term memory as soon as possible.

Question 57
A 50-year-old man perceives his wife has assumed another bodily form, sometimes appearing as a man but sometimes appearing as a young woman. The phenomenon is known as
  a. De Clerambault's syndrome
  b. Capgras syndrome
  c. Fregoli syndrome
  d. Reverse Fregoli syndrome
  e. Subjective double syndrome

Question 58
A 16-year-old African male was studying for his examination. He suddenly had the following symptoms: headache, blurred vision and amnesia for what he had studied. Which one of the following culture-bound syndromes does the man suffer from?
  a. Amok
  b. Brain fag
  c. Dhat
  d. Koro
  e. Latah

Question 59

Based on your understanding about defence mechanisms, avoidance is a defence mechanism that is commonly used by patients with the following psychiatric diagnosis:

a. Depression
b. Schizophrenia
c. Schizoid personality disorder
d. Phobias
e. Post-traumatic stress disorder (PTSD)

Question 60

A medical student was interested in psychodynamic psychotherapy and read more about it. He shared with his supervisor who was a psychotherapist several of the defence mechanisms that he read about. Which one of the following defence mechanisms was not described by Melanie Klein?

a. Projective identification
b. Splitting
c. Denial
d. Introjection (internalization)
e. None of the above

Question 61

A medical student doing his psychiatric posting was spending time attached to the psychologist clinic, to learn what the psychologist does in his daily work. He wonders what the psychology would administer as the most evidence-based and gold standard test for assessment of intelligence. Which of the following measures would it be?

a. Wechsler Adult Intelligence Scale
b. Halstead–Reitan Battery
c. Luria–Nebraska Neuropsychological Battery
d. Repeatable Battery for the Assessment of Neuropsychological Status
e. None of the above

Question 62

Which of the following statements about attribution theory is incorrect?

a. Attribution theory involves making inferences.
b. In attribution theory, people tend to attribute their own behaviour to their personality traits.
c. A dispositional attribution is the inference that the cause of behaviour is due to internal factors.
d. Using an internal attribution to explain other people's behaviour is usual.
e. A person's feelings about the event may influence a particular cause attributed to an event.

Question 63

A 28-year-old female, Pamela, migrated from Bulgaria to London months ago. Her mother has noticed that she has been increasingly withdrawn in her behaviour. Just 2 days ago, her mother has noticed that Pamela is refusing to eat or drink and is totally mute. She is very concerned. What is the most likely clinical diagnosis for Pamela?

a. Manic stupor
b. Depressive stupor
c. Dissociative stupor
d. Transient psychotic episode
e. Adjustment disorder

Question 64

Based on your understanding, déjà vu and jamais vu are considered to be disorders of

a. Orientation
b. Memory
c. Attention
d. Self-awareness
e. Intelligence

Question 65

During an outpatient review, a 20-year-old patient who has chronic schizophrenia and is currently on quetiapine shared that he has been feeling increasingly anxious. He feels that others could have access to his thoughts and that, recently, there have been thoughts that arise elsewhere and are inserted into his head. Which of the following terms best describes the psychopathology that James is experiencing?

a. Made feelings
b. Thought insertion
c. Thought withdrawal
d. Thought control
e. Thought broad-casting

Question 66

Your medical colleague is preparing for the magnetic resonance cholangiopancreato-graphy (MRCP) examination and he complains that he keeps on forgetting the information he has learnt. He wants to seek your advice on the underlying reason for forgetting. The following are established factors which could lead to his forgetfulness, except

a. He forgets the information owing to disuse of information after a 1-year period of unpaid leave.
b. He forgets the information as he spent 6 months learning surgery which has displaced his knowledge of internal medicine.
c. When his consultant asks him questions, the answer is almost at the tip of his tongue but he cannot recall it.

d. He can recite his knowledge perfectly in his bedroom with classical music playing but cannot recall it in the examination hall.

e. When he studies, he usually feels sad. In the examination, he often puts down the answer 'don't know' when answering MCQs as he also feels sad during the examination.

Question 67

All of the following statements about anorexia nervosa are true, with the exception of

a. The condition is relatively rare and occurs in around 1–2 per 1000 women

b. Peak age of onset is 20–29 years.

c. The incidence of the condition is 10 times higher in females as compared to males.

d. It is a condition that is more prevalent in higher socioeconomic classes.

e. Twin studies have revealed higher concordance rates amongst monozygotic twins as compared to dizygotic twins.

Question 68

A 30-year-old is referred to see you for unusual experiences. She complains of recurrent episodes of not being at home or in the office, although she is there. She cannot feel emotions towards people who are close to her. In situations where she supposes to feel angry, she feels numb instead. She also complains that her memories seem pale and she is not certain whether past events really happened. The psychopathology being described is

a. Alexithymia

b. Delusional mood

c. Delusional memory

d. Depersonalization

e. Derealization

Question 69

Which of the following statements regarding the diagnostic criteria for bipolar disorder, manic episode is correct?

a. The DSM-IV-TR and ICD-10 classify bipolar disorder into bipolar I and bipolar II disorder.

b. The DSM-IV-TR and ICD-10 do not require the presence of depressive episode in the past.

c. The DSM-IV-TR and ICD-10 require the presence of depressive episode in the past.

d. The DSM-IV-TR requires the presence of at least one major depressive episode but not ICD-10.

e. The ICD-10 requires the presence of at least one major depressive episode but not DSM-IV-TR.

Question 70

Which of the following is not a special feature for DSM-IV-TR bipolar disorder with depressive episode?

a. Atypical features

b. Catatonic features

c. Melancholic features

d. Postpartum onset

e. Seasonal pattern

Question 71

All of the following statements regarding the aetiology of eating disorder are correct, with the exception of

a. Family studies have shown an increased incidence of eating disorders amongst the first- and second-degree relatives of those suffering from anorexia nervosa.

b. Brain serotonin systems have not been shown to be implicated in the modulation of appetite.

c. An excess of physical illnesses in childhood have been found in those with anorexia nervosa.

d. Relationships in families of anorexics are usually characterized by overprotection and enmeshment.

e. Sociocultural factors such as a cult of thinness might affect the development of the disorder.

Question 72

Which of the following statements about memory and ageing is false?

a. Memory loss of recent events is an early feature of Alzheimer's disease.

b. Procedural memory is affected later than spatial awareness in Alzheimer's disease.

c. Procedural memory is affected later than verbal memory in Alzheimer's disease.

d. In an adult life span, performance for free recall is affected earlier than recognition on a word-list learning.

e. Semantic memory may improve with age until the age of 80.

Question 73

A 25-year-old man is referred to you for visual disturbance that causes images to persist even after their corresponding stimulus has ceased. He often uses lysergic acid diethylamide (LSD). The psychopathology being described is

a. Eidetic imagery

b. Pareidolia

c. Palinopsia

d. Panoramic hallucination

e. Peduncular hallucination

Question 74

Which of the following statements regarding diagnostic criteria for rapid cycling disorder is false?

a. Based on the DSM-IV-TR criteria, at least four episodes of a mood disturbance in the previous 12 months meet criteria.

b. Based on the DSM-IV-TR criteria, episodes are demarcated either by partial or full remission for at least 2 months.

c. Based on the DSM-IV-TR criteria, episodes can switch to an episode of opposite polarity.

d. Rapid cycling disorder is a course specifier in DSM-IV-TR.

e. Rapid cycling disorder is a separate entity in ICD-10.

Question 75

Which of the following statements regarding diagnostic criteria for cyclothymia is false?

a. Based on the DSM-IV-TR and ICD-10 criteria, there must have been a period of at least 2 years of instability of mood involving several periods of both depression and hypomania.

b. Based on the ICD-10 criteria, none of the manifestations of depression or hypomania should be sufficiently severe or long-lasting to meet criteria for manic episode or depressive episode.

c. Based on the DSM-IV-TR and ICD-10 criteria, intervening periods of normal mood should not be present.

d. Based on the DSM-IV-TR criteria, the minimum duration of illness is 1 year for children and adolescents.

e. Based on the DSM-IV-TR criteria, there may be superimposed manic episodes after the initial 2 years.

Question 76

Which of the following statements regarding bipolar mood disorder is incorrect?

a. Male to female ratio is the same.

b. It is a condition that is most common in the lower social classes.

c. The average age of onset is around mid-20s.

d. Being unmarried might account for the higher incidence of bipolar disorder.

e. Common comorbidities might include anxiety disorder, substance misuse disorder and antisocial personality disorder.

Question 77

A 30-year old male surrendered himself at the police station as he feels that he is guilty for causing the war between the United States and Iraq by mixing up the mails. In addition, he shared that he knows that the police are monitoring him each time he sees the colour 'red'. What psychopathology is this?

a. Delusional perception

b. Delusion of poverty

c. Delusion of self-accusation

d. Delusion of doubles

e. Nihilistic delusion

Question 78

Which of the following is not one of the techniques that can be used to measure memory?

a. Paired-associate recall

b. Recognition

c. Memory-span procedure
d. Free recall
e. Memory retrieval procedure

Question 79
Rubin's vase, the Necker cube and Boring's old/young woman are examples of
a. Distortions
b. Ambiguous figures
c. Paradoxical figures
d. Fictions
e. Illusions of shading

Question 80
A mother is concerned that her child might develop autism. Based on the diagnostic criteria for autism, the onset of the disorder is usually before the age of
a. 1 year
b. 2 years
c. 3 years
d. 4 years
e. 5 years

Question 81
A 35-year-old man is suing his company for compensation for his cognitive impairment as a result of a head injury that occurred at his workplace 6 months ago. You have referred him for formal neuropsychological assessment. The neuropsychologist has prepared the report. Which of following findings does not suggest feigned amnesia?
a. Impairment of attention or immediate memory is much worse than impairment of overall learning and memory.
b. Standardized scores on tests of recognition memory are higher than standardized scores on tests of free recall.
c. Reports of severe retrograde amnesia together with intact new learning and absence of neurological abnormality.
d. Gross inconsistency across tests or testing occasions.
e. Evasive or unusual test-taking behaviour.

Question 82
A 20-year-old woman has a history of sexual abuse and you worry that she may develop false memory syndrome. Which of the following statements regarding false memory syndrome is incorrect?
a. The interviewer should avoid leading questions.
b. False memory syndrome may lead to medico-legal problems.
c. False memory syndrome is a recognized diagnostic criterion in ICD-10.
d. False memory syndrome is more common in patients who are prone to fantasy.
e. False memory syndrome is relatively common amongst cases of severe childhood abuse.

Question 83
Schemas are cognitive structures representing knowledge about a concept.
Schemas influence the way people organize knowledge about the social world and
interpret new situations. Which of the following statements about schemas is true?
a. Schemas persist even after evidence for the schema has been discredited.
b. Schemas slow down mental processing.
c. Schemas are not useful in an ambiguous situation.
d. Schemas involve high-effort controlled thinking.
e. Schemas help prevent self-fulfilling prophecy.

Question 84
Which of the following drugs is least likely to cause tremor?
a. Amphetamine
b. B$_2$ agonist
c. B$_2$ antagonist
d. Caffeine
e. Risperidone

Question 85
A 23-year-old male John tells the psychiatrist during the clinical interview that
there are times when he resorts to wearing clothes of the opposite sex to gain
temporary membership and to feel belonged to the opposite sex. He does not have
any desire for any active gender reassignment surgery. Which one of the following
would be the most likely clinical diagnosis?
a. Dual-role transvestism
b. Fetishism
c. Fetishistic transvestism
d. Paedophilia
e. Exhibitionism

Question 86
Schneider proposed the concept of first-rank symptoms. First-rank symptoms
include all of the following, with the exception of
a. Auditory hallucinations
b. Delusions of passivity
c. Somatic passivity
d. Delusional perception
e. Stupor

Question 87
A 22-year-old male has been referred by his GP to see a psychiatrist. He has been
insisting that his GP refers him over to a surgeon for a gender reassignment
surgery. He claims that he feels like a woman and would prefer to undergo gender
reassignment. Which one of the following would be the most likely clinical diagnosis?
a. Dual-role transvestism
b. Fetishistic transvestism

c. Transexualism

d. Exhibitionism

e. Frotteurism

Question 88

Aggression is an intentional behaviour aimed at harming others. There are several explanations of aggression. Which one of the following is incorrect?

a. Aggression is associated with high levels of testosterone.

b. Aggression is a learned response.

c. Aggression is associated with activation of the amygdala.

d. Aggression can be reinforced by operant conditioning.

e. Aggression is associated with high levels of serotonin.

Question 89

A 35-year-old woman has around five episodes of either mania or depression each year and her GP wants to know her diagnosis based on the DSM-IV-TR criteria. Your answer is

a. Bipolar I disorder

b. Bipolar II disorder

c. Bipolar disorder unspecified

d. Rapid cycling bipolar disorder

e. Ultra-rapid cycling bipolar disorder

Question 90

Which of the following conditions is least likely to cause tremor?

a. Degenerative spinal disease

b. Peripheral neuropathy

c. Hypoglycaernia

d. Thyrotoxicosis

e. Wilson's disease

Question 91

Thirty horses galloped out of the riding stables. According to the rescuers, the flock of 20 horses is perceived as together as they are close to each other. There are 10 horses which are far apart and left behind. Which of the following Gestalt's perception theories best describes the rescuers' observation?

a. Closure

b. Continuity

c. Figure ground

d. Proximity

e. Similarity

Question 92

In this clinical condition, the patient actually believes that a familiar person has taken on different appearances. The clinical diagnosis would be

a. Fregoli syndrome

b. Induced psychosis

c. Capgras syndrome
d. Cotard syndrome
e. Erotomania

Question 93
A 20-year-old male has moderate degree of learning disability. Recently, his girlfriend Angela is pregnant and he is increasingly stressed that their baby would be taken away by the social services. He has resorted to exposing his genitalia to others. Which one of the following would be the most appropriate clinical diagnosis?
a. Dual-role transvestism
b. Fetishistic transvestism
c. Transexualism
d. Exhibitionism
e. Frotteurism

Question 94
Which of the following best defines self-fulfilling prophecy?
a. People's expectation of a person causes a person to act in a different way.
b. People's expectation of a person causes a person to act in line with the expectation.
c. People's expectation of a person influences their behaviour towards that person, resulting in an alteration of that person's behaviour.
d. People's expectation of a person influences their behaviour towards that person, resulting in that person acting in line with the expectation.
e. People's expectation of a person influences their behaviour towards that person, causing the person to act in line with the expectation with attempts to modify the expectation.

Question 95
A 24-year-old woman with borderline personality disorder is detained in a gazette ward under the Mental Health Act after a failed suicide attempt. She has politely asked the psychiatrist to discharge her but without success. She suddenly shouted and swore at a health-care assistant with anger. This defence mechanism is known as
a. Displacement
b. Projection
c. Projective identification
d. Reaction formation
e. Splitting

Question 96
A 20-year-old Indian man is referred by an orthopaedic surgeon for psychosomatic complaints. He consulted an orthopaedic surgeon for low back pain and weakness. Physical examination and investigation showed normal findings. When the orthopaedic surgeon tries to explain the normal findings to him, he complains of passage of semen in urine and requests to see an urologist.

On further inquiry, he admits that he is going to get married soon and he fears about sexual performance. This man suffers from which of the following culture-bound syndromes?
a. Amok
b. Brain fag
c. Dhat
d. Koro
e. Khat

Question 97
You were sent to Haiti for volunteer work after the earthquake in 2010. A 30-year-old man is referred to you for sudden outburst of agitation and aggressive behaviour. He had experienced auditory and visual hallucinations for 3 days and then the psychotic experiences disappeared. There is no family history of schizophrenia. Which of the following terms best described his psychopathology in the local context?
a. Folie induite
b. Déjà pensé
c. La belle indifférence
d. La boufféedélirante
e. L'homme qui rit

Question 98
Which of the following statements is true about essential tremor?
a. Early essential tremor is present at rest.
b. Early essential tremor is absent during action.
c. Essential tremor exacerbates with alcohol use.
d. Essential tremor is more common amongst young people.
e. Familial pattern of essential tremor is common.

Question 99
A father is very concerned about his 18-year-old son. He reports to the CAMHS psychiatrist that his son seems to be always withdrawn during social activities. He is not able to partake in a conversation when there are visitors at home. At times, James is noted to be relatively distressed and would be sweating profusely when attending social events. Which one of the following is the most likely clinical diagnosis?
a. Agoraphobia
b. Social phobia
c. Generalized anxiety disorder
d. Obsessive-compulsive disorder
e. Obsessive-compulsive personality disorder

Question 100
A medical student was asked to do a physical examination on a newly admitted psychiatric patient. When the student tried to move the left arm of the patient and asked him to resist against the force applied, he noted that the patient continued to move the arm in the direction of the force applied. The patient later placed his

arm back in its original position. This is an example of which of the following psychopathologies?
a. Automatic obedience
b. Mannerism
c. Mitgehen
d. Mitmachen
e. Negativism

Question 101
Thirty horses galloped out of the riding stables. According to the rescuers, a flock of twenty horses is perceived as together as they are heading to town at the same speed. The other ten horses do not seem to be together and run all over the place. Which of the following Gestalt's perception theories best describes the rescuers' observation?
a. Continuity
b. Common fate
c. Figure ground
d. Proximity
e. Similarity

Question 102
The following laboratory parameters are reduced in patients suffering from anorexia nervosa, except
a. Cortisol-releasing hormone
b. Luteinizing hormone
c. Potassium
d. Sodium
e. Triiodothyronine

Question 103
A 15-year-old female failed a Mathematics examination. She blamed her teacher for setting so many difficult questions that she did not have enough time to answer all the questions. Which of the following best describes the aforementioned phenomenon?
a. Self-serving bias
b. In-group bias
c. Actor/observer bias
d. Hindsight bias
e. Fundamental attribution bias

Question 104
Based on your understanding of the basic ethical principles in psychiatry, deontology refers to
a. Providing a duty-based approach
b. Acting in the patient's best interest
c. Ensuring that the action performed is considered to be morally right if it would lead to the greatest human pleasure, happiness and satisfaction

d. Ensuring that all individuals receive equal and impartial consideration
e. A doctor's native motive to provide morally correct care to his or her patients, and focus solely on the rightness and wrongness of the actions themselves, and not on the consequences of the actions

Question 105

During routine outpatient review, a patient with a diagnosis of schizophrenia, who has been concordant to his medications and has not had a relapse in the past decade, informs the psychiatrist that he wishes to stop medical treatment. The psychiatrist is concerned and cautions him about the risk of relapse as well as the advantage and benefits on staying on the medications. The patient does have mental capacity to understand and formulate a decision; however, his decision in this case would not be the best option. The psychiatrist feels compelled to go along with the wishes of the patient. This is an example of the ethical principle of
a. Utilitarianism
b. Deontology
c. Nonmaleficence
d. Autonomy
e. Beneficence

Question 106

This refers to a duty that needs to be always acted upon unless it conflicts on a particular occasion with an equal or stronger duty. Which of the following is the correct ethical theory for the above?
a. Duty-based approach
b. Paternalism
c. Prima facie duty
d. Fiduciary duty
e. None of the above

Question 107

You are on the liaison psychiatry rotation and a gastroenterologist wants to consult you whether a schizophrenia patient has the capacity to refuse urgent oesophogastroduodenoscopy (OGD). Which of the following statements about capacity is false?
a. Capacity implies that the patient understands the relevant information about OGD given by the gastroenterologist.
b. Capacity is a clinical opinion given by a clinician.
c. Capacity is a legal term.
d. Capacity requires the mental ability from the patient to make and communicate a decision.
e. The gastroenterologist is expected to provide all relevant information about OGD.

Question 108

A 30-year-old pregnant woman presents to the hospital at 12 weeks' gestation with an 8-week history of severe vomiting, 15 kg of weight loss, and new-onset

weakness, dizziness and blurred vision. Examination of the patient shows confusion, papilloedema, ophthalmoplegia, nystagmus, reduced hearing and truncal ataxia. This patient is most likely suffering from
a. Cerebellar hemisphere haemorrhage
b. Delirium tremens
c. Meningitis
d. Wernicke's encephalopathy
e. Status epilepticus

Question 109
A consultant psychiatrist who is lecturing a group of medical students was explaining the concept of a delusional disorder. Which one of the following is not commonly associated or descriptive of a delusional disorder?
a. Bizarre delusions
b. False belief based on incorrect inference about external reality
c. Firmly sustained despite the beliefs of the normal population
d. Firmly sustained despite there being no obvious proof or evidence against
e. Belief system not accepted by members of one's culture

Question 110
A 20-year-old woman presents with bulimia nervosa. Her height and weight are 160 cm and 60 kg, respectively. What is her body mass index (BMI)?
a. Less than 17
b. 18–19
c. 20–21
d. 22–23
e. More than 23

Question 111
There are several conditions that need to be met in order to reduce prejudice. Which one of the following is not one of those conditions?
a. Equal status
b. Interactions with a member of the out-group
c. Social norms favouring equality
d. Co-operative effort
e. The potential for personal acquaintance

Question 112
The following are criteria for a valid consent, except
a. No misrepresentation of beneficial effects of a proposed treatment
b. No coercion
c. No excessive persuasion
d. No implicit consent
e. No inclusion of information, which is irrelevant to a proposed treatment

Question 113
You are able to assess a 20-year-old man who is aggressive and angry towards the staff at the Accident and Emergency Department. Which of the following measures is least useful?
a. Admit own feelings and inform the patient that the staff are frightened of his aggression and anger.
b. Encourage the patient to verbalize his aggression and anger.
c. Inform the patient that restraint or seclusion will be used if necessary.
d. Inform the patient that physical violence is not acceptable in the hospital setting.
e. Offer the option of using psychotropic medication to calm the patient.

Question 114
A 25-year-old woman presents with asymptomatic unequal pupils. During physical examination, her right eye shows pupillary dilatation with poor constriction to light and accommodation. Examination of lower limbs shows depressed deep tendon reflexes. The patient is most likely suffering from?
a. Argyll Robertson pupils
b. Diabetic neuropathy
c. Holmes–Adie syndrome
d. Horner's syndrome
e. Pupillary defect

Question 115
When interviewing a psychotic patient, it is essential to evaluate for delusions, hallucinations and, most importantly, passivity experiences. Passivity experiences, based on your understanding, include all the following, except
a. Thought insertion
b. Thought withdrawal
c. Thought block
d. Thought broadcast
e. Somatic passivity

Question 116
This is one form of suicide that has been previously proposed by Durkheim, in which the individual commits suicide due to feelings of being increasingly distanced from societal norms.
a. Altruistic suicide
b. Egoistic suicide
c. Acute anomic suicide
d. Chronic anomic suicide
e. None of the above

Question 117
Which of the following statements about mental state examination is correct?
a. During the mental state examination, a psychiatrist should ask a large range of psychopathologies to cover every diagnostic possibility.
b. During mental state examination, probe questions about psychopathology are best framed with technical questions.

c. Mental state examination is best conducted as formal exercise which follows a schema.

d. Serial mental state interrogations are extremely reliable methods of judging the progress of treatment or changes in a patient's mental health.

e. The best clinical approach to mental state examination is in a conversational and informal manner.

Question 118

A 25-year-old schizophrenia patient was admitted to the psychiatric ward under the Mental Health Act. He has not been compliant with oral antipsychotics, and you have proposed depot antipsychotics to prevent relapse since he has not been compliant to the oral medication. He strongly refuses depot injection because he is scared of pain. He does not have psychotic features and understands the risks and benefits associated with depot antipsychotics. Which of the following decisions is the best option based on ethical principles?

a. The doctor should inject him with depot antipsychotics under the Common Law.

b. The doctor should inject him with depot antipsychotics because he was admitted under the Mental Health Act.

c. The doctor should inject him with depot antipsychotics based on his best interests.

d. The doctor should postpone the decision to inject him and consult the guardian board.

e. The doctor should not inject him with depot antipsychotics and respect his wish.

Question 119

According to Durkheim, anomie refers to the social disconnectedness of lack of social norms. All of the following are causes of acute anomie, except

a. Migration

b. Bereavement

c. Redundancy

d. Losses

e. Homelessness

Question 120

Which of the following is most likely to be found in patients with carotid artery stenosis?

a. Amaurosis fugax

b. Bitemporal hemianopia

c. Hemianopia

d. Homonymous quadrantanopia

e. Scotoma

Question 121

The terminology 'institutional neurosis' was previously coined by which one of the following individuals?

a. Hecker

b. Bleuler

c. Goffman
d. Barton
e. Pavlov

Question 122
Which of the following is one of the first SSRIs that was introduced?
a. Zimeldine
b. Fluvoxamine
c. Fluoxetine
d. Sertraline
e. None of the above

Question 123
The following are possible explanations as to why certain psychiatric disorders are more prevalent in each of the social classes, with the exception of
a. Downward social drift
b. Environmental stress
c. Differential labelling
d. Differential treatment
e. Breeder's hypothesis

Question 124
A 25-year-old man with schizophrenia hears his thoughts being spoken aloud whenever he hears the sound of a train whistle. This psychopathological phenomenon is known as
a. Echo de la pensée
b. An extracampine hallucination
c. A functional hallucination
d. Gedankenlautwerden
e. A reflex hallucination

Question 125
A 30-year-old expectant father experiences somatic symptoms when his wife is 3-months pregnant. He complains of morning nausea, decreased appetite, weight gain, constipation and labour pain. The psychopathology being described is
a. Capgras syndrome
b. Couvade syndrome
c. Fregoli syndrome
d. Intermetamorphosis syndrome
e. Othello syndrome

Question 126
A 25-year-old female just went for an interview, hoping to get into Psychiatry as a core trainee. Months later, she was informed that she did not get the position and she believes that it must be because she did not perform well enough during the interview. What kind of attribution is she making?
a. Internal attribution
b. External attribution

c. Primary attribution
d. Secondary attribution
e. Fundamental attribution

Question 127
A medical student wonders what terminology would be more consistent with the following definition 'A set of beliefs about an individual, which is based on prior achievements and other social interactions, and this set of beliefs would interact and influence one's own behaviour'. Which terminology would fit the aforementioned description?
  a. Self-concept
  b. Self-esteem
  c. Self-image
  d. Self-evaluation
  e. Self-perception

Question 128
This is a form of memory that involves confabulation and reports of false events. Which one of the following terms best describes this form of memory?
  a. Anterograde amnesia
  b. Retrograde amnesia
  c. Post-traumatic amnesia
  d. Psychogenic amnesia
  e. False memory

Question 129
Which of the following electroencephalogram (EEG) waveforms typically has a frequency between 4 and 7.5 Hz?
  a. Alpha wave
  b. Beta wave
  c. Delta wave
  d. Gamma wave
  e. Theta wave

Question 130
Two main types of conformity, informational social influence and normative social influence, have been proposed. Based on Asch's conformity theory, normative social conformity would most likely be influenced by
  a. Personality traits
  b. Presence of cognitive dissonance
  c. Type of leadership style
  d. Needing to avoid social rejection
  e. Highly intelligent and socially expressive individuals

Question 131
Cognitive dissonance theory comprises all of the following, except
  a. Selective attention
  b. Selective exposure

c. Selective attention
d. Selective perception
e. Selective retention

Question 132
You have been asked to review a 50-year-old man in your dementia clinic for memory problems. Apart from the memory difficulties, the caregivers also vocalized that the patient had been having other difficulties, characterized as abnormal behaviours and movement. Of importance, they shared that one of their close relatives did suffer from a similar movement disorder and passed away at a very young age. It is likely that the patient you are currently assessing has
a. Wilson's disease
b. Early-onset Alzheimer's disease
c. Huntington's disease
d. Fronto-temporal disorder
e. Lewy body dementia

Question 133
A 30-year-old woman is referred by her GP to you for experiencing multiple episodes of unusual experiences at night. She recalls that a sudden loud sound startled her in the middle of the night. Every movement became impossible and she could not speak. She had breathing difficulty and felt her body vibrating. She saw demons staring at her from the ceiling and hands appearing from the wall to strangle her. The psychopathology being described is
a. Cataplexy
b. Nightmare
c. Night terror
d. Sleep paralysis
e. Somnambulism

Question 134
A 40-year-old woman reports that other patients' heads appear to be enlarged as compared to their actual body size. The psychopathology being described is
a. Delusion of doubles
b. Dysmegalopsia
c. Hallucination
d. Hyperaesthesia
e. Xanthopsia

Question 135
You are about to conduct an animal study. The suppliers of animals have a group of mice with reduced expression of glucocorticoid receptors and behavioural

problems. Which of the following psychiatric disorders in humans would this group of mice closely resemble?
a. Anxiety
b. Dementia
c. Depression
d. Learning disability
e. Schizophrenia

Question 136
A 35-year-old woman suffers from a severe depressive episode. She has three young children studying in a primary school. She is unemployed with no confiding relationship. Which of the following works provides an explanation in her case?
a. Brown and Harris: Social Origins of Depression
b. Durkheim E: Anomie
c. Habermas J: The Theory of Communicative Action
d. Parsons T: The Social System
e. Sullivan HS: The Interpersonal Theory of Psychiatry

Question 137
The following are protective factors against depressive disorder in men, except
a. Employment
b. Excessive social support
c. Good parental care when young
d. Social competence
e. Stable marriage

Question 138
The early psychosis intervention team wants to develop a new community support programme to reduce the suicide risk amongst people with schizophrenia. Which of the following groups of patients is the most at risk of suicide?
a. Female schizophrenia patients
b. Nonpsychotic schizophrenia patients
c. Schizophrenia patients who have never been admitted in the past
d. Schizophrenia patients with delusional expectation
e. Schizophrenia patients with low expectation

Question 139
There is evidence that media reports of suicide can be associated with further suicides. The editor of a local newspaper would like to consult you on the appropriate way to report suicide. You would recommend all of the following, except
a. Encourage distressed people to seek help after reading the article
b. Reporting followed by advertisements for helplines
c. Straightforward factual reporting
d. Suppression in suicide reporting
e. Undramatic reporting

Extended matching items (EMIs)

Theme: Clinical assessment and neuropsychological processes
Options:
   a. Sensory memory
   b. Short-term memory
   c. Explicit memory
   d. Implicit memory

Lead in: Select the most appropriate answer for each of the following. Each option may be used once, more than once or not at all.

Question 140
This particular form of memory comprises largely procedural knowledge.

Question 141
Classical and operant learning involve this particular type of memory.

Question 142
This form of memory involves both the visual association cortex and the auditory association cortex.

Question 143
This form of memory involves both the temporal lobe and the occipital area.

Question 144
This particular form of memory requires a deliberate act of recollection and can be reported verbally.

Theme: Clinical assessment and neuropsychological processes
Options:
   a. Anterograde amnesia
   b. Retrograde amnesia
   c. Post-traumatic amnesia
   d. Psychogenic amnesia
   e. False memory
   f. Transient global amnesia
   g. Amnestic syndrome
   h. Amnesia involving episodic memory

Lead in: Select the most appropriate answer for each of the following. Each option may be used once, more than once or not at all.

Question 145
This refers to the memory loss from the time of the accident to the time that the patient can give a clear account of recent events.

Question 146
This particular form of amnesia is usually associated with indifference.

Question 147
This refers to the loss of memory for events that occurred prior to an event or condition.

Question 148
This particular form of memory is associated with confabulation, report of false events and false confessions.

Question 149
This particular form of memory loss is associated with abrupt onset of disorientation, loss of ability to encode recent memories and retrograde amnesia for variable duration.

Theme: Delusional types
Options:
- a. Delusional jealousy
- b. Delusion of infestation
- c. Delusion of poverty
- d. Delusion of pregnancy
- e. Delusion of reference
- f. Doppelganger
- g. Erotomania
- h. Nihilistic delusion
- i. Somatic delusion

Lead in: Select the most appropriate answer for each of the following. Each option may be used once, more than once or not at all.

Question 150
John came into the emergency department demanding to see the nurse who treated him 2 weeks ago. He claimed that she was in love with him.

Question 151
Ross was sent into the emergency services following an attempt to burn herself in the backyard of her garden. She tells the doctors that she is dead and her intestines are rotting.

Question 152
Peter has been feeling that a double of himself exists somewhere.

Question 153
Mary has been avoiding picking up the phone calls and watching the television. She claims that the people on the television are speaking about her.

Question 154
A core trainee was asked to see Samuel who strongly believes that he is pregnant. He has been feeling this way since he learnt of the news that his wife was pregnant 6 months ago.

Question 155
Gillian has been to multiple dermatologists seeking help as she believes that she needs treatment for her skin condition. She believes that her skin is infested by parasites.

Theme: Suicide and risk factors
Options:
a. Schizophrenia
b. Affective psychosis
c. Neurosis
d. Alcoholism
e. Personality disorder

Lead in: Select the most appropriate answer for each of the following. Each option may be used once, more than once or not at all.

Question 156
The high risk factors for this condition are aggressiveness and impulsivity. Which condition is this?

Question 157
There is an estimated 15% mortality from suicide in this condition. Usually it tends to occur later in the course of the illness and especially in those who are depressed.

Question 158
In this condition, nearly 90% of the patients have a history of para-suicide and with a high proportion having threatened suicide in the preceding month.

Question 159
In this condition, there is 15% mortality from suicide. Men who are older, separated, widowed, living alone and not working are predisposed. Which condition is this?

Question 160
In this condition, there is 10% mortality from suicide. Those who commit suicide are usually young, male and unemployed and usually with chronic relapsing illness.

Theme: Prevention of depressive disorders and suicide
Options:
a. Primary prevention
b. Secondary prevention
c. Tertiary prevention

Lead in: Select the most appropriate answer for each of the following. Each option may be used once, more than once or not at all.

Question 161
It is advisable to have close monitoring of patients post discharge.

Question 162
It is advised that people with a strong family history of depression should space out their pregnancies to prevent poor parenting of the child.

Question 163
This refers to the early detection and treatment of psychiatric conditions.

Question 164
It is recommended that there is better community support and enhanced psychiatric outreach efforts. Which form of prevention is this?

Theme: Psychotherapy

Options:
 a. Aversive conditioning
 b. Chaining
 c. Flooding
 d. Habituation
 e. Insight learning
 f. Latent learning
 g. Penalty
 h. Premack's principle
 i. Reciprocal inhibition
 j. Shaping
 k. Systematic desensitization
 l. Token economy

Lead in: From the aforementioned list of behavioural techniques, select the option that best matches each of the following examples. Each option might be used once, more than once or not at all.

Question 165
The staff of a hostel for learning disability patients want to train their clients to clean up the tables after meals. They develop a successive reinforcing schedule to reward their clients. The clients will be rewarded successively over time for removing their utensils from the dining table into the kitchen. Then they need to wash and dry the utensils and put them back into the right drawers. (Choose one option.)

Question 166
A 2-year-old son of a woman is scared of dogs. His mother tries to reduce his fear by bringing him to see the dogs in the park. The fear-provoking situation is coupled and opposed by putting him on her lap and allowing him to drink his favourite juice. (Choose one option.)

Question 167
A 40-year-old woman staying in London develops fear of the tube (underground metro) and she sees a psychologist for psychotherapy. The psychologist has drafted a behavioural programme in which the patient is advised to start with travelling

between two tube stations with her husband and gradually increase this to more stations without her husband. At the end of the hierarchy, she will travel alone on the long journey from Heathrow terminal station to Cockfosters station along almost the entire length of the Piccadilly line. (Choose one option.)

Theme: Pharmacodynamics

Options:

a. $5\text{-}HT_{1A}$ agonist
b. $5\text{-}HT_{1A}$ partial agonist
c. $5\text{-}HT_{1A}$ antagonist
d. $5\text{-}HT_{2A}$ agonist
e. $5\text{-}HT_{2A}$ partial agonist
f. $5\text{-}HT_{2A}$ antagonist
g. $Alpha_2$ agonist
h. $Alpha_2$ partial agonist
i. $Alpha_2$ antagonist
j. D_2 agonist
k. D_2 partial agonist
l. GABA-A agonist
m. GABA-A antagonist
n. NMDA agonist
o. NMDA antagonist

Lead in: Select the most appropriate psychodynamic mechanisms for the following antidepressants. Each option might be used more than once or not at all.

Question 168
Aripiprazole (Choose three options.)

Question 169
Diazepam (Choose one option.)

Question 170
Lofexidine (Choose one option.)

Theme: Antipsychotics

Options:

a. 1
b. 2
c. 5
d. 15
e. 25
f. 35
g. 45
h. 55
i. 65
j. 75

Lead in: A 17-year-old was referred to the early psychosis team for his first episode of schizophrenia. You prescribe risperidone 1 mg nocte. His mother requests an answer from you on the following questions. Each option might be used once, more than once or not at all.

Question 171
His psychotic symptoms are not controlled. His mother wants to know the minimum effective dose (in mg) of risperidone in his case. (Choose one option.)

Question 172
His psychotic symptoms are under control. His mother wants to know duration of antipsychotic treatment (in months) in his case. (Choose one option.)

Question 173
After 18 months of treatment, the patient has decided to stop the medication. His mother wants to know the risk of relapse in percentage. (Choose one option.)

Theme: Ethics
Options:
 a. Accountability
 b. Autonomy
 c. Beneficence
 d. Categorical imperatives
 e. Cultural relativism
 f. Ethical dilemma
 g. Ethical relativism
 h. Justice
 i. Nonmaleficence
 j. Phronesis
 k. Privacy
 l. Utilitarianism

Lead in: Match the above ethical principles to the following descriptions. Each option may be used once, more than once or not at all.

Question 174
A core trainee knows that he has to be an honest doctor and knows how to apply honesty in balance with other considerations in situations when medical errors occur causing suffering to his patients. (Choose one option.)

Question 175
In a multicultural society, different ethnic groups of people are supposed to have different ethical standards for evaluating acts as right or wrong. (Choose one option.)

Question 176

A lay person in the animal ethics research committee says, 'We can judge the heart of a principal investigator by his treatment of animals'. (Choose one option.)

Theme: DSM-IV-TR

Options:
  a. 1–10
  b. 11–20
  c. 21–30
  d. 31–40
  e. 41–50
  f. 51–60
  g. 61–70
  h. 71–80
  i. 81–90
  j. 91–100

Lead in: Choose the appropriate range of Global Assessment Functioning (GAF) Scale score for the following clinical scenarios. Each option might be used once, more than once or not at all.

Question 177

A 20-year-old university student is referred to you for mild anxiety before an examination. She has good functioning in other areas and is involved in a wide range of university activities. (Choose one option.)

Question 178

A 30-year-old woman is referred to you for frequent shoplifting. She cannot control the impulse to steal and fulfil the diagnostic criteria for kleptomania. She was arrested earlier that resulted in serious impairment in social and occupational functioning. (Choose one option.)

Question 179

A 25-year-old man suffers from schizophrenia and stays in a secure setting because of recurrent episodes of violence. He is unkempt with persistent inability to maintain personal hygiene. (Choose one option.)

Theme: Neuropsychological tests

Options:
  a. Clock Drawing Test
  b. Cognitive Estimates Test
  c. Digit Span
  d. Goldstein's Object Sorting Test
  e. Go–No Go Test
  f. Mini Mental State Examination
  g. National Adult Reading Test

h. Raven's Progressive Matrices
i. Rorschach Ink Blot Test
j. Rey–Osterrieth Complex Figure Test
k. Rivermead Behavioural Memory Test
l. Sach's Sentence Completion Test
m. Stroop Test
n. Wechsler Memory Scale
o. Wisconsin Card Sorting Test

Lead in: A 35-year-old woman presents with sexually transmitted disease and promiscuity. Men have taken advantage of her for sexual advancement. She appears to be apathetic and has difficulty to comprehend the risks associated with sexually transmitted diseases. She has a history of epilepsy and has been unemployed for many years. The nurses are concerned about her IQ level. Which of the aforementioned tests is recommended to assess the following? Each option might be used once, more than once or not at all.

Question 180
Her current performance IQ (Choose one option.)

Question 181
Her concrete thinking (Choose one option.)

Question 182
Her executive function (Choose one option.)

Theme: Freud's dream interpretation

Options:
a. Condensation
b. Displacement
c. Latent content
d. Manifest content
e. Symbolism

Lead in: Match the aforementioned Freudian terms to the following definitions. Each option may be used once, more than once or not at all.

Question 183
Secondary elaboration of acceptable images in a narrative manner and those images are often linked to day residue or events prior to sleep. (Choose one option.)

Question 184
The process where impulses are transferred to acceptable images. (Choose one option.)

Question 185
True meaning of the dream in expressing unconscious thoughts and wishes. (Choose one option.)

Theme: Sleep disorders

Options:
- a. Circadian rhythm sleep disorders
- b. Myoclonic jerks
- c. Non-24-hour sleep-wake syndrome
- d. Nonorganic insomnia
- e. Nightmare
- f. Night terror
- g. Restless leg syndrome
- h. Rhythmic movement disorder
- i. Sleep apnoea
- j. Somnambulism

Lead in: Match the aforementioned sleep disorders to the following clinical scenarios. Each option may be used once, more than once or not at all.

Question 186

A 25-year-old man with a history of epilepsy complains of sudden contractions of muscles on both sides of his body while falling asleep. (Choose one option.)

Question 187

A 28-year-old woman complains that she sleeps at 3 AM but wakes up at 10 AM. She has always been late for work, and she has been dismissed by three companies. (Choose one option.)

Question 188

You are working in the Child and Adolescent Mental Health Service. An anxious mother has brought her 10-year-old son to see you. He has body-rocking and head-banging movements at bedtime and naptimes. (Choose one option.)

Question 189

A 55-year-old man complains that it is impossible for him to sleep at normal times and his sleep-wake cycle is changing every day after he developed bilateral blindness as a result of cataracts. (Choose one option.)

Theme: The British history of insanity defence

Options:
- a. First recorded psychiatric testimony
- b. First right versus wrong test
- c. Offspring of a delusion
- d. The irresistible impulse test
- e. Wild beast test

Lead in: Most of the laws in the Western countries originated in England. The British law was built on the principle of precedence. Identify which of the aforementioned descriptions best describes the following trials. Each option may be used once, more than once or not at all.

Question 190
Edward Oxford, who attempted to murder Queen Victoria, was 18 years old when the offence occurred in 1840. He described in his notebooks how he was to be the instrument of a plot of an imaginary secret society, and to this end, had purchased pistols and practised with them. Because of the medical evidence of mental illness, the defence succeeded and a verdict of 'guilty but insane' was issued. After the trial, Oxford was admitted to Bethlem Royal Hospital. (Choose one option.)

Question 191
Earl Ferrers lived with his wife at Stanton Harold in Leicestershire in the mid-1700s. He was an alcoholic, and his chronic drinking led to psychosis and rage. He also made false accusation against a man, Mr Johnson, who lived in his estate for robbery. He ordered Mr Johnson to come to his house and then shot him. Later, Mr Johnson died and Earl Ferrers was charged with murder. He was tried by his fellows in the Tower of London. A plea of insanity was refused and Earl Ferrers was found guilty and sentenced to hang. (Choose one option.)

Question 192
James Hadfield fired a pistol at King George III at the Theatre Royal during the playing of the national anthem on the evening of 15 May 1800. Hadfield was tried for treason and was defended by a prominent barrister. Later, Hadfield pleaded insanity. Three doctors testified that Hadfield had delusions which were the consequence of his earlier head injuries. Hadfield was detained in Bethlem Royal Hospital for the rest of his life. (Choose one option.)

Theme: Piaget's cognitive development
Options:
  a. Accommodation
  b. Animism
  c. Artificialism
  d. Assimilation
  e. Centration
  f. Circular reaction
  g. Egocentrism
  h. Failure of conservation
  i. Finalism
  j. Hypothetico-deductive thinking
  k. Object permanence
  l. Mastery of conservation
  m. Reflective thinking
  n. Seriation
  o. Syncretic thought
  p. Transductive reasoning
  q. Sensorimotor stage
  r. Preoperational stage
  s. Concrete operation stage
  t. Formal operational stage

Lead in: Identify which of the aforementioned terms and stages derived by Piaget best describes the following descriptions. Each option may be used once, more than once or not at all.

Question 193
Children see the world from their own standpoint but cannot appreciate that other people may see things differently. (Choose two options.)

Question 194
An infant can add new information into the existing schema. (Choose two options.)

Question 195
An adolescent can hold several possible explanations in mind for a phenomenon and think of possible outcomes. (Choose two options.)

GET THROUGH MRCPSYCH PAPER A1: MOCK EXAMINATION

Question 1 Answer: b, Thought withdrawal
Explanation: This refers to thought withdrawal. This is the delusion that one's thoughts are being removed from one's mind by an external agency.

Reference: Puri BK, Hall A, Ho R (2014). *Revision Notes in Psychiatry*. London: CRC Press, p. 7.

Question 2 Answer: b, The patient would have repeated regular fixed patterns of movement that are not goal directed.
Explanation: (b) is the correct answer. Stereotypies refer to repeated, regular, fixed patterns of movement, or even speech, which are not goal directed.

Reference: Puri BK, Hall A, Ho R (2014). *Revision Notes in Psychiatry*. London: CRC Press, p. 3.

Question 3 Answer: e, Allow the GP to strengthen the patient and help them to stabilize
Explanation: The key objective of supportive psychotherapy is to help strength defences and help the patient to enhance his or her adaptive capacity. It does help to maintain and improve self-esteem of the patient, but this is not done so by simply agreeing with them. It is helpful in improving symptoms, preventing relapses and also developing adaptive and reasonable behaviour. It also helps patients set goals and have a positive thinking.

Reference: Puri BK, Hall A, Ho R (2014). *Revision Notes in Psychiatry*. London: CRC Press, p. 331.

Question 4 Answer: a, Neuroleptic malignant syndrome
Explanation: The most likely clinical diagnosis would be neuroleptic malignant syndrome. Samuel has some of the signs and symptoms that are characteristic of the condition, and in addition, he was just initiated on a course of antipsychotics. Neuroleptic malignant syndrome is characterized by hyperthermia, fluctuating

level of consciousness, muscular rigidity, autonomic dysfunction such as tachycardia, labile blood pressure, pallor, sweating and urinary continence.

Reference: Puri BK, Hall A, Ho R (2014). *Revision Notes in Psychiatry*. London: CRC Press, p. 253.

Question 5 Answer: d, Confides readily
Explanation: All of the aforementioned are characteristic of paranoid personality disorder, with the exception that the individual usually does not confide readily due to chronic fears of betrayal. The common clinical features are as follows: grudges are usually held without justification; excessive sensitivity to setbacks; threats and hidden meanings are read into benign remarks; fidelity of spouse is unjustifiably doubted; attacks on character or reputation are perceived; confides reluctantly because of fears of betrayal and trustworthiness of others is doubted without due cause.

Reference: Puri BK, Hall A, Ho R (2014). *Revision Notes in Psychiatry*. London: CRC Press, p. 442.

Question 6 Answer: d, There are times when they desire for the presence of close friends.
Explanation: These individuals usually have no desire for or possession of any close friends or confiding relationships. The common clinical features include solitary lifestyle, indifference to praise and criticism, no interest in relationships, no interest in sexual experience, solitary activities and cold and detached emotions.

Reference: Puri BK, Hall A, Ho R (2014). *Revision Notes in Psychiatry*. London: CRC Press, p. 440.

Question 7 Answer: a, Substance abuse
Explanation: Bulimics are more prone to developing substance-related disorders. They are more likely to abuse substance (20%). Their lifetime rates of alcohol dependence are considered to be much higher as well. The presence of these factors also predicts poorer outcomes for bulimics: depression, personality disturbance, greater severity of symptoms, longer duration of symptoms, low self-esteem, substance abuse and childhood obesity.

Reference: Puri BK, Hall A, Ho R (2014). *Revision Notes in Psychiatry*. London: CRC Press, p. 584.

Question 8 Answer: e, The conditioned stimulus is paired with a second conditioned stimulus, which, on presentation, by itself elicits the original condition response.
Explanation: (e) is the correct definition of higher-order conditioning. (a) refers to delayed conditioning, (b) simultaneous conditioning, (c) trace conditioning and (d) backward conditioning.

Reference: Puri BK, Hall A, Ho R (2014). *Revision Notes in Psychiatry*. London: CRC Press, p. 25.

Question 9 Answer: d, Nihilistic delusion
Explanation: Nihilistic delusion or Cotard's syndrome is the belief that one is dead or the external world does not exist. It can also take the form of believing that parts of the body do not exist. Nihilistic delusions can be secondary to severe depression, schizophrenia or an organic disorder.

Reference and Further Reading: Puri BK, Hall AD (2002). *Revision Notes in Psychiatry*. London: Arnold, p. 382.

Question 10 Answer: c, Thought broadcasting
Explanation: Thought broadcasting is the delusion that one's thoughts are being broadcast out loud, for example via a radio or by an external voice, such that others can perceive them. Thought broadcasting is a type of thought alienation under the passivity phenomenon.

Reference and Further Reading: Puri BK, Hall AD (2002). *Revision Notes in Psychiatry*. London: Arnold, p. 153.

Question 11 Answer: d, Premack's principle
Explanation: Premack's principle states that more probable behaviours can be used to reinforce less probable behaviours. If high-probability behaviours (i.e. video games) are made contingent upon lower-probability behaviours (i.e. doing homework), the lower-probability behaviours are more likely to occur.

Reference and Further Reading: Mitchell WS, Stoffelmayr BE (1973). Application of the Premack principle to the behavioral control of extremely inactive schizophrenics. *Journal of Applied Behaviour Analysis*, 6: 419–423.

Question 12 Answer: c, Serotonergic and noradrenergic reuptake inhibitor
Explanation: Duloxetine belongs to the serotonergic and noradrenergic reuptake inhibitor class.

Reference: Puri BK, Hall A, Ho R (2014). *Revision Notes in Psychiatry*. London: CRC Press, p. 239.

Question 13 Answer: a, Amisulpride
Explanation: Amisulpride is the only antipsychotic amongst the options given that belongs to the class of a substituted benzamide.

Reference: Puri BK, Hall A, Ho R (2014). *Revision Notes in Psychiatry*. London: CRC Press, p. 238.

Question 14 Answer: b, Lithium
Explanation: The usage of lithium would result in the aforementioned clinical disorder. Long-term treatment with lithium may give rise to the following: thyroid function abnormalities such as goitre, hypothyroidism and memory impairments, nephrotoxicity, cardiovascular changes such as T-wave flattening on the ECG and also arrhythmias.

Reference: Puri BK, Hall A, Ho R (2014). *Revision Notes in Psychiatry*. London: CRC Press, p. 254.

Question 15 Answer: a, De Clerambault's syndrome
Explanation: De Clerambault's syndrome or erotomania is a condition in which a person holds the delusional belief that someone of a higher social status is in love with him or her. This condition is more common in women than in men.

Reference and Further Reading: Puri BK, Hall AD (2002). *Revision Notes in Psychiatry*. London: Arnold, p. 382.

Question 16 Answer: c, This process was developed in conjunction with both classical conditioning and operant conditioning.
Explanation: This process is known as extinction. Extinction has treatment implication in deconditioning anxiety responses from conditioned stimulus. Extinction applies to both biological and psychological conditioned responses. The conditioned responses usually disappear gradually and return by spontaneous recovery.

Reference and Further Reading: Puri BK, Treasaden I (eds) (2010). *Psychiatry: An Evidence-Based Text*. London: Hodder Arnold, p. 199.

Question 17 Answer: d, 4 days
Explanation: The duration for a manic episode is usually one week. In contrast, the duration for a hypomanic episode is only 4 days. Hypomanic episode has the same requirement of the number of symptoms as manic episode. The only difference is that patients should have no impairment in functioning.

Reference: Puri BK, Hall A, Ho R (2014). *Revision Notes in Psychiatry*. London: CRC Press, p. 378.

Question 18 Answer: a, Pervasive development disorder
Explanation: It has been well established and suggested that the lack of development of a theory of mind has been associated with disorders such as autism. In primate research, theory of mind refers to the abilities of primates to mentalize their fellows. In humans, the theory of mind refers to the ability of most normal people to comprehend the thought processes (such as attention, feelings, beliefs, false beliefs and knowledge) of others. Research into children would tend to suggest that at the age of 3 years, normal human children do not acknowledge false belief as they have difficulty in differentiating belief from world. Formulating a theory of mind appears not to be inevitable, but relies on cognitive changes that happen around the age of 4.

Reference: Puri BK, Hall A, Ho R (2014). *Revision Notes in Psychiatry.* London: CRC Press, p. 59.

Question 19 Answer: a, Bowlby

Explanation: Attachment theory was proposed by Bowlby in 1969. Attachment refers to the tendency of infants to remain close to certain people (attachment figures) with whom they share strong positive emotional ties. Monotropic attachment is when the attachment is to one individual, usually the mother. Polytropic attachment is less common. Attachment usually takes place from infant to mother. In contrast, neonatal–maternal bonding takes place in the opposite direction. Both processes can start immediately after birth.

Reference: Puri BK, Hall A, Ho R (2014). *Revision Notes in Psychiatry.* London: CRC Press, p. 63.

Question 20 Answer: e, Increased tubular secretion

Explanation: All of the aforementioned are pharmacokinetics parameters that are changed in the elderly, with the exception of (e). There would be an increment in the percentage of the total body fat, an increase in the gastric pH, a reduction in the renal clearance as well as a decrease in the serum protein binding. However, it is important to note that the rate of gastrointestinal absorption remains the same. There is no evidence currently that mentions that the rate or the extent of absorption of orally administered psychotropic medications is changed in the elderly. Reduction in clearance may increase the steady-state plasma drug concentration in old people. Hence, because of the lowered renal clearance, lithium doses in the elderly should be approximately 50% lower than in the young. All other psychotropic drugs are cleared by hepatic biotransformation, which is reduced with age. As a result, the half-life of psychotropic medication can be markedly prolonged, having residual effects for weeks after discontinuation.

Reference: Puri BK, Hall A, Ho R (2014). *Revision Notes in Psychiatry.* London: CRC Press, p. 685.

Question 21 Answer: d, Auditory

Explanation: Depression with psychotic features typically is associated with auditory hallucinations. The hallucinations are usually either second person or derogatory in nature. Previous studies (Spiker et al., 1985) have found a superior response when an antidepressant and an antipsychotic are used in combination in psychotic depression.

Reference: Puri BK, Hall A, Ho R (2014). *Revision Notes in Psychiatry.* London: CRC Press, p. 8.

Question 22 Answer: c, It occurs usually in the outer objective space.

Explanation: It is classified as a pseudohallucination and usually would arise from the subjective inner space of the mind. A pseudohallucination lacks the substantiality of normal perceptions. An eidetic image is a vivid and detailed reproduction of a previous perception.

Reference: Puri BK, Hall A, Ho R (2014). *Revision Notes in Psychiatry*. London: CRC Press, p. 8.

Question 23 Answer: c, Classical conditioning
Explanation: In post-traumatic stress disorder, the patient tries to avoid stimuli (e.g. army camp, firearms, the word, 'Iraq') associated with severe trauma by classical conditioning. This is not avoidance or escape conditioning because the aversive event (i.e. gun battle and resulting injury) will not occur in the UK. Escape conditioning, avoidance conditioning and punishments are known collectively as aversive conditioning.

Reference and Further Reading: Puri BK, Treasaden I (eds) (2010). *Psychiatry: An Evidence-Based Text*. London: Hodder Arnold, pp. 197–200.

Question 24 Answer: a, Habituation
Explanation: Habituation is the decrease in response to a stimulus after repeated exposure. This is an essential component in the treatment of OCD using exposure and response prevention. The aim of the exposure technique is to reduce the levels of anxiety associated with the eliciting stimuli through habituation.

Reference and Further Reading: Puri BK, Hall AD (2002). *Revision Notes in Psychiatry*. London: Arnold, p. 7.

Question 25 Answer: c, Delusional perception
Explanation: A delusional perception is a normal perception falsely interpreted by the patient and held as being significant to him. It is one of Schneider's first-rank symptoms.

Reference and Further Reading: Sims A (2003). *Symptoms of the Mind: An Introduction to Descriptive Psychopathology*. London: Saunders, p. 166.

Question 26 Answer: a, An example is when a young animal learns the characteristics of its parents.
Explanation: Psychological imprinting refers to learning occurring at a particular stage of life. The learning process is rapid and independent of the consequences of behaviour. Genetic imprinting is a different concept. When the expression of inheritance is altered, depending upon whether it was passed to the foetus through the egg or the sperm, the phenomenon is known as genetic imprinting. The term 'imprinting' refers to the fact that some genes are stamped with a 'memory' of the parent from whom they came. In the cells of an infant, it is possible to tell which chromosome copy came from the maternal chromosome and which was inherited from the paternal chromosome. This expression of the gene is called a 'parent-of-origin effect' and was first described by Helen Crouse in 1960.

References: Barlow-Stewart K (2007). Genetic imprinting, in *Genetic Fact Sheets* (6th edition). Sydney, AU: Centre for Genetics Education; Crouse HV (1960). The controlling element in sex chromosome behavior in Sciara. *Genetics*, 45: 1429–1443.

Question 27 Answer: d, Antihistaminergic
Explanation: Histamine H_1 and H_3 receptors have been specifically recognized as mediators of energy intake and expenditure, and histamine agonists have been shown to attenuate body weight gain in humans. On the other hand, the first-generation antipsychotics are known to be associated with antihistamine effects. Furthermore, the antihistamine properties of first-generation antipsychotics may sedate the patients and slow down the metabolism. This will contribute to the weight gain.

Reference: Masaki T, Yoshimatsu H (2010). Neuronal histamine and its receptors: Implication of the pharmacological treatment of obesity. *Current Medicinal Chemistry*, 17: 4587–4592.

Question 28 Answer: e, The mild or moderate cognitive impairment due to long-term use of alcohol would not improve with abstinence.
Explanation: All of the aforementioned are true and generally observed in individuals with alcoholic dementia with the exception of (e). Those who have abused alcohol chronically for some years commonly do suffer from mild-to-moderate cognitive impairment. However, these impairments do improve over a number of years of abstinence. Women who are keen to suffer physical complications of alcohol abuse earlier than men also develop cognitive impairment much earlier in their drinking histories. A CT or structural MRI scan of the brain in alcoholics commonly shows ventricular enlargement and sulcal widening, which does not correlate with the degree of cognitive impairment and would also resolve on quitting drinking.

Reference: Puri BK, Hall A, Ho R (2014). *Revision Notes in Psychiatry*. London: CRC Press, p. 518.

Question 29 Answer: c, Avoidant attachment
Explanation: The child seemed to be displaying what might be avoidant attachment. When a child has this form of attachment, he would be keeping a distance from his mother and may even sometimes ignore his mother. Avoidance attachment is usually caused by rejection by his mother and might lead to chronic problems such as poor social functioning later in life.

Reference: Puri BK, Hall A, Ho R (2014). *Revision Notes in Psychiatry*. London: CRC Press, p. 64.

Question 30 Answer: b, Disorganized schizophrenia
Explanation: The ICD-10 only includes the following subtypes for schizophrenia: paranoid, hebephrenic, catatonic, undifferentiated and residual.

Reference: Puri BK, Hall A, Ho R (2014). *Revision Notes in Psychiatry*. London: CRC Press, p. 353.

Question 31 Answer: c, Presence of suggestibility
Explanation: This means that one is easily influenced by others or circumstances. Suggestibility is usually present in the aforementioned disorders.

Reference: Puri BK, Hall A, Ho R (2014). *Revision Notes in Psychiatry*. London: CRC Press, p. 451.

Question 32 Answer: a, Assess attention
Explanation: Serial seven or serial three tests mainly assesses attention. If the patient cannot perform calculation, the interviewer can ask the patient to count the month starting from December in descending order or spell the word, 'WORLD' backwards.

Reference and Further Reading: Puri BK, Treasaden I (eds) (2010). *Psychiatry: An Evidence-Based Text*. London: Hodder Arnold, pp. 92, 179–194, 502–503, 515, 516, 786, 1101.

Question 33 Answer: d, 1 year
Explanation: The ICD-10 classification system states that the diagnosis of alcohol dependence would be made if there are three or more of the classical symptoms that have been present together at some time over the past 1 year.

Reference: Puri BK, Hall A, Ho R (2014). *Revision Notes in Psychiatry*. London: CRC Press, p. 508.

Question 34 Answer: d, 48 hours
Explanation: The onset of withdrawal fits usually occurs within 48 hours of quitting drinking. Oral medications such as lorazepam can be used as first-line treatment for delirium tremens or seizures.

Reference: Puri BK, Hall A, Ho R (2014). *Revision Notes in Psychiatry*. London: CRC Press, p. 516.

Question 35 Answer: c, Fregoli syndrome
Explanation: In Fregoli syndrome, the patient has a delusional belief that a familiar person has taken on different appearances. The patient often believes that he or she is being persecuted by the person in disguise. Primary causes include schizophrenia and organic disorder.

Reference and Further Reading: Puri BK, Hall AD (2002). *Revision Notes in Psychiatry*. London: Arnold, p. 382.

Question 36 Answer: c, Recognition
Explanation: Recognition is the ability to match a stimulus to stored material in memory. Recognition is easier than recall because the cue is the actual object or fact one is trying to recognize. There is often a sense of familiarity because one detects a match between the cue and what is in their memory. An example of recognition is multiple-choice tests, where the answer is present and there is a need to match the answer with what is known in memory.

Reference and Further Reading: Ciccarelli SK, Meyer GE (2006). *Psychology.* Upper Saddle River, NJ: Pearson Education, pp. 227–228; Puri BK, Treasaden I (eds) (2010). *Psychiatry: An Evidence-Based Text.* London: Hodder Arnold, p. 250.

Question 37 Answer: e, 75%

Explanation: If she stops taking the antidepressant, the chance of relapse is 75%. This 32-year-old woman should be reminded that fluoxetine is safe during pregnancy based on a large amount of clinical information on the effects associated with prenatal exposure to fluoxetine. Fluoxetine is not associated with a greater risk of miscarriage or major congenital malformation. Third-trimester use of fluoxetine has been linked with higher rates of perinatal complications (e.g. tachypnea, jitteriness, premature delivery) in some patients.

References: Hendrick V, Altshuler L (2002). Management of major depression during pregnancy. *Am J Psychiatry,* 159: 1667–1673; Cohen LS, Altshuler LL, Stowe ZN (1999). MGH Prospective Study: Depression in pregnancy in women who decrease or discontinue antidepressant medication, in *1999 Annual Meeting Syllabus and Proceedings Summary.* Washington, DC: American Psychiatric Association; Einarson A, Selby P, Koren G (2001). Abrupt discontinuation of psychotropic drugs during pregnancy: Fear of teratogenic risk and impact of counseling. *J Psychiatry Neurosci,* 26: 44–48.

Question 38 Answer: d, Histrionic personality disorder

Explanation: The most likely diagnosis is histrionic personality disorder. In this personality disorder, individuals usually crave to be the centre of attention. They value their own appearances and view certain interpersonal relationships as much closer compared to others. They are seductive in nature and might also have exaggerated expression of emotions.

Reference: Puri BK, Hall A, Ho R (2014). *Revision Notes in Psychiatry.* London: CRC Press, p. 451.

Question 39 Answer: c, Assimilation

Explanation: Assimilation is defined as incorporation of a new or novel information into existing thought patterns. Schemas are cognitive structures or patterns of behaviour or knowledge. Accommodation involves adjustment or modification of existing schemas to facilitate comprehension of new information.

Reference and Further Reading: Puri BK, Treasaden I (eds) (2010). *Psychiatry: An Evidence-Based Text.* London: Hodder Arnold, pp. 113–115.

Question 40 Answer: e, Other neurotic disorder F48

Explanation: Neurasthenia is defined as the persistent complaint of mental tiredness, even after minimal exertion. It is classified under other neurotic disorder F48, in the ICD-10 diagnostic criteria.

Reference: Puri BK, Hall A, Ho R (2014). *Revision Notes in Psychiatry*. London: CRC Press, p. 18.

Question 41 Answer: d, Checking with the patient whether he is able to tell the occupation or the identity of a doctor or an allied health-care staff
Explanation: Orientation is a common aspect covered by the MMSE (Folstein et al., 1975), the ACE-R (Mioshi et al., 2006) and also the MoCA (Nasreddine et al., 2005). Orientation to person would be the best assessment of orientation in an inpatient. It is usually affected much later, as compared to other domains of assessment.

Reference: Puri BK, Hall A, Ho R (2014). *Revision Notes in Psychiatry*. London: CRC Press, p. 689.

Question 42 Answer: c, BPRS
Explanation: For routine screening purposes, the CAGE questionnaire is usually used. Positive answers to two or more of the four questions are indicative of problem drinking. The Clinical Institute Withdrawal Assessment (CIWA) Scale is usually used to quantify the severity of alcohol withdrawal syndrome and monitor patients during detoxification. AUDIT and MAST are also appropriate questionnaires. BPRS is a rating scale that clinicians and researchers usually use to measure psychiatric symptoms such as depression, anxiety and also hallucinations and other psychotic psychopathology.

Reference: Puri BK, Hall A, Ho R (2014). *Revision Notes in Psychiatry*. London: CRC Press, pp. 521–523.

Question 43 Answer: b, Primary memory has been found to have a duration of approximately 7 seconds
Explanation: Short-term (primary or working) memory has a storage duration of 20 seconds, unless the information is rehearsed. Primacy and recency effects are collectively known as the serial position effect and account for the increased probability of correctly recalling information in the beginning and the end of a list of items. Chunking involves rearranging information into chunks such that there is an increased amount of information in each chunk, thereby increasing short-term memory capacity. There is a limited capacity of 7 ± 2 registers.

Reference and Further Reading: Puri BK, Treasaden I (eds) (2010). *Psychiatry: An Evidence-Based Text*. London: Hodder Arnold, pp. 247–249; Puri BK, Hall AD (2002). *Revision Notes in Psychiatry*. London: Arnold, pp. 17, 21.

Question 44 Answer: d, Somatic delusion
Explanation: Somatic delusion is based on false belief being held at absolute conviction in explaining disturbance in an organ. Nihilistic delusion is a delusion of nonexistence of either oneself or the entire world. Hypochondriasis refers to the misinterpretation of physical signs and symptoms unrealistically as indicative of serious disease.

Reference and Further Reading: Campbell RJ (1996). *Psychiatric Dictionary*. Oxford, UK: Oxford University Press.

Question 45 Answer: b, 1%–3%
Explanation: A study of prenatal exposures to sertraline, paroxetine and fluvoxamine found that the rates of major malformations and preterm labour were no higher than those of non-exposed subjects. The rate of major malformation is around 1%–3%.

Reference: Kulin NA, Pastuszak A, Sage SR, Schick-Boschetto B, Spivey G, Feldkamp M, Ormond K, Matsui D, Stein-Schechman AK, Cook L, Brochu J, Rieder M, Koren G (1998). Pregnancy outcome following maternal use of the new selective serotonin reuptake inhibitors: A prospective controlled multicenter study. *JAMA*, 279: 609–610.

Question 46 Answer: b, The remission rate was 20%.
Explanation: The remission rate was noted to be around 30%, instead of 20%. It is correct that one-third of participants reached a remission or virtual absence of symptoms during the initial phase of the study, with an additional 10%–15% experiencing some improvement. There were consistent findings across both standard and patient-rated depression rating scales. It was noted that one in three depressed patients who previously did not achieve remission using an antidepressant became symptom-free with the help of augmenting with another antidepressant. One in four achieved remission after switching to a different antidepressant. At level 3, 20% of participants became symptom-free after 9 weeks. Patients taking T3 complained of fewer side effects than those taking lithium.

Reference: Puri BK, Hall A, Ho R (2014). *Revision Notes in Psychiatry*. London: CRC Press, p. 392.

Question 47 Answer: a, Schizotypal personality disorder
Explanation: Schizotypal personality disorder is classified differently in the ICD-10. It is clustered under Schizophrenia, Schizotypal and delusional disorders are given a code of F21 Schizotypal personality disorder.

Reference: Puri BK, Hall A, Ho R (2014). *Revision Notes in Psychiatry*. London: CRC Press, p. 24.

Question 48 Answer: d, Lewy body dementia
Explanation: The aetiology given the clinical presentation and the scan results are suggestive of Lewy body dementia. Dementia with Lewy bodies is the third most common causes of dementia. Lewy bodies are usually found located in the cingulated gyrus, the cortex and the substantia nigra. They contain eosinophilic inclusion with high amyloid content but absence of tau pathology. The specialized scan refers to the DaTSCAN.

Reference: Puri BK, Hall A, Ho R (2014). *Revision Notes in Psychiatry*. London: CRC Press, p. 702.

Question 49 Answer: c, Onset is usually gradual and slow
Explanation: Onset is usually rapid, intense and unexpected. According to ICD-10 criteria, koro is not just restricted to men but also applies to women.

Reference and Further Reading: Puri BK, Treasaden I (eds) (2010). *Psychiatry: An Evidence-Based Text*. London: Hodder Arnold, pp. 309–318; World Health Organisation (1994). ICD-10 Classification of Mental and Behavioural Disorders. Edinburgh, UK: Churchill Livingstone.

Question 50 Answer: e, Taijinkyofusho
Explanation: This is a common culture-bound syndrome that occurs in Japan. The individual is afraid that he would make others uncomfortable through his inappropriate behaviour or self-presentation (such as offensive odour or physical blemish).

Reference: Puri BK, Hall A, Ho R (2014). *Revision Notes in Psychiatry*. London: CRC Press, p. 462.

Question 51 Answer: d, K-SADS
Explanation: Around 6.6% of adolescents have been diagnosed with depression at the age of 15 years; 60%–70% of depressive symptoms are associated with adverse life events. Symptoms are largely similar to an adult's presentation, with a minimum of 2 weeks of sadness, irritability, loss of interest and loss of pleasure. The diagnostic interview that is recommended would be the Kiddie-Sads-Present and Lifetime Version. It helps to provide information about current diagnosis as well as symptoms over the past one year.

Reference: Puri BK, Hall A, Ho R (2014). *Revision Notes in Psychiatry*. London: CRC Press, p. 648.

Question 52 Answer: c, Social role
Explanation: Social role is the behaviour expected of a person who is in a particular social position. The experiment demonstrated that social roles can be so powerful that the personal identities and personalities can get lost. Social identity is part of an individual's self-concept based on one's view of self in a particular social group. Social categorization is the assignment of people to groups based on common characteristics the new person has with the people in a particular category. Social norms are the acceptable behaviours, values and beliefs of a group. Social influence is the effect of words, actions or presence of others on a person's thoughts, feelings and behaviour.

Reference and Further Reading: Aronson E, Wilson TD, Akert RM (2007). *Social Psychology*. Upper Saddle River, NJ: Prentice Hall, pp. 274–275.

Question 53 Answer: c, Those in a couple relationship
Explanation: Induced psychosis is a delusional disorder shared by two people who are usually closely linked together emotionally. Usually, one of the individuals has

a genuine psychotic disorder, and his or her psychotic disorder is then transferred or induced in the other individual. The other individual may be dependent or less intelligent than the first person.

Reference: Puri BK, Hall A, Ho R (2014). *Revision Notes in Psychiatry*. London: CRC Press, p. 373.

Question 54 Answer: b, Convert the phone number into six items: 18-00-33-77-92–4

Explanation: Working memory holds 7±2 bits of information. The difficulty arises because there are eleven items or digits in this phone number. By chunking, the 11-item phone number is converted into smaller number of pieces of information. The working memory should be able to handle six items or six bits. Option (a) is not easy to remember because there are too many digits in each item.

Reference and Further Reading: Puri BK, Treasaden I (eds) (2010). *Psychiatry: An Evidence-Based Text*. London: Hodder Arnold, pp. 247-248, 504, 505, 507.

Question 55 Answer: c, occur in stage 1 of non-REM sleep

Explanation: Hypnagogic hallucinations are usually auditory and occur at the point of falling asleep. Hypnagogic hallucinations do not require antipsychotic medication.

Reference and Further Reading: Rechtschaffen A, Kales A (1968). A Manual of Standardized Terminology, Techniques and Scoring System for Sleep Stages of Human Subjects. Washington, DC: Public Health Service, U.S. Government Printing.

Question 56 Answer: d, The course organizer should emphasize the participants to store the information in their brain and advise them to reduce access to the information during the course.

Explanation: Option (a) is useful. The lecturer can either present information in small segments or use chunking to convert larger amounts into smaller number of pieces of information. Option (b) is useful. The lecturer should project information onto a screen; this will minimize the demand on working memory. Option (c) is useful and course organizers should rehearse key points often enough to keep them active in working memory. Option (d) is not useful. The course organizer should allow the participants to have access to the information whenever it is needed. Option (e) is useful. Information is temporarily stored in working memory for 15–30 seconds and needs to be transferred to long-term memory as soon as possible. The course organizer should also help the participants to retrieve the information to working memory whenever it is needed.

Reference and Further Reading: Puri BK, Treasaden I (eds) (2010). *Psychiatry: An Evidence-Based Text*. London: Hodder Arnold, pp. 247–248, 504, 505, 507.

Question 57 Answer: c, Fregoli syndrome
Explanation: In Fregoli syndrome, a patient perceives that a familiar person has assumed another bodily form. In reverse Fregoli syndrome, a patient believes that other people are suffering from Fregoli syndrome and misidentifying himself or herself. In Capgras syndrome, a familiar person is perceived as being replaced by identical doubles. There are two types of subjective double syndrome. In subjective double syndrome, a patient perceives that his or her own double is projected onto another person but cannot see himself or herself in the mirror.

Reference and Further Reading: Puri BK, Hall AD (2002). *Revision Notes in Psychiatry*. London: Arnold, p. 382.

Question 58 Answer: b, Brain fag
Explanation: This is considered to be a widespread low-grade stress syndrome that has been described in many parts of Africa. It is commonly encountered among students. Five symptom types have been described: head symptoms, eye symptoms, difficulties in grasping the meaning of the spoken or written words, poor reactivity and sleepiness on studying.

Reference: Puri BK, Hall A, Ho R (2014). *Revision Notes in Psychiatry*. London: CRC Press, p. 463.

Question 59 Answer: d, Phobias
Explanation: The common defence mechanism used in phobia includes displacement, projection and denial.

Reference: Puri BK, Hall A, Ho R (2014). *Revision Notes in Psychiatry*. London: CRC Press, p. 137.

Question 60 Answer: c, Denial
Explanation: Klein believed that the infant was capable of object relations. Klein believed and proposed the concept of paranoid-schizoid position, which developed as a result of the frustration during the first year of life with pleasurable objects such as the good breast. The paranoid-schizoid position, characterized by isolation and persecutory fears, developed as a result of the infant viewing the world as part objects, using the following defence mechanisms: introjection, projective identification and splitting.

Reference: Puri BK, Hall A, Ho R (2014). *Revision Notes in Psychiatry*. London: CRC Press, p. 135.

Question 61 Answer: a, Wechsler Adult Intelligence Scale
Explanation: The Wechsler Adult Intelligence Scale (WAIS-IV) was released in 2008. It allows for four index scores to be derived: the verbal comprehension index, the perceptual reasoning index, the working memory index and the

processing speed index. It is regarded as the most evidenced based and the gold standard in the assessment of intelligence. It is important to note that the Full Scale IQ follows a normal distribution with a mean of 100 and a standard deviation of 15.

Reference: Puri BK, Hall A, Ho R (2014). *Revision Notes in Psychiatry*. London: CRC Press, p. 91.

Question 62 Answer: b, In attribution theory, people tend to attribute their own behaviour to their personality traits.
Explanation: In attribution theory, people tend to attribute their own behaviour to situational factors and attribute other people's behaviour to dispositional factors. This is known as fundamental attribution error. A person's feelings can influence attribution. For example, in a happy marriage, the spouse tends to attribute positive events to an internal attribution and negative events to an external cause. In an unhappy marriage, the reverse is true.

Reference and Further Reading: Puri BK, Hall AD (2002). *Revision Notes in Psychiatry*. London: Arnold, p. 52.

Question 63 Answer: b, Depressive stupor
Explanation: The most likely clinical diagnosis is depressive stupor. The patient might be unresponsive, akinetic, mute and fully conscious. Following the episode, the patient can recall the events that have taken place. It is essential to note that there might be periods of excitement that might occur between episodes of stupor.

Reference: Puri BK, Hall A, Ho R (2014). *Revision Notes in Psychiatry*. London: CRC Press, p. 380.

Question 64 Answer: d, Self-awareness
Explanation: Déjà vu refers to how an individual feels that the current situation has been seen or previously experienced. Jamais vu refers to the illusion of failure to recognize a familiar situation.

Reference: Puri BK, Hall A, Ho R (2014). *Revision Notes in Psychiatry*. London: CRC Press, p. 9.

Question 65 Answer: b, Thought insertion
Explanation: James is experiencing what is known as thought insertion. This is a delusional ideation that an individual's thoughts are no longer one's own, but are inserted into the mind by some external agency.

Reference: Puri BK, Hall A, Ho R (2014). *Revision Notes in Psychiatry*. London: CRC Press, p. 6.

Question 66 Answer: e, When he studies, he usually feels sad. In the examination he often puts down the answer 'don't know' when answering MCQs as he also feels sad during the examination.
Explanation: The state-dependent effect should theoretically facilitate recall. His low mood during the examination may lead to low motivation. The patient has poor motivation to attempt the questions rather than memory deficit or forgetfulness. Option (a) refers to the decay or trace decay theory. Option (b) refers to displacement theory. Option (c) refers to cue-dependent forgetting, and option (d) refers to context-dependent forgetting.

Reference and Further Reading: Puri BK, Treasaden I (eds) (2010). *Psychiatry: An Evidence-Based Text*. London: Hodder Arnold, pp. 256–262.

Question 67 Answer: b, Peak age of onset is 20–29 years.
Explanation: All of the following statements are true, with the exception that the peak age of onset is 20–29 years. The peak age of onset should be 15–19 years. Based on the ECA study, it has been found that there are approximately 11 cases in 20,000 persons studied. The incidence is noted to be 10 times higher in females as compared to males. There is a higher prevalence in higher socioeconomic classes and Western Caucasians and a significant association with greater parental education.

Reference: Puri BK, Hall A, Ho R (2014). *Revision Notes in Psychiatry*. London: CRC Press, p. 575.

Question 68 Answer: d, Depersonalization
Explanation: Depersonalization is the experience of change in awareness of oneself, as though one is 'unreal'. Some associated characteristics include emotional numbing, changes in body/visual/auditory experiences and changes in the subjective experience of memory and loss of feelings of agency. It is associated with unpleasant emotion. Derealization is the feeling of unreality in objects of the outer perceptual field, whereas depersonalization applies to the person feeling that he/she is 'unreal'.

Reference and Further Reading: Sims A (2003). *Symptoms of the Mind: An Introduction to Descriptive Psychopathology*. London: Saunders, pp. 83, 95, 230–233.

Question 69 Answer: b, The DSM-IV-TR and ICD-10 do not require the presence of depressive episode in the past.
Explanation: The presence of past depressive episode is not required to fulfil the DSM-IV-TR and ICD-10 diagnostic criteria for bipolar disorder, manic episode. Only DSM-IV-TR classifies bipolar disorder into bipolar I and bipolar II disorder but not the ICD-10.

References and Further Reading: American Psychiatric Association (2000). *Diagnostic Criteria from DSM-IV-TR*. Washington, DC: American Psychiatric Association; World Health Organisation (1994). ICD-10 *Classification of Mental and Behavioural Disorders*. Edinburgh, UK: Churchill Livingstone; Puri BK, Treasaden I (eds) (2010). *Psychiatry: An Evidence-Based Text*. London: Hodder Arnold, pp. 624–634.

Question 70 Answer: e, Seasonal pattern
Explanation: Seasonal pattern is a special feature for DSM-IV-TR bipolar disorder with manic episode.

Reference and Further Reading: American Psychiatric Association (2000). *Diagnostic Criteria from DSM-IV-TR*. Washington, DC: American Psychiatric Association; Puri BK, Treasaden I (eds) (2010). *Psychiatry: An Evidence-Based Text*. London: Hodder Arnold, pp. 624–634.

Question 71 Answer: b, Brain serotonin systems have not been shown to be implicated in the modulation of appetite.
Explanation: Brain serotonin systems have been shown to be implicated in the modulation of appetite, mood, personality variables and neuroendocrine function. In fact, an increase in the intrasynaptic serotonin would cause a reduction in food consumption. A reduction in serotonin activity increases food consumption and promotes weight gain.

Reference: Puri BK, Hall A, Ho R (2014). *Revision Notes in Psychiatry*. London: CRC Press, p. 575.

Question 72 Answer: c, Procedural memory is affected later than verbal memory in Alzheimer's disease.
Explanation: Episodic memory (early loss of recent events) deficits are an early feature of Alzheimer's disease. Certain parts of the brain show volume reductions with age, especially the prefrontal cortex and hippocampus. Both are important for the functioning of episodic memory, which plays a critical role in remembering past events. Verbal memory depends on episodic memory and is affected earlier than semantic and procedural memories. In contrast to the steady declines in episodic memory across all decades of life, semantic memory (e.g. languages, objects, places, spatial relationships, social norms) is not only preserved, but also shows improvement until around the eighth decade of life. The preservation of a wide variety of semantic memory (i.e. knowledge about objects and their relationships) has been demonstrated for both healthy elderly adults and patients with Alzheimer's disease. Spatial awareness (e.g. remembering visuospatial information) is part of the semantic memory and affected later than procedural memory (e.g. bicycle riding) because procedural memory is affected by speed and reaction time. Elderly with or without dementia may perform these tasks more slowly owing to other factors such as arthritis and muscle weakness.

There is a difference between recall and recognition. Recall is affected earlier than recognition in aging. The dissociation between recall and recognition is why we often fail to recall the name of a movie we saw whereas we can easily recognize when the movie is presented to us.

Reference and Further Reading: Ober BA (2010) Memory, brain and aging: The good, the bad and the promising. *California Agriculture*, 64: 174–182.

Question 73 Answer: c, Palinopsia
Explanation: Palinopsia is a reoccurrence or prolongation of visual perception after the stimulus has been removed. Palinopsia is associated with mania, depression and substance dependence. LSD is a hallucinogen that causes this phenomenon.

Reference and Further Reading: Abert B, Ilsen PF (2010). Palinopsia. *Optometry*, 81: 394–404.

Question 74 Answer: e, Rapid cycling disorder is a separate entity in ICD-10.
Explanation: Rapid cycling disorder is not a separate entity or course specifier in ICD-10.

References and Further Reading: American Psychiatric Association (2000). *Diagnostic Criteria from DSM-IV-TR*. Washington, DC: American Psychiatric Association; World Health Organisation (1994). ICD-10 Classification of Mental and Behavioural Disorders. Edinburgh, UK: Churchill Livingstone; Puri BK, Treasaden I (eds) (2010). *Psychiatry: An Evidence-Based Text*. London: Hodder Arnold, pp. 611, 625, 628.

Question 75 Answer: c, Based on the DSM-IV-TR and ICD-10 criteria, intervening periods of normal mood should not be present.
Explanation: The DSM-IV-TR and ICD-10 criteria allow intervening periods of normal mood. DSM-IV-TR specifies that the duration of normal mood cannot be longer than 2 months.

References and Further Reading: American Psychiatric Association (2000). *Diagnostic Criteria from DSM-IV-TR*. Washington, DC: American Psychiatric Association; World Health Organisation (1994). ICD-10 Classification of Mental and Behavioural Disorders. Edinburgh: Churchill Livingstone; Puri BK, Treasaden I (eds) (2010). *Psychiatry: An Evidence-Based Text*. London: Hodder Arnold, pp. 610, 634.

Question 76 Answer: b, It is a condition that is most common in the lower social classes.
Explanation: Bipolar affective disorder is a condition that is most common in the upper social classes. The sex ratio has been shown to be the same. The point prevalence in Western countries is 0.4%–1.2% in the adult population. In the

general population of Western countries, the lifetime risk of suffering from a bipolar disorder is 0.6%–1.1%. The average age of onset is around the mid-twenties. Being unmarried is associated with higher rates of bipolar disorder.

Reference: Puri BK, Hall A, Ho R (2014). *Revision Notes in Psychiatry*. London: CRC Press, p. 384.

Question 77 Answer: a, Delusional perception
Explanation: The psychopathology is delusional perception. It is important to bear in mind that a delusion is a false belief that is based on incorrect inference about external reality that is firmly sustained despite what almost everyone else believes and despite what constitutes incontrovertible and obvious proof or evidence to the contrary.

Reference: Puri BK, Hall A, Ho R (2014). *Revision Notes in Psychiatry*. London: CRC Press, p. 6.

Question 78 Answer: e, Memory retrieval procedure
Explanation: Option (a) involves participants learning a list of paired words (e.g. 'table' and 'shoe'). They are then presented with one of the words (e.g. 'table') and the participant must recall the word pair ('shoe').

Option (b) involves matching a stimulus to what is already stored in memory. An example would be a multiple-choice test.

Option (c) and (d) are recall techniques used to measure memory. In free recall, participants have to actively search their memory stores to retrieve information. An example would be examinations in the form of essays. There are little retrieval cues available, unlike recognition. Memory-span procedure is similar to serial recall. Participants are given a list of digits or letters and asked to immediately repeat the same digit span in the same order that was presented to them. This technique is called digit span, which is one of the subtests in the Wechsler Adult Intelligence Scale.

Option (e) is the correct answer; there is no such procedure.

Reference and Further Reading: Puri BK, Treasaden I (eds) (2010). *Psychiatry: An Evidence-Based Text*. London: Hodder Arnold, p. 250.

Question 79 Answer: b, Ambiguous figures
Explanation: These are examples of ambiguous figures. Rubin's vase is a common example of the figure-ground reversal. The Necker's cube illustrates depth reversal, and Boring's old/young woman illustrates object reversal.

Reference and Further Reading: Puri BK, Treasaden I (eds) (2010). *Psychiatry: An Evidence-Based Text*. London: Hodder Arnold, pp. 234–236.

Question 80 Answer: c, 3 years
Explanation: Based on the existing ICD-10 diagnostic criteria, the diagnosis is only made if there is the presence of abnormal development manifested before

the age of 3 years. This might include abnormal receptive or expressive language, abnormal selective or reciprocal social interaction and abnormal functional or symbolic play.

Reference: Puri BK, Hall A, Ho R (2014). *Revision Notes in Psychiatry*. London: CRC Press, p. 624.

Question 81 Answer: b, Standardized scores on tests of recognition memory are higher than standardized scores on tests of free recall.
Explanation: Standardized scores on tests of recognition are lower than standardized scores on tests of free recall in people with feigned amnesia. Furthermore, people with feigned amnesia have a forced-choice recognition test performance that is worse than chance.

References and Further Reading: Cercy SP, Schretlen DJ, Brandt J (1997). Simulated amnesia and the pseudo-memory phenonmena, in Rogers R (ed) *Clinical Assessment or Malingering and Deception*. New York: Guilford Press; Trimble M (2004). *Somatoform Disorders – A Medico-Legal Guide*. Cambridge, UK: Cambridge University Press; Puri BK, Treasaden I (eds) (2010). *Psychiatry: An Evidence-Based Text*. London: Hodder Arnold, pp. 93–95, 149, 252–254, 260, 557–559, 581, 667, 1160, 1165.

Question 82 Answer: c, False memory syndrome is a recognized diagnostic criterion in ICD-10.
Explanation: False memory syndrome describes a condition in which a person's identity and relationships are affected by memories that are factually incorrect but strongly believed. During clinical interview and psychotherapy, the interviewer or therapist should avoid leading questions which may suggest false memory. It is not a recognized diagnostic criterion in ICD-10.

Reference: McHugh PR (2008). *Try to Remember: Psychiatry's Clash over Meaning, Memory and Mind*. New York: Dana Press.

Question 83 Answer: a, Schemas persist even after evidence for the schema has been discredited.
Explanation: Schemas persist after evidence for the schema has been discredited because the old schema has been activated more times than the new, modified schema and would be reactivated when there are little cognitive resources or time to activate the new schema and suppress the old one. Automatic, low-effort thinking involves schemas as people make use of previous knowledge, stored as schemas, to quickly process a new situation. Thus, schemas help speed up mental processing. Schemas are used to resolve ambiguity when a situation can be interpreted in various ways. When people act on their schemas, their actions can affect the way they treat other people, changing how the person reacts to them and, as a result, supporting their schema. This cycle illustrates self-fulfilling prophecy.

Reference and Further Reading: Aronson E, Wilson TD, Akert RM (2007). *Social Psychology*. Upper Saddle River, NJ: Prentice Hall, pp. 58–72.

Question 84 Answer: c, B₂ antagonist

Explanation: B_2 antagonist is not associated with tremor but B_2 agonist does. Amphetamine, B_2 agonist and caffeine are associated with physiological tremor. Risperidone is associated with extrapyramidal side effects.

Reference and Further Reading: Ward N, Frith P, Lipsedge M (2001). *Medical Masterclass Neurology, Ophthalmology and Psychiatry*. London: Royal College of Physicians; Puri BK, Treasaden I (eds) (2010). *Psychiatry: An Evidence-Based Text*. London: Hodder Arnold, p. 523.

Question 85 Answer: a, Dual role transvestism

Explanation: This includes the wearing of clothes of the opposite sex for part of the time in order to enjoy temporary membership or experience of the opposite sex. This occurs without the desire for a more permanent sex change. There is usually no sexual excitement that is derived from the cross-dressing.

Reference: Puri BK, Hall A, Ho R (2014). *Revision Notes in Psychiatry*. London: CRC Press, p. 603.

Question 86 Answer: e, Stupor

Explanation: Schneider has identified the following to be first-rank symptoms: auditory hallucinations, delusions of passivity, somatic passivity and delusional perception. Auditory hallucinations include the following: repeating the thoughts out loud, in third person, or in the form of a running commentary. Delusions of passivity include thought insertion, withdrawal and broadcasting. They include made feelings, impulses and actions as well.

Reference: Puri BK, Hall A, Ho R (2014). *Revision Notes in Psychiatry*. London: CRC Press, p. 351.

Question 87 Answer: c, Transexualism

Explanation: This refers to the desire to live as a member of the opposite sex, with intense discomfort about one's anatomical sex and a wish to change bodily features into those of the preferred sex. In order to make this diagnosis, the symptoms must have persisted for 2 years and it should not be attributed to any other mental health disorder.

Reference: Puri BK, Hall A, Ho R (2014). *Revision Notes in Psychiatry*. London: CRC Press, p. 603.

Question 88 Answer: e, Aggression is associated with high levels of serotonin.

Explanation: Aggression is associated with low levels of serotonin and high levels of testosterone. Serotonin has an inhibiting effect on impulsive aggression.

According to the social learning theory, aggression is a learned response, acquired through observation, imitation and operant conditioning. Aggression can also be learnt through positive reinforcements.

Reference and Further Reading: Puri BK, Hall AD (2002). *Revision Notes in Psychiatry*. London: Arnold, p. 55; Puri BK, Treasaden I (eds) (2010). *Psychiatry: An Evidence-Based Text*. London: Hodder Arnold, pp. 293, 1130, 1173, 1175.

Question 89 Answer: d, Rapid cycling bipolar disorder
Explanation: This woman suffers from at least four episodes of mood disturbance in the previous year and she meets the criteria of rapid cycling disorder based on the DSM-IV-TR criteria. Ultra-rapid cycling bipolar disorder requires at least four episodes of mood disturbance per month.

Reference and Further Reading: American Psychiatric Association (2000). *Diagnostic Criteria from DSM-IV-TR*. Washington, DC: American Psychiatric Association; Puri BK, Treasaden I (eds) (2010). *Psychiatry: An Evidence-Based Text*. London: Hodder Arnold, pp. 611, 625, 628.

Question 90 Answer: a, Degenerative spinal disease
Explanation: Degenerative spinal disease is associated with back and leg pain. Option (b) is correct because fine distal tremor is occasionally seen as part of a peripheral neuropathy. Options (c) and (d) are associated with physiological tremor. Physiological tremor is a small-amplitude, higher-frequency tremor, enhanced by fear or anxiety. Option (e) is correct because tremor may be an early feature in 30% of Wilson's disease.

Reference and Further Reading: Ward N, Frith P, Lipsedge M (2001). *Medical Masterclass Neurology, Ophthalmology and Psychiatry*. London: Royal College of Physicians; Puri BK, Treasaden I (eds) (2010). *Psychiatry: An Evidence-Based Text*. London: Hodder Arnold, pp. 523, 548.

Question 91 Answer: d, Proximity
Explanation: The closer the objects or events are to one another, the more likely they are to be perceived as belonging together.

Reference and Further Reading: Puri BK, Treasaden I (eds) (2010). *Psychiatry: An Evidence-Based Text*. London: Hodder Arnold, pp. 229–232.

Question 92 Answer: a, Fregoli syndrome
Explanation: This is a very rare delusional disorder in which the patient believes so. Primary causes would include schizophrenia as well as other associated organic causes. In this condition, the patient believes that a familiar person who is often believed to be the patient's persecutor has taken on different appearances. It is

important to differentiate this from (c), which is also a rare condition, but the essential feature of that condition is that a person who is familiar to the patient is believed to have been replaced by a double.

Reference: Puri BK, Hall A, Ho R (2014). *Revision Notes in Psychiatry*. London: CRC Press, p. 373.

Question 93 Answer: d, Exhibitionism
Explanation: In this clinical diagnosis, it is defined as the recurrence or the persistent tendency to expose the genitalia to strangers or people of the opposite sex in public places. There is usually sexual excitement, and this is often followed by masturbation.

Reference: Puri BK, Hall A, Ho R (2014). *Revision Notes in Psychiatry*. London: CRC Press, p. 605.

Question 94 Answer: d, People's expectation of a person influences their behaviour towards that person, resulting in that person acting in line with the expectation.
Explanation: Self-fulfilling prophecy is the process whereby a person's expectations of another affects his/her behaviour towards that person, resulting in the person acting in line with the expectation and hence confirming the 'prophecy'. An example would be a teacher who thinks a certain student is academically gifted and might give the student more opportunities to answer challenging questions during class, resulting in the student performing better.

Reference and Further Reading: Aronson E, Wilson TD, Akert RM (2007). *Social Psychology*. Upper Saddle River, NJ: Prentice Hall, pp. 67–70, 440.

Question 95 Answer: a, Displacement
Explanation: This 24-year-old woman has displaced her anger from the psychiatrist to the health care assistant.

Reference and Further Reading: Puri BK, Hall AD (2002). *Revision Notes in Psychiatry*. London: Arnold, pp. 168–169.

Question 96 Answer: c, Dhat
Explanation: The four core symptoms of dhat syndrome include excessive loss of semen, specific sexual dysfunction, anxiety about present or future sexual function and multiple physical/psychological symptoms. Most of the empirical studies on dhat syndrome have emerged from Asia (India), whereas its concepts have been described historically in other cultures, including Britain, the USA and Australia.

Reference: Sumathipala A, Siribaddana SH, Bhugra D (2004). Culture-bound syndromes: The story of dhat syndrome. *The British Journal of Psychiatry*, 184: 200–209.

Question 97 Answer: d, La boufféedélirante
Explanation: Haiti was previously a French colony. In French psychiatric nomenclature, la boufféedélirante refers to acute delusional psychosis with a favourable outcome. This condition has no genetic link to schizophrenia.

Reference: Campbell RJ (1996). *Psychiatric Dictionary*. Oxford, UK: Oxford University Press.

Question 98 Answer: e, Familial pattern of essential tremor is common
Explanation: Essential tremor is defined as uncontrollable shaking of part of the body that lasts for at least a few seconds. It is a common movement disorder among old people that usually affects the arms and hands, but can affect the head, jaw, face, feet and tongue. It is inherited in autosomal dominant manner. Essential tremor attenuates with alcohol use and puts patients at risk for alcohol misuse. Early essential tremor is absent at rest but present during action.

Reference and Further Reading: Puri BK, Treasaden I (eds) (2010). *Psychiatry: An Evidence-Based Text*. London: Hodder Arnold, p. 523.

Question 99 Answer: b, Social phobia
Explanation: The clinical diagnosis would be social phobia. Based on the ICD-10 diagnostic criteria, social phobia is defined as anxiety that is restricted to or predominates in a particular social situation. The phobic situation is usually avoided whenever possible. There is marked fear of being the focus of attention and marked avoidance of being the focus of attention.

Reference: Puri BK, Hall A, Ho R (2014). *Revision Notes in Psychiatry*. London: CRC Press, p. 408.

Question 100 Answer: c, Mitgehen
Explanation: This is an example of mitgehen. There is usually excessive limb movement in response to even the slightest amount of applied pressure, even when the person is told to resist movement. In another example, the examiner wants to move the patient's arm upward and asks the patient to resist movement. However, even with a slight touch, the person continued to move his or her arm upwards and then return to the original position after the test.

Reference: Puri BK, Hall A, Ho R (2014). *Revision Notes in Psychiatry*. London: CRC Press, p. 2.

Question 101 Answer: b, Common fate
Explanation: Objects moving in the same direction (common fate) at the same speed are perceived together.

Reference and Further Reading: Puri BK, Treasaden I (eds) (2010). *Psychiatry: An Evidence-Based Text*. London: Hodder Arnold, pp. 229–232.

Question 102 Answer: a, Cortisol-releasing hormone
Explanation: Cortisol-releasing hormone is usually increased in patients suffering from anorexia nervosa because of the central activation of the hypothalamus–pituitary and adrenal axis.

Reference and Further Reading: Puri BK, Treasaden I (eds) (2010). *Psychiatry: An Evidence-Based Text London: Hodder Arnold,* pp. 687–703, 1063.

Question 103 Answer: a, Self-serving bias
Explanation: Self-serving bias refers to the tendency to attribute our successes to internal, dispositional factors and failures to external, situational factors. In-group bias is the positive feelings towards people belonging to one's in-group and negativity towards one's out-group. Actor/observer bias refers to the tendency to attribute other people's behaviour to internal, dispositional factors, and to use external, situational factors to explain our own. Hindsight bias is the tendency to see events as more predictable after the event has occurred. Fundamental attribution error is the tendency to overestimate the extent to which a person's behaviour is due to internal, dispositional factors and to underestimate the role of external, situational factors.

Reference and Further Reading: Aronson E, Wilson TD, Akert RM (2007). *Social Psychology.* Upper Saddle River, NJ: Prentice Hall, pp. 30, 109, 116–117, 120, 424–426.

Question 104 Answer: e, A doctor's native motive to provide morally correct care to his or her patients, and focus solely on the rightness and wrongness of the actions themselves, and not on the consequences of the actions
Explanation: The deontological theories emphasize on a doctor's motive to provide morally correct care to his or her patients. They focus solely on the rightness and wrongness of the doctor's actions and not on the consequences of the actions themselves.

Reference: Puri BK, Hall A, Ho R (2014). *Revision Notes in Psychiatry.* London: CRC Press, p. 146.

Question 105 Answer: d, Autonomy
Explanation: This is an example of autonomy. Autonomy refers to the obligation of the doctor to respect his or her patients' rights to make their own choices in accordance to their beliefs and wishes. Nonmaleficence refers to the obligation of a doctor to avoid harm to his or her patients. Beneficence refers to the commitment of a doctor to provide benefits to patients and balance benefits against risks when making such decisions.

Reference: Puri BK, Hall A, Ho R (2014). *Revision Notes in Psychiatry.* London: CRC Press, p. 146.

Question 106 Answer: c, Prima Facie Duty

Explanation: The ethical theory that is being referred to would be the 'Prima Facie Duty'. This refers to a duty that is always to be acted upon unless it conflicts on a particular occasion with an equal or stronger duty. For example, a psychiatrist would have to maintain his or her own patient's confidentiality (this is a Prima Facie Duty). However, if one day one of his patients mentions that he or she has a plan to harm others, then the psychiatrist would have to consider carefully the various ethical principles involved and decide whether it would be appropriate to breach confidentiality.

Reference: Puri BK, Hall A, Ho R (2014). *Revision Notes in Psychiatry*. London: CRC Press, p. 146.

Question 107 Answer: c, Capacity is a legal term

Explanation: Capacity is not a legal term but competence is. A person is deemed to be competent if he or she has the capacity to understand and act reasonably. Competence is a legal term and determined by the legal system.

Reference and Further Reading: Puri BK, Treasaden I (eds) (2010). *Psychiatry: An Evidence-Based Text*. London: Hodder Arnold, pp. 1226–1227.

Question 108 Answer: d, Wernicke's encephalopathy

Explanation: Hyperemesis gravidarum in the first trimester may cause thiamine deficiency and result in Wernicke's encephalopathy. Wernicke's encephalopathy is characterized by confusion, ataxia and ophthalmoplegia.

Reference and Further Reading: Puri BK, Treasaden I (eds) (2010). *Psychiatry: An Evidence-Based Text*. London: Hodder Arnold, pp. 531, 697, 716, 1028.

Question 109 Answer: a, Bizarre delusions

Explanation: The delusions involved in a delusional disorder are usually non-bizarre in nature. A delusion is defined as a false belief based on incorrect inference about external reality that is firmly sustained despite what everyone else believes and despite what constitute as incontrovertible and obvious proof or evidence to the contrary. The belief is usually also not accepted by members of one's culture.

Reference: Puri BK, Hall A, Ho R (2014). *Revision Notes in Psychiatry*. London: CRC Press, p. 6.

Question 110 Answer: e, More than 23

Explanation: A patient with bulimia nervosa may have normal or even high BMI. BMI = Weight/Height (in metres)^2 = $60/1.6^2$ = 23.44.

Reference and Further Reading: Puri BK, Treasaden I (eds) (2010). *Psychiatry: An Evidence-Based Text*. London: Hodder Arnold, pp. 694–695, 1063.

Question 111 Answer: b, Interactions with a member of the out-group
Explanation: Option (b) is incorrect as interacting with only one member of an out-group would lead to no change in the stereotype. This is because the single out-group member would be seen as an exception to the stereotype. Exposure to multiple non-stereotypical members of the out-group would help to reduce prejudice.

Reference and Further Reading: Puri BK, Hall AD (2002). *Revision Notes in Psychiatry*. London: Arnold, pp. 54–55.

Question 112 Answer: d, No implicit consent
Explanation: Both explicit and implicit consent can be considered as valid consent. Implicit consent is used to describe situations where it is judged that the nature and risk of a procedure (e.g. blood taking) are such that a less formal or retrospective transfer of information about the intervention is considered sufficient. The use of explicit and implicit consent is also dependent upon the building up of rapport and trust between clinicians and patients.

Reference and Further Reading: Puri BK, Treasaden I (eds) (2010). *Psychiatry: An Evidence-Based Text*. London: Hodder Arnold, pp. 1224–1225.

Question 113 Answer: a, Admit own feelings and inform the patient that the staff are frightened of his aggression and anger
Explanation: Option (a) may confuse the patient and give the wrong impression to the patient that the staff are incompetent in handling his aggression and anger. Patients with antisocial personality disorder may see this as weakness of the team and manipulate the situation by escalating his aggression and anger. Psychiatrist in this situation should deliver a clear and correct message to inform the patient that physical violence is not acceptable and there are chemical and physical interventions to help him calm down.

Reference: Poole R, Higgo R (2006). *Psychiatric Interviewing and Assessment*. Cambridge, UK: Cambridge University Press.

Question 114 Answer: c, Holmes–Adie syndrome
Explanation: The triad of Holmes–Adie syndrome is classically described as unilateral pupillary dilatation, poor constriction to light and accommodation and depressed deep tendon reflexes. This syndrome commonly affects young women. The pupil may become small over time.

Reference: Ward N, Frith P, Lipsedge M (2001). *Medical Masterclass Neurology, Ophthalmology and Psychiatry*. London: Royal College of Physicians.

Question 115 Answer: c, Thought block
Explanation: Passivity phenomenon refers to a delusional belief that an external agency is controlling aspects of self that are normally entirely under one's own

control. Passivity phenomena include thought alienation (which includes thought insertion, thought withdrawal, and thought broadcasting. In addition, made impulses, made feelings, made actions and somatic passivity are also part of the passivity phenomenon.

Reference: Puri BK, Hall A, Ho R (2014). *Revision Notes in Psychiatry*. London: CRC Press, p. 7.

Question 116 Answer: b, Egoistic suicide
Explanation: This is commonly referred to as egoistic suicide. This usually results when individuals feel that they are being socially further distanced from social norms and restraints, such that meaning in life is being questioned.

Reference: Puri BK, Hall A, Ho R (2014). *Revision Notes in Psychiatry*. London: CRC Press, p. 118.

Question 117 Answer: e, The best clinical approach to mental state examination is in a conversational and informal manner.
Explanation: Option (e) is correct because unskilled interviewers often conduct the mental state examination in a rigid schema with a lot of technical questions. It will prevent the patient from opening up and volunteering new information. This also explains why option (d) is incorrect. Option (a) is incorrect because the psychiatrist should focus on possible psychopathology based on information obtained in history-taking. Option (b) is incorrect because probe questions about psychopathology are best framed with reference to activities and ideas that are familiar to the patient. Option (d) is incorrect because state interrogations are unreliable methods of judging the progress of treatment or changes in patient's mental health.

Reference and Further Reading: Poole R, Higgo R (2006). *Psychiatric Interviewing and Assessment*. Cambridge, UK: Cambridge University Press; Puri BK, Treasaden I (eds) (2010). *Psychiatry: An Evidence-Based Text*. London: Hodder Arnold, pp. 91–92.

Question 118 Answer: e, The doctor should not inject him with depot antipsychotics and respect his wish.
Explanation: This man has the capacity to make decisions and is able to communicate his preference. His wish should be respected and the doctor should not inject him with depot antipsychotics.

Reference and Further Reading: Puri BK, Treasaden I (eds) (2010). *Psychiatry: An Evidence-Based Text*. London: Hodder Arnold, pp. 1094, 1226–1227.

Question 119 Answer: e, Homelessness
Explanation: An acute anomie is caused by a sudden change or crisis that leaves the individual in an unfamiliar situation. The causes of an acute anomie would include

migration, bereavement, redundancy and losses. It does not include homelessness. Homelessness and long-term employment are causes of chronic anomie.

Reference: Puri BK, Hall A, Ho R (2014). *Revision Notes in Psychiatry*. London: CRC Press, p. 118.

Question 120 Answer: a, Amaurosis fugax

Explanation: Amaurosis fugax is defined as a transient monocular visual loss. Carotid artery stenosis causes transient ischemic attacks (TIAs). TIAs usually last less than 24 hours and the patient presents with unilateral motor weakness or sensory loss and amaurosis fugax in one eye.

Scotoma is defined as an area of reduced vision (e.g. central scotoma) and is commonly caused by demyelinating diseases such as multiple sclerosis or macular degeneration. Hemianopia is defined as loss of half of visual field of both eyes (either left side or right side). Damage to the right posterior portion of the brain usually causes a loss of the left half of visual fields in both eyes. Similarly, damage to the left posterior brain usually causes a loss of right half of visual fields in both eyes. Homonymous quadrantanopia is defined as loss of either outer upper or lower quadrant of visual field of one eye. For example, left superior homonymous quadrantanopia is caused by right temporal lobe lesion. Bitemporal hemianopia is defined as loss of outer half of visual fields in both eyes and is commonly caused by pituitary tumour.

Reference and Further Reading: Hoya K, Morikawa E, Tamura A, Saito I (2008). Common carotid artery stenosis and amaurosis fugax. *Journal of Stroke and Cerebrovascular Diseases*, 17: 1–4.

Question 121 Answer: d, Barton

Explanation: Barton (1959) first used the term to describe a syndrome which he considered to be caused by institutions in which individuals show marked apathy, inability to plan for the future, submissiveness, withdrawal and low self-esteem.

Reference: Puri BK, Hall A, Ho R (2014). *Revision Notes in Psychiatry*. London: CRC Press, p. 124.

Question 122 Answer: a, Zimeldine

Explanation: Zimeldine was one of the first SSRIs introduced. It was withdrawn later as it caused an increased incidence of hypersensitivity syndrome and also demyelinating disease.

Reference: Puri BK, Hall A, Ho R (2014). *Revision Notes in Psychiatry*. London: CRC Press, p. 237.

Question 123 Answer: e, Breeder's hypothesis

Explanation: All of the aforementioned are possible explanations for the existence of a relationship between social classes and a given psychiatric diagnosis with the exception of Breeder's hypothesis. Downward social drift proposes that there might be increased prevalence of schizophrenia in the lower social classes as a result of social drift. Environmental stress theory proposes that the lower social class is associated with adverse life situations, material deprivation and lower self-esteem that manual job entails. Differential labelling implies that individuals of certain origin are more likely to be detained under mental health legislation and diagnosed as suffering from schizophrenia. Differential treatment theory proposes that there are likely to be differences in the type of psychiatric treatment received by those who are from different social classes.

Reference: Puri BK, Hall A, Ho R (2014). *Revision Notes in Psychiatry*. London: CRC Press, p. 116.

Question 124 Answer: c, A functional hallucination
Explanation: A functional hallucination is defined as the hallucination that occurs when a patient simultaneously receives a real stimulus in the same perceptual field as the hallucination.

Reference and Further Reading: Hunter MD, Woodruff PWR (2004). Characteristics of functional auditory hallucinations. *American Journal of Psychiatry*, 161: 923.

Question 125 Answer: b, Couvade syndrome
Explanation: Couvade syndrome refers to the abnormal obstetric symptoms the husband experiences during his wife's pregnancy.

Reference and Further Reading: Sims A (2003). *Symptoms of the Mind: An Introduction to Descriptive Psychopathology*. London: Saunders, pp. 288, 290.

Question 126 Answer: a, Internal attribution
Explanation: Sandra has made what is known as an internal attribution. Attribution in itself refers to the rules that people use to infer and assume the cause of particular observed behaviours. An internal attribution is made when the person feels that he or she is primarily responsible for their behaviour. An external attribution is made when the cause of a behaviour is assumed to be due to other factors that are external to the person. Primary or fundamental error refers to the bias towards dispositional causes rather than situational causes when asked about the underlying motivation for other's behaviour.

Reference: Puri BK, Hall A, Ho R (2014). *Revision Notes in Psychiatry*. London: CRC Press, p. 59.

Question 127 Answer: c, Self-Image
Explanation: This refers to self-image. It is important to have a general understanding of the rest of self-psychology. Self-concept usually refers to the set of attitudes that one has about himself or herself. Self-esteem refers to one's own evaluation of self-worth and the associated feelings of being accepted by others.

Self-perception states that an individual would infer what his or her attitude should be through observation of his or her own behaviour.

Reference: Puri BK, Hall A, Ho R (2014). *Revision Notes in Psychiatry*. London: CRC Press, p. 58.

Question 128 Answer: e, False memory
Explanation: The concept test here is false memory. The false memory syndrome is a condition in which an individual's identity and interpersonal relationships are centred around the memory of a traumatic experience, which in itself is false. However, the individual would still have a firm belief that the experience did actually take place. It is important to note that false confessions might not always have an underlying psychiatric cause.

Reference: Puri BK, Hall A, Ho R (2014). *Revision Notes in Psychiatry*. London: CRC Press, p. 104.

Question 129 Answer: e, Theta wave
Explanation: Theta wave has a frequency between 4 and 7.5 Hz. Increase in theta wave is found in organic psychosis, Alzheimer's disease and hypoxia.

Reference and Further Reading: Puri BK, Treasaden I (eds) (2010). *Psychiatry: An Evidence-Based Text*. London: Hodder Arnold, pp. 400–409, 536.

Question 130 Answer: d, Needing to avoid social rejection
Explanation: In particular for normative social influence, the individual might openly conform to the ideas of a group, but might have a varying opinion deep within his self. The underlying rationale for conforming is largely to avoid social rejection.

Reference: Puri BK, Hall A, Ho R (2014). *Revision Notes in Psychiatry*. London: CRC Press, p. 60.

Question 131 Answer: e, Selective retention
Explanation: When cognitive dissonance occurs, the individual feels uncomfortable, may experience increased arousal and is motivated to achieve cognitive consistency. This may occur usually by changing one or more of the cognitions involved in the dissonant relationship, changing the behaviour that is inconsistent with the cognition or adding new cognitions that are consonant with the pre-existing ones. Cognitive consistency can also be achieved when attitude and behaviour are inconsistent by altering attitude.

Reference: Puri BK, Hall A, Ho R (2014). *Revision Notes in Psychiatry*. London: CRC Press, p. 58.

Question 132 Answer: c, Huntington's disease
Explanation: The patient is likely to have Huntington's disease. This is a genetic disorder that affects 5 in 100,000 individuals in the UK. It is characterized by a

slowly progressive dementia and associated continuous involuntary movement. Genetic studies have found out that transmission is usually due to a fully penetrant single autosomal dominant mutation, which is located on chromosome 4, and this might affect 50% of the offspring.

Reference: Puri BK, Hall A, Ho R (2014). *Revision Notes in Psychiatry*. London: CRC Press, p. 706.

Question 133 Answer: d, Sleep paralysis
Explanation: Sleep paralysis is the inability to move during the period between sleep and wakefulness and vice versa. Somnambulism refers to sleep walking.

Reference and Further Reading: Sims A (2003). *Symptoms of the Mind: An Introduction to Descriptive Psychopathology*. London: Saunders, p. 58.

Question 134 Answer: b, Dysmegalopsia
Explanation: Dysmegalopsia is also known as the Alice in Wonderland effect. Illusory change in the size and shape (both reduction and increase in size) is perceived visually. In this example, the objects (i.e. the heads) appear to be enlarged. This phenomenon is specifically known as macropsia. When the object is perceived as smaller than it actually is, this is known as micropsia.

Reference and Further Reading: Campbell RJ (1996). *Psychiatric Dictionary*. Oxford, UK: Oxford University Press.

Question 135 Answer: c, Depression
Explanation: The glucocorticoid receptor hypothesis is associated with depression.

Reference and Further Reading: Puri BK, Treasaden I (eds) (2010). *Psychiatry: An Evidence-Based Text*. London: Hodder Arnold, pp. 391–392, 612.

Question 136 Answer: a, Brown and Harris: Social Origins of Depression
Explanation: Brown and Harris stated that women with three young children under the age of 14, unemployed and with no confiding relationship are more likely to develop depression.

Reference and Further Reading: Brown, G, Harris T (1978). *Social Origins of Depression. A Study of Psychiatric Disorder in Women*. London: Tavistock.

Question 137 Answer: b, Excessive social support
Explanation: Excessive social support reduces the sense of personal control and this may be as damaging as little support. Hence, excessive social support may cause depression.

Reference: Krause N (1987). Understanding the stress process: linking social support and locus of control beliefs. *Journal of Gerontology*, 42: 589–593.

Question 138 Answer: b, Nonpsychotic schizophrenia patients
Explanation: Among the five groups, nonpsychotic schizophrenia patients are at maximum risk of suicide. Other high-risk groups include young male schizophrenia patients, high level of education status, unemployed, those with high and non-delusional expectations of themselves and those who are relatively nonpsychotic.

Reference: Paykel ES, Jenkins R (1994). *Prevention in Psychiatry*. London: Gaskell.

Question 139 Answer: d, Suppression in suicide reporting
Explanation: Appropriate reporting may be an important element in education of the public about suicide, and suppression in suicide reporting is not an appropriate recommendation

Reference: Paykel ES, Jenkins R (1994). *Prevention in Psychiatry*. London: Gaskell.

Extended matching items (EMIs)

Theme: Clinical assessment and neuropsychological processes

Question 140 Answer: d, Implicit memory
Explanation: Implicit memory is automatically recalled without effort and is learned slowly through repetition. It is usually not readily amenable to verbal reporting. It comprises of procedural knowledge, that is knowing how.

Question 141 Answer: d, Implicit memory
Explanation: Both classical and operant learning involve the implicit memory.

Question 142 Answer: a, Sensory memory
Explanation: The anatomical correlate of the iconic memory is probably the visual association cortex, while that of the echoic memory is the auditory association cortex.

Question 143 Answer: b, Short-term memory
Explanation: The anatomical correlate of auditory verbal short-term memory is the left (dominant) parietal lobe, whilst that of visual verbal short-term memory is possibly the left temporo-occipital area. The anatomical correlate of nonverbal short-term memory is possibly the right (nondominant) temporal lobe.

Question 144 Answer: c, Explicit memory
Explanation: This particular form of memory requires a deliberate act of recollection and can be reported verbally. It includes declarative memory and episodic memory, which are stored separately, since it is possible to lose one type of memory while retaining the other.

Reference: Puri BK, Hall A, Ho R (2014). *Revision Notes in Psychiatry*. London: CRC Press, p. 103.

Theme: Clinical assessment and neuropsychological processes

Question 145 Answer: c, Post-traumatic amnesia

Explanation: Post-traumatic amnesia, once present, tends to remain unchanged. Post-traumatic amnesia is confounded by sedatives that are given during admission and prolonged sleep. It does not correlate with the duration of consciousness loss.

Question 146 Answer: d, Psychogenic amnesia

Explanation: Psychogenic amnesia is part of the dissociative disorder consisting of a sudden inability to recall important personal data. The amnesia may be localized or generalized. The amnesia may be selective or continuous. The clinical presentation is usually atypical and cannot be explained by ordinary forgetfulness. It is associated with indifference and has a highly unpredictable course.

Question 147 Answer: b, Retrograde amnesia

Explanation: Retrograde amnesia refers to the loss of memory for events that occurred prior to an event or a condition. Such an event is presumed to cause the memory disturbances in the first place. Retrograde memory related to public events is more likely to be subjected to a greater memory loss than personal events.

Question 148 Answer: e, False memory

Explanation: False memory involves confabulation, report of false events (such as childhood sexual abuse) and false confessions. The false-memory syndrome is a condition in which a person's identity and interpersonal relationships are centred around a particular traumatic event.

Question 149 Answer: f, Transient global amnesia

Explanation: In transient global amnesia, the person presents with an abrupt onset of disorientation, loss of ability to encode recent memories and retrograde amnesia for a variable duration. The patient has a remarkable degree of alertness and responsiveness. This episode usually lasts for a few hours and is never repeated. The pathophysiology is a result of transient ischemia.

Reference: Puri BK, Hall A, Ho R (2014). *Revision Notes in Psychiatry*. London: CRC Press, p. 104.

Theme: Delusional types

Question 150 Answer: g, Erotomania

Explanation: This is a delusion that another person, usually of a higher status, is deeply in love with the individual.

Question 151 Answer: h, Nihilistic delusion

Explanation: This refers to a delusion of death, disintegration of organs and nonexistence.

Question 152 Answer: f, Doppelganger
Explanation: This is a delusion that a double of a person or place exists somewhere else.

Question 153 Answer: e, Delusion of Reference:
Explanation: The theme is that events, objects or other people in one's immediate environment have a particular and unusual significance.

Question 154 Answer: d, Delusion of pregnancy
Explanation: This is also commonly known as couvade syndrome and it is a delusion that one is pregnant. It usually involves the husband of a pregnant wife.

Question 155 Answer: b, Delusion of infestation
Explanation: This is also known as Ekbom's syndrome and it is a delusion that one is infested by parasites.

Reference: Puri BK, Hall A, Ho R (2014). *Revision Notes in Psychiatry*. London: CRC Press, p. 7.

Theme: Suicide and risk factors

Question 156 Answer: e, Personality disorder
Explanation: The risk factors for suicide in those with personality disorder include lability of mood, aggressiveness, impulsivity, being isolated from peers and associated alcohol and substance misuse.

Question 157 Answer: d, Alcoholism
Explanation: There is an estimated 15% mortality from suicide if there is an underlying disorder such as alcoholism. It tends to occur later in the course of the illness, and those affected tend to be also depressed. Associated with completed suicide are poor physical health, poor work record, previous para-suicide and also a recent loss of a close relationship.

Question 158 Answer: c, Neurosis
Explanation: Nearly 90% have a history of para-suicide with a high proportion having threatened suicide in the preceding month. There is a tendency after a failed attempt to resort to more violent means. There is a high risk in depressive neurosis and panic disorder, but a lower risk of obsessive-compulsive disorder.

Question 159 Answer: b, Affective psychosis
Explanation: There is a 15% mortality from suicide in affective psychosis. Men who are older, separated, widowed or divorced, living alone and not working are predisposed. Women who are middle-aged, middle class, with a history of para-suicide and threats made in the last month are predisposed.

Question 160 Answer: a, Schizophrenia
Explanation: There is a 10% mortality from suicide. Schizophrenics who commit suicide tend to be young, male and unemployed and have chronic relapsing illness.

It should be noted that fewer schizophrenic patients give warning of their intention to commit suicide as compared to patients in other age groups. The suicide is usually after recent discharge, with good insight.

Reference: Puri BK, Hall A, Ho R (2014). *Revision Notes in Psychiatry*. London: CRC Press, p. 398.

Theme: Prevention of depressive disorders and suicide

Question 161 Answer: a, Primary prevention
Explanation: The aim of primary prevention is to reduce the incidence of the disorder. Hence, close monitoring during the post-discharge period is essential, especially so for young men with schizophrenia and high educational background who have regained insight. Depressed elderly with somatic complaints should also be monitored closely.

Question 162 Answer: a, Primary prevention
Explanation: The aim of primary prevention is to reduce the incidence of the disorder. It is advised that people with strong family history of depression should space out their pregnancies to avoid poor parenting of the child. In addition, other interventions in parent–child relationship with a special focus on depressed mothers to improve parenting would also be crucial towards reducing the incidence of the disorder. Events centered interventions that target life events would also reduce the incidence of depressive disorder.

Question 163 Answer: b, Secondary prevention
Explanation: In secondary prevention, the aim is early detection and treatment of hidden morbidity in order to prevent the progress of the disorder. For depressive disorder, early detection of depressive disorders by GPs or through public education and use of screening instruments and psychiatric outreach services can help with this.

Question 164 Answer: c, Tertiary prevention
Explanation: The aim of tertiary prevention is to reduce the disabilities arising as a consequence of the disorder.

Reference: Puri BK, Hall A, Ho R (2014). *Revision Notes in Psychiatry*. London: CRC Press, p. 400.

Theme: Psychotherapy

Question 165 Answer: j, Shaping
Explanation: This phenomenon is known as shaping.

Reference and Further Reading: Puri BK, Treasaden I (eds) (2010). *Psychiatry: An Evidence-Based Text*. London: Hodder Arnold, p. 204.

Question 166 Answer: i, Reciprocal inhibition
Explanation: Reciprocal inhibition is a concept developed by Joseph Wolpe. Opposing emotions cannot exist simultaneously.

Reference and Further Reading: Puri BK, Treasaden I (eds) (2010). *Psychiatry: An Evidence-Based Text*. London: Hodder Arnold, pp. 655, 990.

Question 167 Answer: k, Systematic desensitization
Explanation: Systemic desensitization was developed by Wolpe.

Reference and Further Reading: Puri BK, Treasaden I (eds) (2010). *Psychiatry: An Evidence-Based Text*. London: Hodder Arnold, p. 990.

This question has been modified from the 2008–2010 examination.

Theme: Pharmacodynamics

Question 168 Answer: b, 5-HT$_{1A}$ partial agonist, f, 5-HT$_{2A}$ antagonist, k, D$_2$ partial agonist
Explanation: Aripiprazole is a 5-HT$_{1A}$ partial agonist, 5-HT$_{2A}$ antagonist and D$_2$ partial agonist.

Reference and Further Reading: Puri BK, Treasaden I (eds) (2010). *Psychiatry: An Evidence-Based Text*. London: Hodder Arnold, pp. 425, 426, 604, 904.

Question 169 Answer: l, GABA-A agonist
Explanation: Diazepam is a GABA-A agonist.

Reference and Further Reading: Puri BK, Treasaden I (eds) (2010). *Psychiatry: An Evidence-Based Text*. London: Hodder Arnold, pp. 648, 873, 905.

Question 170 Answer: g, Alpha$_2$ agonist
Explanation: Lofexidine is an alpha$_2$ agonist.

Reference and Further Reading: Puri BK, Treasaden I (eds) (2010). *Psychiatry: An Evidence-Based Text*. London: Hodder Arnold, p. 1040.

This question has been modified from the 2008 examination.

Theme: Antipsychotics

Question 171 Answer: b, 2
Explanation: 2 mg is the minimum effective dose in this case.

Question 172 Answer: d, 15
Explanation: This patient needs to continue for 2–24 months.

Reference: Taylor D, Paton C, Kapur S (2009). *The Maudsley Prescribing Guidelines*. London: Informa Healthcare.

Question 173 Answer: j, 75
Explanation: This risk of relapse is around 75%.

Reference and Further Reading: Puri BK, Treasaden I (eds) (2010). *Psychiatry: An Evidence-Based Text*. London: Hodder Arnold, pp. 632, 601, 602.

This question has been modified from the 2008–2010 examination.

Theme: Ethics

Question 174 Answer: j, Phronesis
Explanation: Phronesis is defined as the action of a person in a particular situation based on ethical principle. Phronesis was proposed by Aristotle and it is one of the appeals to character. The other two appeals are good will and virtue. Phronesis is a prerequisite for virtue.

Question 175 Answer: g, Ethical relativism
Explanation: Ethical relativism prescribes the way different groups of people ought to behave. In contrast, cultural relativism describes how different groups of people actually hold different moral standards for evaluating acts as right or wrong in a society.

Question 176 Answer: d, Categorical imperatives
Explanation: Immanuel Kant (1724–1804) proposed the concept of categorical imperatives. According to this theory, human beings occupy a special place among all categories of organisms. The views or proposition of a human being towards the other animals (i.e. the imperatives) determine his or her actions or morality.

Theme: DSM-IV-TR

Question 177 Answer: i, 81–90
Explanation: Her score is between 81 and 90 because her symptoms are mild and she demonstrates good functioning in wide range of areas.

Question 178 Answer: e, 41–50
Explanation: Her score is between 41 and 50 because the kleptomania results in serious impairment in social and occupational functioning.

Question 179 Answer: a
Explanation: This man got the lowest GAF score because he cannot maintain personal hygiene.

Reference and Further Reading: American Psychiatric Association (2000). *Diagnostic Criteria from DSM-IV-TR*. Washington, DC: American Psychiatric Association; Puri BK, Treasaden I (eds) (2010). *Psychiatry: An Evidence-Based Text.* London: Hodder Arnold, pp. 493, 494.

Theme: Neuropsychological tests

Question 180 Answer: h, Raven's Progressive Matrices
Explanation: The Raven's Progressive Matrices assess her performance IQ. In each test item of the Raven Progressive Matrices test, one is asked to find the missing pattern in a series and this is a nonverbal test of intelligence.

Question 181 Answer: d, Goldstein's Object Sorting Test
Explanation: The Goldstein's Object Sorting Test assesses her concrete thinking.

Question 182 Answer: o, Wisconsin Card Sorting Test
Explanation: The Wisconsin Card Sorting Test assesses her executive function.

Reference and Further Reading: Puri BK, Treasaden I (eds) (2010). *Psychiatry: An Evidence-Based Text*. London: Hodder Arnold, pp. 96, 509, 536.

This question has been modified from the 2008–2010 examination.

Theme: Freud's dream interpretation

Question 183 Answer: d, Manifest content
Explanation: Manifest content is the secondary elaboration of acceptable images in a narrative manner and these images are often linked to day residue or events prior to sleep.

Question 184 Answer: a, Condensation
Explanation: Condensation is the process where impulses are transferred to acceptable images.

Question 185 Answer: c, Latent content
Explanation: Latent content refers to the true meaning of the dream in expressing unconscious thoughts and wishes.

Theme: Sleep disorders

Question 186 Answer: b, Myoclonic jerks
Explanation: Myoclonic jerks are caused by sudden muscle contractions. Myoclonic jerks are seen in people with neurological disorders such as Creutzfeldt–Jakob disease, Parkinson's disease and epilepsy.

Reference and Further Reading: Puri BK, Treasaden I (eds) (2010). *Psychiatry: An Evidence-Based Text*. London: Hodder Arnold, p. 523.

Question 187 Answer: a, Circadian rhythm sleep disorders
Explanation: She suffers from circadian rhythm sleep disorders because she cannot sleep and wake up at the time, which correspond to normal routine in the general population and result in decline in occupational function.

Reference and Further Reading: Puri BK, Treasaden I (eds) (2010). *Psychiatry: An Evidence-Based Text*. London: Hodder Arnold, pp. 142–143, 398; Puri BK, Treasaden I (eds) (2010). *Psychiatry: An Evidence-Based Text*. London: Hodder Arnold, pp. 541–552.

Question 188 Answer: h, Rhythmic movement disorder
Explanation: Rhythmic movement disorder (RMM) includes a group of stereotyped movements such as body rocking and head banging is usually seen in early childhood. When the movements occur, they usually last less than 15 minutes. The large muscles of the body, often in the head and neck, are usually involved. RMM occurs during the transition between sleep and wake states, at bedtime and naptimes, during arousals from sleep at night and sometimes during light sleep.

Question 189 Answer: c, Non-24-hour sleep-wake syndrome
Explanation: In non-24-hour sleep-wake syndrome, patients feel that a day is longer than 24 hours and there is 1- to 2-hour daily delay in sleep onset and wake times compared to other individuals in the society. This condition is common among blind people who cannot see light.

Theme: British history of insanity defence
Question 190 Answer: d, The irresistible impulse test
Explanation: The Edward Oxford trial (1840) is associated with the irresistible impulse test.

Question 191 Answer: a, First recorded psychiatric testimony
Explanation: The Earl Ferrers trial was the first recorded psychiatric testimony in the history of British law.

Question 192 Answer: c, Offspring of a delusion
Explanation: James Hadfield was known as the offspring of a delusion.

Reference: Bewley T (2008). *Madness to Mental Illness. A History of the Royal College of Psychiatrists*. London: Gaskell.

Theme: Piaget's cognitive development

Question 193 Answer: g, Egocentrism, r, Preoperational stage
Explanation: Egocentrism occurs in preoperational stage (2–7 years).

Question 194 Answer: d, Assimilation, q, Sensorimotor stage
Explanation: Assimilation occurs in sensorimotor stage (0–2 years).

Question 195 Answer: j, Hypothetico-deductive thinking, t, Formal operational stage
Explanation: Hypothetical–detective thinking occurs in formal operational stage (older than 11 years).

Reference and Further Reading: Puri BK, Treasaden I (eds) (2010). *Psychiatry: An Evidence-Based Text*. London: Hodder Arnold, pp. 113–115.

GET THROUGH MRCPSYCH PAPER A1: MOCK EXAMINATION

Total number of questions: 193 (133 MCQs, 60 EMIs)
Total time provided: 180 minutes

Question 1
A 70-year-old woman is referred by her general practitioner (GP) to you for psychiatric assessment. She mistakes her husband for her deceased father and later for her elder brother. She believes that she has never married. She also mistakes her daughter for her younger sister. The psychopathology being described is
a. De Clerambault's syndrome
b. Capgras syndrome
c. Fregoli syndrome
d. Intermetamorphosis syndrome
e. Othello syndrome

Question 2
The community mental health team visits a 40-year-old man who describes the experience of being able to hear conversations from the police station in the neighbouring town. The psychopathology being described is
a. Autoscopy
b. Doppelgänger
c. Extracampine hallucination
d. Hypnagogic hallucination
e. Hypnopompic hallucination

Question 3
When the condition response seems more prominent after multiple exposure to the original conditioned stimulus, it is typically known as
a. Generalization
b. Discrimination
c. Incubation
d. Stimulus preparedness
e. Extinction

Question 4
Based on your understanding of pharmacology, neuroleptic malignant syndrome is classified under which of the following particular type of side effect?
a. Idiosyncratic reaction to medication
b. Time-dependent side effect
c. Dose-dependent side effect
d. Toxicity side effect
e. Withdrawal side effect

Question 5
Which of the following statements regarding the neurodevelopment and the neurochemistry of attention deficit hyperactivity disorder (ADHD) is incorrect?
a. September is considered to be the peak month for births of children with ADHD and without comorbid learning disorders.
b. Early infection, inflammation, toxins and trauma would cause circulatory, metabolic and physical brain damage, which might lead to ADHD in adulthood.
c. Psychosocial adversity is not one of the key factors associated with ADHD in childhood.
d. A dysfunction in noradrenaline might lead to negative feedback to the locus coeruleus.
e. A dysfunction in noradrenaline might lead to a reduction of noradrenaline in the central nervous system (CNS).

Question 6
A 30-year-old man is suspected to be a malingerer who tries to avoid court hearing and admitted himself to an orthopaedic ward for sudden paralysis. You want to examine his gait. Which of the following features strongly suggest that this man is indeed a malingerer?
a. Bending forward and advancing with rapid shuffling gait
b. Gait improves with suggestion
c. Reeling clownish gait
d. Unable to commence gait during examination
e. Walking like a pigeon

Question 7
In this form of dysphasia, there are difficulties with comprehension. Which form of dysphasia would this be?
a. Receptive dysphasia
b. Expressive dysphasia
c. Conduction dysphasia
d. Global dysphasia
e. Paraphasia

Question 8
A 60-year-old male suffered from a stroke recently, and after treatment, he is left with some speech difficulties. He is able to comprehend and understand what

others are saying, but he is not able to formulate and say a sentence such that others would understand. Which form of dysphasia would this be?
a. Receptive dysphasia
b. Expressive dysphasia
c. Conduction dysphasia
d. Global dysphasia
e. Paraphasia

Question 9
A 25-year-old man with a history of cocaine misuse feels bugs on his skin. He scratches at the 'bugs' trying to remove them, gouging his skin and leaving scars. The psychopathology being described is
a. Formication
b. Functional hallucination
c. Gustatory hallucination
d. Reflex hallucination
e. Visceral hallucination

Question 10
The concept of systematic desensitization that is being used in the treatment of anxiety-related disorders are based on which of the following behavioural models?
a. Reciprocal inhibition
b. Habituation
c. Chaining
d. Shaping
e. Cueing

Question 11
A 30-year-old male has had a history of bipolar disorder and he has been on lithium monotherapy. He just returned from a trip to Singapore, where he did a lot of outdoor activities in the sun. He just also developed diarrhoea. Currently, he noticed that he has hand tremors. Which of the following side effect is he suffering from?
a. Idiosyncratic reaction
b. Time dependent
c. Dose dependent
d. Toxicity
e. Withdrawal

Question 12
Which of the following is not considered to be a core symptom of adult ADHD?
a. Hyperactivity
b. Impatient
c. Forgetfulness
d. Distractibility
e. Chronic procrastination

Question 13

A 50-year-old man has been diagnosed with acquired immunodeficiency syndrome (AIDS). He is concerned about getting other infections. Which opportunistic infection is the commonest life-threatening opportunistic infection seen in patients with AIDS?

a. Leishmaniasis
b. Pneumocystis carinii
c. *Streptococcus pneumoniae*
d. *Toxoplasma gondii*
e. Tuberculosis

Question 14

A 60-year-old man has just suffered from an acute stroke. Immediately after the stroke, he realized that he is unable to understand written materials. However, when his care-giver spells the words out loud, he can immediately recognize them. He is still able to write. Which of the following is the most appropriate diagnosis?

a. Alexia without agraphia
b. Alexia with agraphia
c. Apraxia
d. Acalculia
e. Anarithmetria

Question 15

Which of the following is the most characteristic and consistent abnormality in delirium?

a. Agitation
b. Disturbance in attention
c. Disorientation to place
d. Short- or long-term memory loss
e. Visual hallucination

Question 16

Which of the following is the most lethal combination of medications in causing serotonin syndrome?

a. Phenelzine and fluoxetine
b. Phenelzine and amitriptyline
c. Phenelzine and meperidine
d. Methylphenidate and MDMA
e. Moclobemide and paroxetine

Question 17

The local dual addictions services just introduced a new programme aimed at promoting cocaine abstinence. The new programme would last for 12 weeks, and for the initial 6 weeks, the participants would earn cash vouchers if their urine sample showed a 25% decrease in the amount of cocaine, and in the next 6 weeks, they would continue to earn cash vouchers if their urine sample was entirely

negative. This method of promoting cocaine abstinence is based on which of the following psychological theories?
a. Cueing
b. Chaining
c. Shaping
d. Gradual approximation
e. Variable reinforcement scheduling

Question 18
A 60-year-old man, Peter, is referred by his GP to you for auditory hallucinations before he falls asleep. Which of the following is the most common presentation of such psychopathology?
a. Hearing classical music
b. Hearing, 'Peter, Peter'
c. Hearing, 'You are useless'
d. Seeing flash lights
e. Seeing a view of wide area

Question 19
A 3-year-old boy has a fear of dogs. When he sees a dog around, he experiences marked tachycardia and increased arousal and then he feels an intense feeling of fear. His experience of fear would be best described by which one of the following theories?
a. James–Lange theory
b. Cannon–Bard theory
c. Cognitive labelling theory
d. Cognitive appraisal theory
e. Emotion-regulation theory

Question 20
A medical student is puzzled as to why there are so many different subtypes of schizophrenia. She wonders which one of the following terminologies best describes a form of schizophrenia that is characterized by the development of prominent negative symptoms, without much positive symptoms.
a. Paranoid schizophrenia
b. Hebephrenia schizophrenia
c. Simple schizophrenia
d. Post-schizophrenia depression
e. Residual schizophrenia

Question 21
The core trainee on examination of a patient noticed that the patient has been having difficulties with performing movements involving that of the face, lips, tongue and cheek. The patient is not able to pretend to blow out a match. What specific type of apraxia is this?
a. Ideational apraxia
b. Ideomotor apraxia

c. Orobuccal apraxia

d. Construction apraxia

e. None of the above

Question 22

When a 2-year-old child is separated from his mother, it will lead to all of the following emotions except

a. Protesting by crying

b. Searching behaviour

c. Marked apathy and misery

d. Detachment

e. Anger

Question 23

Which of the following is not included under 'Mental Retardation' International Classification of Diseases (ICD) classification system?

a. Mild mental retardation

b. Moderate mental retardation

c. Severe mental retardation

d. Profound mental retardation

e. Mental retardation not otherwise specified

Question 24

Which of the following symptoms is not a part of the Diagnostic and Statistical Manual of Mental Disorders (DSM)-IV-TR diagnostic criteria for melancholia?

a. Distinct quality of depressed mood

b. Depression regularly worse in the evening

c. Marked psychomotor agitation

d. Significant anorexia or weight loss

e. Excessive or inappropriate guilt

Question 25

A 25-year-old woman presents with anxiety. You order a thyroid function test. Her serum thyroid-stimulating hormone (TSH) level is 0.3 mU/L (normal range: 0.5–5 mU/L) and her total thyroxine is 90 mmol/L (normal range: 70–140 mmol/L). The patient does not have a non-thyroidal illness and is not on drug treatment that could suppress TSH. Physical examination shows no goitre. What is your next step?

a. Check serum free thyroxine (FT4) and free triiodothyronine (FT3).

b. Order isotope scan.

c. Refer for specialist management.

d. Recheck TSH in 1 week.

e. Start levothyroxine therapy.

Question 26

In order to make the diagnosis of post-schizophrenia depression, the schizophrenic illness must have occurred within which of the following duration of time?

a. Last 3 months

b. Last 6 months

c. Last 8 months
d. Last 12 months
e. Last 24 months

Question 27
A 60-year-old woman complained of depression and her GP started her on citalopram. After 2 weeks of treatment, she complains of lethargy, muscle weakness and nausea. The GP wants to know the most likely cause for her symptoms. Your answer is
   a. Acute confusional state
   b. Generalized anxiety disorder
   c. Hyponatraemia
   d. Serotonin syndrome
   e. Somatization disorder

Question 28
You have been asked to interview a prisoner, as the prison officers have noticed abnormalities in his behaviour. It was noted that he would not eat his food unless they were packaged, and at times, he attempted to cover his head with his clothes. When the officers asked him the reasons for doing so, he told them he needed to do so as he believed that there were people around who could get to know what he was thinking. What psychopathology does this represent?
   a. Passivity experience
   b. Hallucinations
   c. Delusional ideations
   d. Thought broadcasting
   e. Thought echo

Question 29
A 45-year-old man is recently diagnosed with Huntington's disease. He is very concerned about the diagnosis. He has read information from the Internet about Huntington's disease. Which of the following statements is false?
   a. Patients with Huntington's disease may suffer from akinetic mutism at late stage.
   b. Patients with Huntington's disease have a higher risk of committing suicide compared to the general population.
   c. Patients with Huntington's disease will die in 5–10 years after the onset of visible symptoms.
   d. Most patients with Huntington's disease die of pneumonia.
   e. The longer length of trinucleotide repeats is associated with faster progression of symptoms.

Question 30
The core trainee was administering the Mini Mental State Examination for one of the patients. It was noted that the patient was unable to draw the interconnected double pentagon. What form of apraxia is this?
   a. Ideational apraxia
   b. Ideomotor apraxia

c. Orobuccal apraxia

d. Construction apraxia

e. Dressing apraxia

Question 31

An 11-month-old baby is shown his favourite toy. His mother then covers the toy with a cloth. The baby reaches out to remove the cloth and grasps the toy. According to Piaget, which concept best describes the aforementioned phenomenon?

a. Invisible displacement

b. Conservation

c. Problem solving

d. Circular reaction

e. Object permanence

Question 32

A 25-year-old man is referred by his GP for depression after the death of his father. Based on the DSM-IV-TR diagnostic criteria, which of the following symptoms favours the diagnosis of bereavement rather than major depressive disorder?

a. Auditory hallucination of hearing voices from his father

b. Guilt about delay in sending his father to the hospital

c. Marked psychomotor retardation

d. Thought of dying with his father

e. Worthlessness

Question 33

Based on Parsons's model, the role of doctors includes all of the following, with the exception of

a. Defining the underlying illness

b. Legitimizing the illness

c. Imposing an illness diagnosis

d. Offering help when needed

e. Imposing the appropriate cost

Question 34

The Camberwell Family Interview has been used to assess expressed emotions. Which combination of factors has been identified to be predictive of relapse?

a. Critical comments, hostility, emotional over-involvement

b. Critical comments, hostility, warmth

c. Critical comments, emotional over-involvement, warmth

d. Hostility, emotional over-involvement, warmth

e. Emotional over-involvement, warmth, positive remarks

Question 35

Based on the Holmes and Rahe Social Readjustment Scale, which of the following is associated with the highest life change value?
a. Marital separation
b. Marriage
c. Pregnancy
d. Birth of a child
e. Problems with boss

Question 36

All of the following statements accurately reflect the similarities between depression in the young and depression in the old, with the exception of
a. Sleep disturbances (such as early morning awakening, subjective poor sleep quality)
b. Poor appetite
c. Weight loss
d. Depressive pseudo-dementia
e. Reduction in interest

Question 37

A junior doctor is having her first night call. She sees a man walking alone in the hospital corridor at 3:00 AM. Based on her experience, there should be staff working in the hospital in the middle of the night. She deduced this man is either a medical or nursing staff. Which of the following types of processing is she most likely using in her deduction?
a. Bottom-up processing
b. Central processing
c. Control processing
d. Information processing
e. Top-down processing

Question 38

A core trainee was asked to review a newly admitted patient prior to the ward rounds. During physical examination, he noted that on attempting to move the patient's arm upwards, it stays in the same position thereafter. He is unable to ask the patient to relax his arm and this lasted for a total duration of 2 hours. This sign is commonly referred to as
a. Posturing
b. Stereotypies
c. Waxy flexibility
d. Tics
e. Parkinsonism

Question 39

A 25-year-old man drinks alcohol every morning before going to the office and he is often late to work due to slowness. He drinks again during lunchtime. After coming home, he usually needs to drink at least 8 units of alcohol before he sleeps because he has repeated thoughts that alcohol calms his nerves. His drinking habit has been the same for the past 5 years. A medical student wants to describe his behaviour. Which of the following description is incorrect?

a. Compulsion to drink
b. Lack of resistance to control drinking
c. Obsession with alcohol
d. Rationalization of the need to drink
e. Tolerance to the effects of alcohol

Question 40

The following are signs and symptoms indicative of an insult to the dominant parietal lobe, with the exception of

a. Gerstmann's syndrome
b. Astereognosis
c. Ideomotor apraxia
d. Impairment in two-point discrimination
e. Asomatognosia

Question 41

A 25-year-old man is referred by his GP for depression after the death of his father. He exhibits almost all symptoms of depression except worthlessness and active suicidal ideation. Based on the DSM-IV-TR criteria, what is the maximum duration of symptoms to meet the diagnostic criteria of uncomplicated bereavement rather than major depression?

a. 1 month
b. 2 months
c. 3 months
d. 4 months
e. 6 months

Question 42

A widely used toolkit for further research into life events and associated psychiatric disorder would be the Life Events and Difficulties Schedule (LEDS) proposed by Brown and Harries (1978). All of the following statements regarding LEDS are true, with the exception of

a. It is based on a semi-structured interview.
b. Forty areas are being probed during the interview.
c. Detailed narratives are obtained regarding events, including their circumstances.
d. It has a high level of reliability.
e. It has a high level of validity.

Question 43

Which one of the following toolkits would be most useful for evaluating damage to the brain?

a. Mini Mental State Examination
b. Halstead–Reitan Battery

c. Luria Neuropsychological Battery
d. Nebraska Neuropsychological Battery
e. Repeatable Battery for the Assessment of Neuropsychological Status

Question 44
Which of the following statements about Piaget's cognitive development theory is correct?
  a. In the preoperational stage, rules are believed to be inviolable.
  b. The preoperational stage is linked to circular reactions.
  c. Piaget held that conservation was established in the preoperational stage.
  d. Object permanence gets fully developed during the preoperational stage.
  e. The preoperational stage is linked to conservation of fluid volume.

Question 45
A 30-year-old pregnant woman finds it difficult to not drink at all throughout pregnancy. She is currently 10-weeks pregnant. She wants to know the upper limits of units of alcohol she can take per week. Your answer is
  a. Absolutely 0 units
  b. 1–4 units
  c. 3–6 units
  d. 5–8 units
  e. 7–10 units

Question 46
A 45-year-old female is here to seek help from the CAMHS psychiatrist. She shared that her son James has been too much for her to handle. He not only skips school for no reason, but has been getting himself into bad company and has been recently using drugs too. What diagnosis do you think the CAMHS consultant would label James with?
  a. ADHD
  b. Pervasive development disorder
  c. Conduct disorder
  d. Oppositional defiant disorder
  e. School refusal

Question 47
Which of the following antidepressants exhibit alpha-receptor antagonism and serotonin receptor inhibition?
  a. Amitriptyline
  b. Duloxetine
  c. Mirtazapine
  d. Reboxetine
  e. Venlafaxine

Question 48
A 25-year-old male has been referred by his GP to the mental health service. Over the past 3 months or so, he has been feeling increasingly troubled by his neighbours. He

believes that they are deliberately sending in radiation to harm him and his mother. In addition, he claims that he is able to hear his neighbours making demeaning remarks by the wall. At times, he is even more troubled as they seemed to be commenting on his every action. What form of psychopathology does he present with?

a. Extracampine hallucinations
b. Pseudo-hallucination
c. Thought interference
d. Passivity phenomenon
e. Running commentary

Question 49

A junior doctor is having her first night call. She sees a man walking alone in the hospital corridor at 3:00 AM. He wears a white coat and holds a stethoscope. She deduces that he must be a medical doctor. Which of the following types of processing is she most likely using in her deduction?

a. Bottom-up processing
b. Central processing
c. Control processing
d. Information processing
e. Top-down processing

Question 50

A 25-year-old male has been seen by the addiction services and he has since been abstinent from alcohol for the past 3 months. However, he is still bothered by recurrent auditory hallucinations. Which of the following is the most likely clinical diagnosis?

a. Alcohol withdrawal
b. Delirium tremens
c. Alcoholic hallucinosis
d. Delusional disorder
e. Schizophrenia

Question 51

A 42-year-old man is referred by his GP for depression, memory impairment, fidgety hands and flycatcher's tongue. His father committed suicide at the age of 47. His grandfather suffered from behavioural problems and died at the age of 50. Which of the following is the most likely diagnosis?

a. Cervical myelopathy
b. Huntington's disease
c. Malignant spinal disease
d. Parkinson's disease
e. Wilson's disease

Question 52

Which stage of Kohlberg theory of moral development is achieved at the conventional stage?

a. Universal ethical principle orientation
b. Social-order-maintaining orientation

c. Instrumental purpose orientation
d. Punishment and obedience orientation
e. Social-contract orientation

Question 53
A 21-year-old female medical student was brought in by the university counsellor as she was in shock and anger after being informed that she had failed in all subjects in her examinations and that she would need to repeat the first year. When you examined her, she was in a daze with purposeless overactivity. The counsellor would like to know when her symptoms would start to disappear. Based on the ICD-10 criteria, the answer is
a. 1 hour
b. 12 hours
c. 24 hours
d. 48 hours
e. 60 hours

Question 54
A 22-year-old university student has decided that he needs to see a psychiatrist as he has a fear of darkness since youth. However, he tells the psychiatrist that he is not overtly distressed when he is in the dark and he does not take measures to avoid being in darkness. Which one of the following statements is true?
a. He has a specific phobia, as the fear of darkness is out of proportion to the norm.
b. He has a specific phobia, as the fear of darkness cannot be reasoned or explained away.
c. He has a specific phobia, as the feelings of fear are way beyond his own voluntary control.
d. He has no specific phobia, as the fear of darkness is not included in the list of specific phobia.
e. He does not have specific phobia, as there is no avoidance behaviour in his case.

Question 55
A 30-year-old woman suffers from bipolar disorder and she has been treated with lithium. She is concerned about renal and thyroid dysfunction. She wants to change the mood stabilizer. Which of the following medications has the least prophylactic effect against future manic episodes?
a. Carbamazepine
b. Olanzapine
c. Risperidone
d. Sodium valproate
e. Topiramate

Question 56
A medical student is puzzled and confused about the signs and symptoms associated with mania and hypomania. Which of the following is not one of the classical signs and symptoms of someone with a diagnosis of mania?
a. Elevated energy level
b. Marked irritability, out of keeping with character

c. Elevated mood
d. Spending more than usual
e. Memory disturbances

Question 57
Which of the following metabolic causes is least likely to cause chorea?
a. Hypercalacaemia
b. Hyperglycaemia
c. Hyponatraemia
d. Hypoglycaemia
e. Hypomagnesaemia

Question 58
Nondominant temporal lobe damage could potentially lead to impaired performance on this particular test:
a. Object learning test
b. Synonym learning test
c. Paired associated learning test
d. Rey–Osterrieth Test
e. Benton Visual Retention Test

Question 59
With regards to the aetiology of schizophrenia, which of the following statements is true about the risk of developing schizophrenia among immigrants?
a. Social factors are less in importance in predisposing individuals towards schizophrenia as compared to biological factors.
b. Afro-Caribbean immigrants to the United Kingdom have a higher risk of schizophrenia.
c. Afro-Caribbean immigrants have the same risk as the population in their native countries.
d. First-generation immigrants are more likely to develop schizophrenia and hence efforts should be focused on them.
e. The higher rates of schizophrenia in urban areas is mainly due to migration.

Question 60
A mother is worried that her child will develop bipolar disorder. Which of the following genes has been found to be associated with an increased risk of developing bipolar disorder?
a. Tryptophan hydroxylase gene
b. Serotonin transporter gene
c. COMT gene
d. APOE3 gene
e. Presenilin-2

Question 61

This is a psychiatric disorder that is characterized by the following cluster of symptoms: cataplexy and excessive daytime sleepiness. The most likely clinical diagnosis would be

a. Narcolepsy
b. Circadian rhythm disorder
c. Primary hypersomnia
d. Secondary hypersomnia
e. Sleep terror

Question 62

Which particular subtypes of schizophrenia has been believed to have an increased rate of suicide?

a. Paranoid schizophrenia
b. Hebephrenic schizophrenia
c. Catatonic schizophrenia
d. Post-schizophrenia depression
e. Simple schizophrenia

Question 63

A 30-year-old woman suffers from depression and she is very concerned about gastrointestinal side effects. Which of the following antidepressants causes the most intense gastrointestinal side effects?

a. Citalopram
b. Mirtazapine
c. Paroxetine
d. Sertraline
e. Venlafaxine

Question 64

Which of the following statements about emotion is true?

a. According to the James–Lange theory, emotions have primacy over physiology.
b. Distress is a primary emotion.
c. According to the Cannon–Bard theory, the emotion-arousing stimulus is processed by the hypothalamus.
d. According to Lazarus, emotions can be without cognition.
e. Facial expression can affect emotional response.

Question 65

A patient who has a long-standing history of schizophrenia has been on continuous follow-up with the community psychiatric nurse. He has been concordance to treatment. However, lately he vocalizes that some of his symptoms seem to be coming back. He is complaining of having difficulties in thinking as he

believes that the every black car that passes by his house has an electronic device within to jam up his thoughts. What form of psychopathology is this?
a. Thought insertion
b. Thought withdrawal
c. Passivity phenomenon
d. Hallucinations
e. Delusional perception

Question 66
The triad of narcolepsy is classically defined as
a. Daytime sleep attacks, catalepsy, hypnogogic hallucination
b. Daytime sleep attacks, catalepsy, hypnopompic hallucination
c. Daytime sleep attacks, cataplexy, hypnogogic hallucination
d. Daytime sleep attacks, cataplexy, hypnopompic hallucination
e. Night-time sleep attacks, cataplexy, hypnopompic hallucination

Question 67
Which of the following statements regarding diagnostic criteria for panic disorder is false?
a. Based on the DSM-IV-TR, panic disorder is classified into panic disorder with agoraphobia and panic disorder without agoraphobia.
b. Based on the DSM-IV-TR, agoraphobia is classified into agoraphobia without history of panic disorder and panic disorder with agoraphobia.
c. Based on the ICD-10, agoraphobia is classified into agoraphobia without history of panic disorder and panic disorder with agoraphobia.
d. Based on the ICD-10, panic disorder is classified into panic disorder with agoraphobia and panic disorder without agoraphobia.
e. Based on the ICD-10 criteria further define severe panic disorder of having at least 4 panic attacks per week over a 4-week period.

Question 68
The following statements about the Mini Mental State Examination (MMSE) are true, with the exception of
a. It is a relatively brief test that could be routinely used to rapidly detect possible underlying dementia.
b. It could help to estimate the relative degree of severity of dementia.
c. It could help to follow up on dementia and progression over a period of time.
d. It cannot be used to differentiate between dementia and delirium.
e. It includes tests of short-term memory and immediate recall memory.

Question 69
Which one of the following dementia rating scales could be given to caregivers for an assessment of the cognitive functions of an individual?
a. Blessed Dementia Scale
b. Information-Memory-Concentration Test
c. Geriatric Mental State Schedule

d. Cambridge Neuropsychological Test Automated Battery
e. Gresham Ward Questionnaire

Question 70

There has been much media attention about how dangerous patients with schizophrenia could be. What is the actual estimated risk of violence amongst patients with schizophrenia?
   a. 0.01
   b. 0.05
   c. 0.08
   d. 0.10
   e. 0.20

Question 71

A 50-year-old man, after brain injury to the nondominant parietal lobe, came to believe that he has seen himself on a number of occasions while travelling to different cities in his country. He is aware of himself both inside and outside his body. He feels that his office has been copied and exists in two different cities. Which of the following statements is false?
   a. The knowledge of having a double is occasionally a delusion, or hallucination but more commonly is a variant of depersonalization.
   b. This condition can occur in other people without psychiatric illness.
   c. This condition consists of a delusion that a double of a person or place exists somewhere else.
   d. This condition is known as reduplicative paramnesia.
   e. This condition is a perceptual rather than ideational or cognitive disturbance.

Question 72

Which of the following is not one of Cannon's critiques of the James–Lange theory?
   a. Physiological arousal is not sufficient.
   b. Emotions can be independent of bodily responses.
   c. Similar visceral changes can accompany different emotions.
   d. Overt behaviour can lead to emotions without visceral changes.
   e. Emotions can occur before somatic responses.

Question 73

Which of the following is the most common type of violence demonstrated by patients with schizophrenia?
   a. Verbal aggression
   b. Physical aggression towards objects
   c. Physical aggression towards others
   d. Self-directed violence
   e. None of the above

Question 74

Restless leg syndrome is most commonly associated with
   a. Calcium deficiency
   b. Iron deficiency

c. Potassium deficiency
d. Sodium deficiency
e. Zinc deficiency

Question 75

Which of the following is an assessment scale that involves a structured interview with a relative?
a. Geriatric Mental State Schedule
b. Cambridge Examination for Mental Disorders
c. Crichton Geriatric Behavior Rating Scale
d. Stockton Geriatric Rating Scale
e. Clifton Assessment Schedule

Question 76

Which of the following statements about Amok is incorrect?
a. This is a condition that was initially described in Malays in the mid-sixteenth century.
b. It occurs only in Malays and there have not been reports of Amok from any other countries.
c. It consists of a period of withdrawal, followed by a sudden outburst of homicidal aggression in which the sufferer will attack anyone within reach.
d. The attack usually lasts for several hours until the sufferer is overwhelmed.
e. Following the attack, the person typically passes into a deep sleep or stupor for several days, and would have subsequent amnesia of the event.

Question 77

Which of the following statements regarding diagnostic criteria for post-traumatic stress disorder is true?
a. The DSM-IV-TR and the ICD-10 specify acute and chronic PTSD.
b. The DSM-IV-TR and ICD-10 specify PTSD with delayed onset.
c. The DSM-IV-TR specifies the minimum duration of disturbance of PTSD is more than 2 months.
d. If duration of symptoms is less than 4 months, it will be specified as acute PTSD.
e. The ICD-10, but not the DSM-IV-TR, specifies acute and chronic PTSD.

Question 78

You are a core trainee who has just started out your inpatient psychiatry posting. The consultant asked you to review a patient prior to the ward rounds. When speaking to the patient, you noticed that the patient appeared to keep repeating whatever word you have just mentioned. The phrase that correctly describes this form of psychopathology is
a. Approximate answer (Vorbeireden)
b. Cryptolalia
c. Echolalia
d. Perseveration
e. Neologism

Question 79

A 26-year-old man was exercising at the neighbourhood park at night. He was sweating profusely, and his heart was palpitating. The lights were out at one section of the park, and he became aware of how dark and quiet the surroundings were. The awareness of his surroundings made him feel scared. Which of the following theories best describes the aforementioned phenomenon?'

a. Cannon–Bard theory
b. Ekman–Paul theory
c. Plutchik theory
d. James–Lange theory
e. Schachter–Singer theory

Question 80

A 30-year-old woman attempts suicide after ingesting 25 50-mg tablets of amitriptyline prescribed by her GP. The patient looks alert. The Accident and Emergency Department consultant asks you to admit this patient to the psychiatric ward, as he thinks that the psychiatric risk is higher than the medical risk. You are concerned about her medical condition. Which part of the ECG would be most significant in assessing her cardiac risk?

a. Length of P wave
b. Length of QRS interval
c. Length of RR interval
d. T wave inversion
e. Pathological U wave

Question 81

A 50-year-old man presents with a 6-month history of forgetfulness and urinary incontinence. Physical examination shows gait disturbance. Which of the following conditions is the most likely?

a. Chronic subdural haematoma
b. Hypothyroidism
c. Normal pressure hydrocephalus
d. Neurosyphilis
e. Vitamin B_{12} deficiency

Question 82

In clinical practice, it is often difficult to differentiate obsession from delusion. Which of the following strongly indicates that a patient suffers from obsessive-compulsive disorder (OCD) rather than delusional disorder?

a. Better occupational functioning.
b. No other psychotic phenomenon such as hallucinations.
c. The thought content is less bizarre.
d. The patient believes that the origin of thoughts is from his or her own mind.
e. The patient tries to resist his thoughts.

Question 83

A 44-year-old man suffers from depression. He had severe aortic regurgitation, and aortic valve replacement was performed after percutaneous coronary intervention. He takes warfarin 2 mg every morning. The prothrombin time (PT) is 24.5 seconds (normal range: 12.0–14.5 seconds) and the international normalized ratio (INR) is 3.60 (normal range: 2.50–3.50). Based on the National Institute of Clinical Excellence (NICE) guidelines, which of the following antidepressants would you recommend?

a. Citalopram
b. Fluoxetine
c. Fluvoxamine
d. Mirtazapine
e. Sertraine

Question 84

In Alzheimer's disease, the most common EEG pattern is

a. Loss of alpha activity and decrease in diffuse slow waves
b. Loss of alpha activity and increase in diffuse slow waves
c. Loss of delta activity and decrease in diffuse slow waves
d. Loss of delta activity and increase in diffuse slow waves
e. Loss of theta activity and decrease in fast activity

Question 85

Which one of the following statements about the culture-bound condition 'Dhat' is incorrect?

a. It is most prevalent in Nepal, Sri Lanka, Bangladesh and Pakistan.
b. This is a condition that strictly affects individuals of the Indian culture.
c. It includes vague somatic symptoms.
d. It includes sexual dysfunction.
e. Individuals usually attribute the passage of semen as a consequence of excessive indulgence in masturbation or intercourse.

Question 86

A recent immigrant from Inuit suddenly presents with a marked change of behaviour in public. From the information obtained, she went wild for no reason and started to roll around shouting obscenities. She is now referred to the psychiatrist for assessment. The culture-bound syndrome that the patient is likely to have is

a. Amok
b. Latah
c. Koro
d. Piblotoq
e. Frigophobia

Question 87

A 44-year-old man suffers from depression. He has a history of myocardial infarction and takes aspirin 100 mg every morning. Based on the NICE guidelines, which of the following antidepressants would you recommend?

a. Citalopram
b. Fluoxetine

c. Fluvoxamine
d. Mirtazapine
e. Sertraline

Question 88

A callus on a tree resembled a monkey, and villagers flocked to the tree to pay homage to the 'Monkey God'. Which of the following statements about the aforementioned phenomenon is true?
  a. This phenomenon appears in villagers' vision after the exposure to the tree has ceased.
  b. This phenomenon is a form of pseudo-hallucination.
  c. This phenomenon is increased by attention.
  d. This phenomenon is associated with delusion shared by villagers.
  e. This phenomenon occurs the first time villagers look at the tree and does not persist.

Question 89

A 30-year-old woman has informed the psychologist that she is not coming for the psychotherapy session and intends to leave the world. The psychologist gives you a call and you have decided to contact the patient. Her colleagues mention that she has just swallowed a large amount of medication in the office and she is sent to the hospital. Later, you are informed that this patient is admitted to the Accident and Emergency Department. On admission, her arterial blood gas result is as follows: pH = 7.0 (normal: 7.35–7.45), HCO_3 = 20 (normal: 22–26) and CO_2 >40 (normal: 35–45). Her QTC interval is 600 ms. The consultant from the intensive care unit wants to consult you because they want to know which of the following agents is most likely to contribute to her clinical picture. Your answer is
  a. Diazepam
  b. Fluoxetine
  c. Haloperidol
  d. Imipramine
  e. Risperidone

Question 90

A 60-year-old man with a history of depression complains of vertigo and tinnitus. The tinnitus has worsened his depression. Which of the following condition is the most likely?
  a. Anxiety
  b. Cervical spondylosis
  c. Epilepsy
  d. Postural hypotension
  e. Meniere's disease

Question 91

A patient has requested to have a word with her psychiatrist regarding the therapy session that she has been undergoing. She has undergone four sessions and decided that she needs to stop the sessions. She claims that she is not comfortable with

the therapist and finds the therapist to be harsh and critical, much like what her parents used to be like. Which one of the following best explains her negative experiences?
a. Transference
b. Countertransference
c. Therapeutic resistance
d. Acting out behaviour
e. Learned helplessness

Question 92
In terms of prevention of genetic conditions such as Down's syndrome, genetic screening at what number of weeks would show the presence of raised human chorionic gonadotropin, lowered alpha-fetoprotein and lowered unconjugated estriol?
a. 4 weeks
b. 6 weeks
c. 8 weeks
d. 12 weeks
e. 16 weeks

Question 93
Which one of the following is true with regards to the risk of inheriting bipolar disorder amongst first-degree relatives of patients with bipolar disorder?
a. 1%–2% increment
b. 2%–4% increment
c. 5%–10% increment
d. 15%–20% increment
e. More than 30% increment

Question 94
Which one of the following is not one of the phases of psychosexual development proposed by Freud?
a. Oral phase
b. Anal phase
c. Phallic phase
d. Stagnant phase
e. Genital phase

Question 95
A 28-year-old mother has been very concerned about Tom, her 4-year-old son. He has developmental delays and poor communication skills. He is unable to reciprocate and interact with others and occasionally does have stereotype mannerisms. Which of the following would be the most likely clinical diagnosis?
a. Learning disability
b. Autistic disorder
c. Hyperkinetic disorder
d. Separation anxiety disorder
e. Emotional disorders of childhood

Question 96
Elective mutism usually occurs amongst which of the following age groups?
a. 3–4 years old
b. 5–6 years old
c. 10–12 years old
d. 15–17 years old
e. 18–20 years old

Question 97
A 28-year-old female is at a welcoming cocktail party for new psychiatric trainees. While she is talking to a consultant, she suddenly hears that someone calls her name. Which of the following attention allows Lucy to recognize her name is called?
a. Automatic attention
b. Controlled attention
c. Divided (dual) attention
d. Focused (selective) attention
e. Sustained attention

Question 98
Which of the following statements regarding alcoholic hallucinosis is false?
a. Auditory hallucinations are more common than visual hallucinations.
b. The hallucinations may be fragmentary in the beginning.
c. The hallucinations are characteristically fragmented.
d. The hallucinations can lead to persecutory delusions.
e. The hallucinations respond favourably to antipsychotics.

Question 99
A 25-year-old man informs you that he took an antidepressant from a GP and developed priapism. Which of the following antidepressants is most likely to be associated with the aforementioned phenomenon?
a. Imipramine
b. Moclobemide
c. Paroxetine
d. Trazodone
e. Venlafaxine

Question 100
A teacher has requested Tom's parents to bring him to the CAMHS service. He has been extremely difficult and disruptive in class. He does not wait for his turns, is impulsive and is always on the go. He is also not performing well in his school work, as he is not able to concentrate well. Which one of the following would be the most likely clinical diagnosis?
a. Conduct disorder
b. Oppositional defiant disorder
c. Hyperkinetic disorder
d. Separation anxiety disorder
e. Normal behaviour of childhood

Question 101
Based on Freud's psychosexual developmental theory, which is the phase during which the sex drive remains relatively stable and latent?
a. Oral phase
b. Anal phase
c. Phallic phase
d. Latency phase
e. Genital phase

Question 102
A core trainee was asked during his weekly tutorial about the differences between ICD-10 and DSM-5 in the classification of personality disorder. Which one of the following personality disorders could be found on the DSM-5 and not on the ICD-10?
a. Paranoid personality disorder
b. Schizoid personality disorder
c. Histrionic personality disorder
d. Narcissistic personality disorder
e. Dependent personality disorder

Question 103
Based on the Holmes and Rahe Social Readjustment Rating Scale, which one of the following events has been considered to be the most stressful, which may precipitate a psychiatric illness?
a. Death of a close spouse
b. Death of a close family member
c. Poor martial relationship
d. Separation from children
e. Imprisonment

Question 104
A 60-year-old Irish man staying in the countryside of Ireland complains of seeing wide views of huge skyscrapers and great avenues in front of him and he feels like he is suddenly in New York City. He has history of epilepsy. The lesion is most likely to be found in which of the following neuroanatomical areas?
a. Cingulate gyrus
b. Frontal lobe
c. Occipital lobe
d. Parietal lobe
e. Temporal lobe

Question 105
All of the following are factors that might predispose one to acquire schizophrenia, with the exception of
a. Residing in the urban settings
b. Being of Afro-Caribbean ethnicity
c. High level of expressed emotions within the family
d. Winter excess of birth in schizophrenics
e. Being of high birth weight

Question 106
Carl Jung founded the psychoanalytic school of analytic psychology. He has proposed five different archetypes. Which one of the following correctly describes 'the masculine prototype within each person?'
a. Anima
b. Animus
c. Persona
d. Shadow
e. Self

Question 107
Which of the following statements about panic attacks is incorrect?
a. It usually involves recurrent unpredictable attacks of severe anxiety.
b. These attacks usually last only for a few minutes only.
c. There might be a sudden onset of palpitation, chest pain, choking, dizziness, depersonalization, and together with a secondary fear of dying, losing control or going mad.
d. It does not result in subsequent avoidance of similar situations.
e. It may be followed by persistent fear of another attack.

Question 108
A 70-year-old woman is referred to old-age psychiatric service. She reports several incidents when she suddenly saw several four-inch-high beings wearing hats parading in front of her. She tried to catch one, but could not. She has no past psychiatric history. Her only medical problem is macular degeneration. The patient is most likely to be suffering from
a. Behcet's syndrome
b. Charles Bonnet syndrome
c. Leber's syndrome
d. Horner's syndrome
e. Reiter's syndrome

Question 109
A 20-year-old woman seeks outpatient treatment for her binge eating and self-induced vomiting. Which of the following antidepressants is contraindicated?
a. Bupropion
b. Citalopram
c. Fluoxetine
d. Fluvoxamine
e. Sertraline

Question 110
The following are aetiological factors that might predispose a child to have conduct disorder, with the exception of
a. Conduct disorder is associated with the inheritance of antisocial traits from parents who have demonstrated criminal activities.
b. Biological factors include the presence of elevated plasma dopamine levels.

c. Psychological factors include the difficult temperament and a poor fit between temperament and emotional needs.

d. There has been an association with parental criminality.

e. There has been an association with repeated physical and sexual abuse.

Question 111

A 25-year-old woman is referred by her lawyer after a road traffic accident which occurred one month ago. Her lawyer wants you to certify that she suffers from post-traumatic stress disorder (PTSD). Which of the following clinical features is not a predisposing factor in PTSD?

a. Childhood trauma

b. Inadequate family support

c. Low premorbid intelligence

d. Lack of control of the accident

e. Recent stressful life events

Question 112

A 30-year-old woman developed depression 2 weeks after delivery. Which of the following is not a risk factor for her condition?

a. Ambivalence towards pregnancy prior to delivery

b. Age

c. Episiotomy during vaginal delivery

d. Lack of support from her husband

e. Obstetric complications

Question 113

Which of the following statements is false?

a. Acculturation is a cultural change.

b. Culture has a pathoplastic effect on psychopathology.

c. Personality is not shaped by culture.

d. The ethnic-minority patients may not perceive the practice of psychiatry as benign.

e. The nosological systems employed by psychiatry are largely anglocentric and eurocentric.

Question 114

Which one of the following co-morbidities is known to increase the incidences of mortality amongst women with anorexia nervosa?

a. Alcohol dependence

b. Depressive disorder

c. Anxiety disorder

d. Younger age of onset

e. Poor social support

Question 115

A 23-year-old male came for his routine outpatient appointment and tells the psychiatrist that he is no longer keen to continue on his selective serotonin reuptake inhibitor (SSRI) antidepressant, as it has affected the sexual side of his relationship. This is commonly due to the action of SSRI on which of the following receptors?

a. GABA receptors
b. Histamine receptors
c. 5-HT2A/2C receptors
d. Noradrenaline receptor
e. Adrenaline receptors

Question 116

A 50-year-old with a history of mitral valve replacement takes warfarin on a daily basis. Her GP has recently prescribed fluoxetine to treat her depression. The interaction between fluoxetine and warfarin will cause which of the following symptoms?

a. Bruising
b. Headache
c. Palpitation
d. Tremor
e. Vomiting

Question 117

A 45-year-old woman complains of seeing herself outside her body. Which of the following statements about this phenomenon is false?

a. The double image typically appears as semi-transparent.
b. The experience rarely lasts longer than a few seconds.
c. The mean age of onset of this phenomenon is 40.
d. The most common emotional reactions after seeing her double are sadness and bewilderment.
e. This phenomenon is more common in women.

Question 118

Which of the following is not a typical cause of olfactory hallucination?

a. Alcohol withdrawal syndrome
b. Amphetamine intoxication
c. Cocaine withdrawal
d. Migraine
e. Temporal lobe epilepsy

Question 119

A 25-year-old man suffering from schizophrenia committed suicide one day after discharge from the psychiatric hospital. He killed himself under the influence of command hallucinations. The hospital sentinel event committee found that the patient was discharged prematurely, psychosis was not fully treated and no proper suicide assessment was conducted. The sentinel event committee concluded that this could be a case of negligence. The following constitutes negligence in this case, except

a. Family members did not agree with the premature discharge and their opinions were not sought.
b. Other psychiatrists would have conducted a proper suicide assessment before discharge.
c. The premature discharge caused physical damage (i.e. death).
d. The premature discharge is one of the direct causes of suicide.
e. The psychiatrist-in-charge must act in the patient's best interests before discharge.

Question 120
The first textbook in psychiatry, *Medical Inquiries and Observations,* was authored by

a. Celsus
b. King George III
c. Philippe Pinel
d. Willhelm Griesinger
e. Benjamin Rush

Question 121
The terminology 'schizophrenia' was first invented by

a. Morel
b. Hecker
c. Emil Kraepelin
d. Bleuler
e. Langfeldt

Question 122
The individual who was responsible for coining the term catatonic was

a. Ewald Hecker
b. Karl Ludwig Kahlbaum
c. Paul Broca
d. Sir William Gall
e. Theodor Meynert

Question 123
The core principles of medical ethics include

a. Autonomy, nonmaleficence, beneficence, justice
b. Autonomy, nonmaleficence, beneficence, paternalism
c. Autonomy, nonmaleficence, beneficence, virtue
d. Autonomy, nonmaleficence, beneficence, deontology
e. Autonomy, nonmaleficence, beneficence, confidentiality

Question 124
A 35-year-old female has been visiting the emergency department at least three times each week. She has been telling the doctors that she has been feeling unwell

and she would need more detailed investigations. She is willing to go for any surgery. The emergency doctors referred her to see the psychiatrist, to whom she eventually confessed that she has been lying and giving the doctors a soiled urine specimen many a times. What do you think is her most likely clinical diagnosis?
a. Malingering disorder
b. Factitious disorder
c. Munchausen syndrome
d. Conversion disorder
e. No specific mental health disorders

Question 125
Which of the following anticonvulsants is the least likely to cause visual side effects?
a. Carbamazepine
b. Gabapentin
c. Sodium valproate
d. Topiramate
e. Vigabatrin

Question 126
A core trainee has been asked to perform a suicide risk assessment for a patient who has just been admitted to the emergency department following an overdose on 60 tablets of lamotrigine. Which of the following questioning techniques should he not use when he performs the assessment?
a. Open-ended questions
b. Reflective listening
c. Summarizing
d. Silence
e. Suggestive probes

Question 127
Mood is often assessed during psychiatric interview. Which of the following statements about mood is incorrect?
a. Mood can change over a short period of time.
b. Mood has a complex and multi-faceted quality.
c. Mood is reactive to circumstances.
d. Mood refers to a static unidimensional emotion on a depression–mania spectrum with depression and mania at the extremes and euthymia in the middle.
e. Within normal experiences, happiness can include blissfulness, contentment and playfulness.

Question 128
Dementia praecox was a term coined by
a. Morel
b. Kahlbaum
c. Sommer
d. Emil Kraepelin
e. Bleuler

Question 129

You are able to assess a 20-year-old man who is aggressive and angry towards the staff at the Accident and Emergency Department. Which of the following measures is least useful?

a. Admit own feelings and inform the patient that the staff are frightened of his aggression and anger.
b. Encourage the patient to verbalize his aggression and anger.
c. Inform the patient that restraint or seclusion will be used if necessary.
d. Inform the patient that physical violence is not acceptable in the hospital setting.
e. Offer the option of using psychotropic medication to calm the patient.

Question 130

Plato and Aristotle were responsible for proposing the virtue theory. Which one of the following statements correctly describes what the theory encompasses?

a. The theory emphasizes that a doctor needs to be caring, compassionate, committed and conscientious in nature.
b. The theory emphasizes the importance of the doctor in provision of morally correct care to his or her patients.
c. The theory emphasizes the need to maximize the benefits for the greatest number and also minimize the risks involved.
d. The theory emphasizes that all parties involved should receive equal consideration.
e. The theory emphasizes that all parties involved should receive impartial consideration.

Question 131

A 38-year-old female mother reports to the CAMHS psychiatrist that she has been having problems with her son. She claims that James, her son, gets angry very easily and would argue with her frequently. He does not obey any of the house rules. Which one of the following would be the most likely clinical diagnosis?

a. Conduct disorder
b. Oppositional defiant disorder
c. Emotional disturbances in childhood
d. Bipolar disorder
e. Normal behaviour of childhood

Question 132

The emergency trainee is seeing a patient who has complaints of having vivid, unpleasant dreams and improved appetite after consuming a certain drug. Which one of the following drugs should the trainee suspect that the patient has consumed?

a. Cocaine
b. Benzodiazapine
c. Amphetamines
d. Opiate
e. Caffeine

Question 133
A 30-year-old woman suffers from first episode of bipolar disorder and her psychiatrist has started lithium. She wants to find out the onset of action of lithium. Your answer is
- a. 5–10 hours
- b. 18–24 hours
- c. 2–3 days
- d. 5–14 days
- e. 21–28 days

Extended matching items (EMIs)

Theme: Psychosexual development
Options:
- a. Oral phase
- b. Anal phase
- c. Phallic phase
- d. Latency phase
- e. Genital phase

Lead in: Select the most appropriate answer for each of the following. Each option may be used once, more than once or not at all.

Question 134
This phase occurs around 30–36 months of age.

Question 135
This is the phase in which boys pass through the Oedipal complex.

Question 136
This is the phase in which the sexual drive remains relatively latent.

Question 137
This is the phase in which successful resolution of conflicts would lead to a mature well-integrated adult identity.

Theme: Psychodynamic theory of defence mechanisms
Options:
- a. Repression
- b. Reaction formation
- c. Isolation
- d. Undoing
- e. Projection
- f. Projective identification
- g. Identification
- h. Introjection
- i. Incorporation

j. Turning against the self
k. Rationalization
l. Sublimation
m. Regression

Lead in: Select the most appropriate answer for each of the following. Each option may be used once, more than once or not at all.

Question 138
This refers to how an impulse which is meant to express to another is turned against oneself.

Question 139
This refers to how sexual instincts are being used to motivate creative activities.

Question 140
This refers to how one returns to an earlier level of maturational functioning.

Question 141
This is a common defence mechanism seen in paranoid patients.

Question 142
This is a common defence mechanism seen in patients with OCD.

Theme: Competency and capacity

Options:
a. Competency
b. Capacity
c. Testamentary capacity
d. Capacity for informed consent
e. Advocacy
f. Appointeeship
g. Powers of attorney
h. Court of protection

Lead in: Select the most appropriate answer for each of the following. Each option may be used once, more than once or not at all.

Question 143
A person needs to have this in order to prove that he/she is of sound disposing mind to be able to make a will.

Question 144
A person is deemed to have this if he or she is able to weight the information in balance to arrive at a choice.

Question 145
This refers to a legal concept and construct and refers to the capacity to act and understand.

Question 146
This refers to a person who would speak on the patient's behalf, but has no legal status.

Question 147
This refers to someone who has been authorized by the department of social security to receive and administer benefits on the behalf of someone else.

Theme: Basic psychology

Options:
- a. Acceptance
- b. Multi-perspective internalization
- c. Naivety
- d. Redefinition and reflection
- e. Resistance and naming

Question 148
A 20-year-old African-Caribbean man was born in the UK and his parents migrated to the UK 30 years ago. He was brought up and received education in the UK. From the aforementioned list of five stages of culture consciousness development, select the stage that best matches with each of the following examples. Each option might be used once, more than once or not at all.

He has no awareness of African-Caribbean and British cultural influences on his own self. The colour of skin, ethnicity and cultural identity play no role in his life. (Choose one option.)

Question 149
His cultural identity is defined by his friends and partner. (Choose one option.)

Question 150
He identifies himself as a 'black' man and understands the full meaning of his identity in society. He feels that it is more difficult for him to climb up the social ladder compared to white British. (Choose one option.)

Question 151
After repeated thoughts and analysis, he establishes a personal consciousness of cultural identity in his own right. (Choose one option.)

Question 152
He is able to see himself as having a 'black' identity and take pride in himself. (Choose one option.)

Theme: Psychopathology

Options:
- a. Audible thoughts
- b. Hearing voices arguing
- c. Command hallucination
- d. Écho de pensee
- e. Elementary hallucination

f. Gediankenlautwerden
g. Running commentary
h. Second person hallucination
i. Third person hallucination

Lead in: Identify which of the aforementioned terms best describes the following clinical scenarios. Each option may be used once, more than once or not at all.

Question 153
'Look at what he's doing now, he's sitting in the library and reading a book. Now he's walking to the counter to borrow the book.' (Choose two options.)

Question 154
'You should take the knife from the kitchen and get the fish from the refrigerator. You should cut the fish and then smell the fish's head for 10 times.' (Choose two options.)

Question 155
Female voice: 'She will fail the exam. She is an idiot and cannot focus in her study.'
    Male voice: 'Shut up, leave her alone. She will pass the exam. Susan, you should reject her and not listen.'
    Female voice: 'Don't tell me to shut up. My prediction is always correct' (Choose two options.)

Theme: Abnormal experiences

Options:
a. Elementary hallucination
b. Extracampine hallucination
c. Functional hallucination
d. Haptic hallucination
e. Hygric hallucination
f. Hypnagogic hallucination
g. Hypnopompic hallucination
h. Kinaesthetic hallucination
i. Lilliputian hallucination
j. Reduplicative hallucination
k. Reflex hallucination

Lead in: Identify which of the aforementioned terms best describes the following clinical scenarios. Each option may be used once, more than once or not at all.

Question 156
A 30-year-old woman is admitted to the hospital after an attempt to stab herself. She feels that her abdomen is filled with a large amount of fluid and she needs to

release the fluid. Physical examination shows a soft, non-tender abdomen without any distension or presence of air-fluid level. (Choose one option.)

Question 157
A 25-year-old man with schizophrenia describes the sensation that somebody is touching his body in intimate areas. (Choose one option.)

Question 158
A 40-year-old man asks the orthopaedic surgeon to arrange for the amputation of a third lower limb that he feels he has developed. (Choose one option.)

Theme: Psychopathology
Options:
   a. Complex visual hallucination
   b. Dysmegalopsia
   c. Illusion
   d. Macropsia
   e. Micropsia
   f. Pareidolia
   g. Peduncular hallucination
   h. Pseudohallucination
   i. Simple visual hallucination
   j. Visual hyperaesthesia

Lead in: A 65-year-old woman is found to be disorientated in time and place. During your assessment, she gives a history of the following experiences. Identify which of the aforementioned psychopathological terms best describes the following clinical scenarios. Each option may be used once, more than once or not at all.

Question 159
She is terrified and shouts, 'White Lady, White Lady, Go away.' She perceives the curtain as a female ghost. (Choose one option.)

Question 160
She finds the colour in the ward appears to her to be brighter and more vivid than usual. (Choose one option.)

Question 161
She mentions that the bed and other furniture look smaller or larger than they should be. (Choose one option.)

Question 162
She feels that her body size is smaller than that of a foot tall compared with the size of the wardrobe. (Choose one option.)

Question 163
She sees the face of Jesus Christ in the callus of a tree outside the ward. (Choose one option.)

Question 164
She reports that she saw a colourfully dressed clown and children dancing in the ward last night. (Choose one option.)

Theme: Type of prevention
Options:
 a. Primary prevention
 b. Secondary prevention
 c. Tertiary prevention

Lead in: Identify which of the aforementioned type of prevention best describes the following scenarios. Each option may be used once, more than once or not at all.

Question 165
An early psychosis programme involves efforts to reduce the prevalence of first episode of schizophrenia by reducing the duration of untreated psychosis. (Choose one option.)

Question 166
The Department of Health promotes an alcohol misuse treatment programme specifically targeting at women of childbearing age. This programme aims at reducing the number of new cases of foetal alcohol syndrome in the community. (Choose one option.)

Question 167
A rehabilitation programme is designed to reduce the severity and disability associated with head injury. (Choose one option.)

Theme: Prevention strategies in schizophrenia
Options:
 a. Listen to loud stimulating music to drown out the auditory hallucinations not responding to antipsychotic treatment
 b. Maintenance in antipsychotic treatment
 c. Psychoeducation about schizophrenia
 d. Reduction in perinatal trauma
 e. Reduction in stress associated with migration
 f. Successful treatment of middle ear disease in childhood
 g. Teaching problem-solving skill

Lead in: The Department of Health have devised various strategies to prevent schizophrenia in the UK. Classify the aforementioned prevention strategies into the following type of prevention. Each option may be used once, more than once or not at all.

Question 168
Primary prevention (Choose three options.)

Question 169
Secondary prevention (Choose two options.)

Question 170
Tertiary prevention (Choose one option.)

Theme: Neurology

Options:
   a. Classical migraine
   b. Cluster headache
   c. Costen's syndrome
   d. Cranial arteritis
   e. Orbital onset migraine
   f. Occipital onset migraine
   g. Post-herpetic neuralgia
   h. Tension headache

Lead in: A 50-year-old woman with a history of depression complains of chronic pain in her face. Match the aforementioned lesions or neurological conditions to the following descriptions. Each option might be used once, more than once or not at all.

Question 171
The pain is centred around her right eye, right forehead and usually extends to involve the whole right head. She also sees zigzag lines and feels nauseated (Choose one option.)

Question 172
The pain starts around the right orbit and may extend across to the opposite eye and to the adjacent facial, frontal and temporal areas but the main pain remains in the right orbit. (Choose one option.)

Question 173
The pain starts as a tightness in the occipital area and extends forward around the temporal area or over the top of the head. The ultimate location of the headache is around her right eye. (Choose one option.)

Question 174
The pain has a quality like a tight band around her head, coming forwards to the forehead. (Choose one option.)

Options:
   a. 3–5 years
   b. 6–8 years
   c. 9–11 years

d. 12–14 years
   e. 15–17 years

Lead in: A young person's grandmother recently died of cancer. Identify which of the aforementioned age ranges best resembles the following grief reactions. Each option might be used once, more than once or not at all.

Question 175
He needs more information about his grandmother's death to gain sense of control. (Choose one option.)

Question 176
He is confused and asks repetitive questions about his grandmother. He struggles to understand the abstract concept of death. (Choose one option.)

Question 177
He understands death and talks openly about his grandmother. He has magical thinking that grandmother will come back. (Choose one option.)

Question 178
He exhibits similar grief reaction compared to other adults. (Choose one option.)

Theme: Clinical diagnosis (I)
Options:
   a. Acute stress disorder
   b. Adjustment disorder
   c. Avoidant personality disorder
   d. Asperger's syndrome
   e. Bipolar disorder – manic episode
   f. Catatonic schizophrenia
   g. Depressive episode
   h. Delirium tremens
   i. Disorganized schizophrenia
   j. Dysthymic disorder
   k. Malignant catatonia
   l. Manic stupor
  m. Neuroleptic malignant syndrome
   n. OCD
   o. Obsessive-compulsive personality disorder
   p. Paranoid schizophrenia
   q. Postnatal psychosis
   r. Post-traumatic stress disorder
   s. Psychotic depression
   t. Separation anxiety disorder
   u. Social phobia

Lead in: Match the aforementioned diagnoses to the following clinical scenarios. Each option might be used once, more than once or not at all.

Question 179
A 30-year-old man is admitted to the psychiatric ward and he appears to be stiff. Prior to admission, he was standing in the Oxford Street for 3 hours. His wife described him as still as a 'statue'. When he was asked the purpose of standing in the Oxford Street, he replied, 'Satan sent me there and I was controlled by Satan'. He has been hearing multiple voices for the past 6 months. (Choose one option.)

Question 180
A 23-year-old British solider goes missing in action in Afghanistan and is found collapsed on a bridge. When the medics examine him, he has no wounds and there is no sign of recent crossfire. He is unconscious and appears to be rigid and dehydrated. His body temperature is 39°C, and his blood pressure is 150/90. (Choose one option.)

Theme: Clinical diagnosis (II)
Options:
- a. Acute stress disorder
- b. Adjustment disorder
- c. Avoidant personality disorder
- d. Asperger's syndrome
- e. Bipolar disorder – manic episode
- f. Catatonic schizophrenia
- g. Depressive episode
- h. Delirium tremens
- i. Disorganized schizophrenia
- j. Dysthymic disorder
- k. Malignant catatonia
- l. Manic stupor
- m. Neuroleptic malignant syndrome
- n. OCD
- o. Obsessive-compulsive personality disorder
- p. Paranoid schizophrenia
- q. Postnatal psychosis
- r. Post-traumatic stress disorder
- s. Psychotic depression
- t. Separation anxiety disorder
- u. Social phobia

Lead in: Match the aforementioned diagnoses to the following clinical scenarios. Each option might be used once, more than once or not at all.

Question 181
A 30-year-old mother gave birth to her first baby 6 months ago. She has been coping well initially. She starts feeling down, loses weight, complains of tiredness, eats poorly, wakes up before dawn and expresses guilt in her poor care to the baby.

Her husband also notices that she worries constantly that accident will happen to her baby after she read the news on a baby who died of choking after breastfeeding. She begins checking her baby every 5 minutes. (Choose one option.)

Question 182
A 40-year-old unemployed man is admitted after he was arrested by police for dangerous driving. He drove in the opposite direction at 120 km/hr on the M5 southbound because he firmly believed that the paparazzi tried to harm him. He informs you that he wants to pursue a PhD degree at this moment. He has incurred £100,000 in food business, although he worked as a technician before. He also sent email to the Prime Minister to advise him on how to attract investments for the UK from overseas investors. He first consulted a psychiatrist 10 years ago and he developed psychiatric complications after taking an antidepressant. He firmly believes that he suffers from schizophrenia because he hears voices when nobody is around. (Choose one option.)

Question 183
A 50-year-old man is referred by a gastroenterologist. He firmly believes that his gut has rotted and he is already dead. The gastroenterologist is very concerned as he has ceased to eat or drink. (Choose one option.)

Theme: Defence mechanisms
Options:
- a. Isolation
- b. Intellectualization
- c. Displacement
- d. Splitting
- e. Idealization
- f. Sublimation
- g. Repression
- h. Undoing
- i. Denial
- j. Regression
- k. Projection

Lead in: Match the aforementioned defence mechanisms to the following. Each option may be used once, more than once or not at all.

Question 184
A man is passed over for promotion at work. He does not get upset while at work but loses his temper at another driver on the way home. (Choose one option.)

Question 185
It is suggested to him that perhaps some of his anger is related to his relationship with his boss. He denies this saying that 'She's like a mother to me – always kind and supportive.' (Choose one option.)

Question 186
He suggests that his anger is due to his childhood and then begins to speak about all the books he has recently read on child rearing across different cultures. (Choose one option.)

Theme: Concepts of dynamic psychotherapy
Options:
a. Acting-out
b. Affirmation
c. Boundary violation
d. Counter-transference
e. Empathetic failure
f. Holding environment
g. Metaphor
h. Mirroring
i. Parallel process
j. Process interpretation
k. Resistance
l. Transference

Lead in: A 30-year-old man is seeing a core trainee for brief dynamic psychotherapy. You are supervising the core trainee. Identify which of the aforementioned terminology resembles the following clinical examples encountered by the core trainee. Each option might be used once, more than once or not at all.

Question 187
The patient is very forthcoming during the session but he only talks about superficialities. The core trainee tries to probe further but without success. (Choose one option.)

Question 188
The core trainee was on leave for one month. After his return, the patient is in a withdrawn state in a session and the core trainee feels that the patient is angry because of his leave. (Choose one option.)

Question 189
The core trainee reflects on his positive qualities when he was confronted with a challenge to self-esteem at work. (Choose one option.)

Theme: General adult psychiatry
Options:
a. Allport's theory
b. Cattell's theory
c. Eysenck's theory
d. Type A personality

Lead in: Identify which of the aforementioned resembles the following descriptions. Each option may be used once, more than once or not at all.

Question 190
Personality comprises of common traits and individual traits. (Choose one option.)

Question 191
Personality has four dimensions: introversion, extroversion, neuroticism and psychoticism. (Choose one option.)

Question 192
Personality has three sources of data: L-data, Q-data and T-data. (Choose one option.)

Question 193
Personality comprises of achievement strivings and impatience irritability. (Choose one option.)

GET THROUGH MRCPSYCH PAPER AI: MOCK EXAMINATION

Question 1 Answer: d, Intermetamorphosis syndrome
Explanation: Intermetamorphosis syndrome is a misidentification syndrome and the patient develops the delusional conviction that various people have been transformed physically and psychologically into other people.

Reference and Further Reading: Campbell RJ (1996). *Psychiatric Dictionary*. Oxford, UK: Oxford University Press.

Question 2 Answer: c, Extracampine hallucination
Explanation: Extracampine hallucinations are hallucinations that occur beyond the limits of the sensory field. In this case, 'hearing' conversations from the neighbouring town is an auditory extracampine hallucination. Autoscopy is a visual hallucination of seeing a 'double' image of oneself viewed from within one's physical body. The Doppelgänger phenomenon is the subjective feeling of doubling, where the person feels like his exact 'double' is present both outside alongside and inside oneself.

Options (d) and (e) involve hallucinations that occur when one is falling asleep and waking up from sleep respectively.

Reference and Further Reading: Sims A (2003). *Symptoms of the Mind: An Introduction to Descriptive Psychopathology*. London: Saunders, pp. 105–106, 112, 217–220.

Question 3 Answer: c, Incubation
Explanation: Incubation refers to the increase in strength of the conditioned response, resulting from multiple repeated brief exposures to the conditioned stimulus. Generalization refers to the process whereby a CR has been established to a given stimulus; that response can also be evoked by other stimuli that are similar to the original CS. Discrimination is the differential recognition of and response to two or more similar stimuli.

Reference: Puri BK, Hall A, Ho R (2014). *Revision Notes in Psychiatry*. London: CRC Press, p. 26.

Question 4 Answer: a, Idiosyncratic reaction to medication
Explanation: Neuroleptic malignant syndrome has been classified as an idiosyncratic reaction to medication. Idiosyncratic reactions to mediations are adverse drug reactions that are not characteristic or predictable and that are associated with an individual human difference not present in members of the general population.

Reference: Puri BK, Hall A, Ho R (2014). *Revision Notes in Psychiatry*. London: CRC Press, p. 252.

Question 5 Answer: c, Psychosocial adversity is not one of the key factors associated with ADHD in childhood.
Explanation: Psychosocial adversity is one of the factors associated with ADHD in childhood. This might include factors such as maternal psychopathology, large family sizes, parental conflict and emotional deprivation.

Reference: Puri BK, Hall A, Ho R (2014). *Revision Notes in Psychiatry*. London: CRC Press, p. 631.

Question 6 Answer: d, Unable to commence gait during examination
Explanation: A malingerer is unable to commence gait during examination when he is being watched by the examiner. Option (a) refers to festinant gait found in Parkinson's disease. Option (b) is found in hysteria. Option (c) is found in Huntington's disease.

Reference and Further Reading: Puri BK, Treasaden I (eds) (2010) *Psychiatry: An Evidence-Based Text*. London: Hodder Arnold, pp. 682, 684.

Question 7 Answer: a, Receptive dysphasia
Explanation: This is an example of receptive dysphasia. This usually involves underlying damage to the Wernicke's area and this would thus result in a disruption of the ability to comprehend language, either written or even spoken. In addition, the individual might be unaware that his or her speech, though normal in rhythm and intonation, has abnormal content.

Reference: Puri BK, Hall A, Ho R (2014). *Revision Notes in Psychiatry*. London: CRC Press, p. 105.

Question 8 Answer: b, Expressive dysphasia
Explanation: This is an example of inherent damage to the Broca's area, thus resulting in the loss of the rhythm, intonation and grammatical aspects of speech. Comprehension is normal, and the individual is usually aware that his or her speech is difficult for others to follow.

Reference: Puri BK, Hall A, Ho R (2014). *Revision Notes in Psychiatry*. London: CRC Press, p. 105.

Question 9 Answer: a, Formication

Explanation: Formication is the sensation of insects crawling under the skin and is a form of haptic (tactile) hallucination. Haptic hallucinations are superficial sensations on or under the skin in the absence of a real stimulus. Option (e), visceral hallucination, on the other hand, is a deep sensation involving inner organs without any real stimuli.

Reference and Further Reading: Puri BK, Hall AD (2002). *Revision Notes in Psychiatry*. London: Arnold, p. 154.

Question 10 Answer: a, Reciprocal inhibition

Explanation: The concept of systematic desensitization is largely based on the concept of reciprocal inhibition. The theory of reciprocal inhibition states that relaxation would help to reduce the anxiety levels, and that the two states cannot coexist. This has been proven to be a useful technique to treat patients with a lot of anticipatory anxiety, for example, in specific phobias. Patients, with the guidance of their therapist, are encouraged to identify increasingly greater anxiety-provoking stimulus and then to form a hierarchy of anxiety situations. During treatment, they are gradually exposed to situations lower in the hierarchy, with each exposure being paired with appropriate relaxation exercises.

Reference: Puri BK, Hall A, Ho R (2014). *Revision Notes in Psychiatry*. London: CRC Press, p. 28.

Question 11 Answer: d, Toxicity

Explanation: He has developed what is commonly known as lithium toxicity. This usually occurs due to dehydration. It is important to note that the therapeutic index of lithium is low, and therefore regular plasma lithium level monitoring would be required. At lithium plasma levels of greater than 2mM, the following effects could occur: hyper-reflexes, toxic psychosis, convulsions, syncope, oliguria, circulatory failure, coma and death.

Reference: Puri BK, Hall A, Ho R (2014). *Revision Notes in Psychiatry*. London: CRC Press, p. 254.

Question 12 Answer: a, Hyperactivity

Explanation: Hyperactivity is not considered to be one of the core symptoms of adult ADHD. In adult ADHD, the symptoms of ADHD tend to focus on the inattentive symptoms. The symptoms of hyperactivity would have improved with time.

Reference: Puri BK, Hall A, Ho R (2014). *Revision Notes in Psychiatry*. London: CRC Press, p. 631.

Question 13 Answer: b, Pneumocystis carinii

Explanation: Pneumocystis carinii is the commonest life-threatening opportunistic infection seen in patients with AIDS.

Reference and Further Reading: Puri BK, Treasaden I (eds) (2010). *Psychiatry: An Evidence-Based Text*. London: Hodder Arnold, p. 789.

Question 14 Answer: a, Alexia without agraphia

Explanation: He has alexia without agraphia. The explanation for the clinical presentation is as follows: after the stroke, the patient starts off with right hemianopia and he cannot read in the right visual field. Then, the words have to be seen on the left side, and are projected to onto the right hemisphere. There is a lesion in the splenium that prevents the transfer of information from the right to the left. As a result, the patient is unable to comprehend any written materials, although he can write. As time goes by, he develops a strategy of identifying the individual letters in the right hemisphere. Saying each letter aloud enables him to access the pronunciation of words in the left hemisphere.

Reference: Puri BK, Hall A, Ho R (2014). *Revision Notes in Psychiatry*. London: CRC Press, p. 107.

Question 15 Answer: b, Disturbance in attention

Explanation: Disturbance in attention is the most characteristic and consistent abnormality in delirium.

Reference and Further Reading: Puri BK, Treasaden I (eds) (2010). *Psychiatry: An Evidence-Based Text*. London: Hodder Arnold, pp. 94, 503, 511–513.

Question 16 Answer: c, Phenelzine and meperidine

Explanation: All combinations will lead to serotonin syndrome but there are reports that the combination of phenelzine and meperidine has led to death on several occasions. Meperidine is a narcotic pain killer.

Reference and Further Reading: Sharav VH (2007). Serotonin syndrome: A mix of medicines that can be lethal. *The New York Times*. New York: The New York Times Company; Puri BK, Treasaden I (eds) (2010). *Psychiatry: An Evidence-Based Text*. London: Hodder Arnold, pp. 874–875.

Question 17 Answer: c, Shaping

Explanation: The underlying psychological theory is shaping. Shaping refers to the successive closer approximations to the intended behaviour (in this case, not using cocaine at all) which are reinforced gradually in order to achieve the intended behaviour. This is in contrast to chaining, which teaches aspects of a more complicated behaviour, and in the later stages, the individual learned behaviours are then connected to achieve the desired response.

Reference: Puri BK, Hall A, Ho R (2014). *Revision Notes in Psychiatry*. London: CRC Press, p. 29.

Question 18 Answer: b, hearing, 'Peter, Peter'

Explanation: This condition is hypnagogic hallucination. Hypnagogic hallucinations are false perceptions that occur when falling asleep. These can be auditory, visual or tactile. These hallucinations usually occur suddenly and the person believes it wakes him or her up. Hearing one's name being called is the most common hypnagogic hallucination. These phenomena may be considered normal even though they are real hallucinations.

Reference and Further Reading: Sims A (2003). *Symptoms of the Mind: An Introduction to Descriptive Psychopathology*. London: Saunders, p. 112.

Question 19 Answer: a, James–Lange theory
Explanation: James–Lange theory would best explain what James has had experienced. Based on the theory, the experience of emotion is secondary to the somatic responses that an individual experiences. Thus, in the case of James, when he sees the dog, there will be an increased activity of his sympathetic nervous system and his feelings of anxiety and fear are due to the result of the increased sympathetic activity. This is in contrast to Cannon–Bard theory, which proposes that both somatic responses and the experience of the emotions would occur concurrently.

Reference: Puri BK, Hall A, Ho R (2014). *Revision Notes in Psychiatry*. London: CRC Press, p. 53.

Question 20 Answer: c, Simple schizophrenia
Explanation: In simple schizophrenia, there is an insidious onset of decline in functioning. Negative symptoms develop without preceding positive symptoms. Diagnosis usually requires changes in behaviours for over at least 1 year, with marked loss of interest and social withdrawal.

Reference: Puri BK, Hall A, Ho R (2014). *Revision Notes in Psychiatry*. London: CRC Press, p. 355.

Question 21 Answer: c, Orobuccal apraxia
Explanation: This is an example of orobuccal apraxia. The patient usually has difficulties in performing learned, skilled movements of the face, lips, tongue, cheek, larynx and pharynx on command. This might be due to a lesion involving the left inferior frontal lobe and insula.

Reference: Puri BK, Hall A, Ho R (2014). *Revision Notes in Psychiatry*. London: CRC Press, p. 109.

Question 22 Answer: e, Anger
Explanation: All of the aforementioned are correct, with the exception of anger. With separation, the child initially responds by protesting. This might include crying and searching behaviour. In the second stage, the child would be in despair. This presents itself as marked apathy and misery from a belief that the mother would not be returning. Finally, detachment occurs, in which the child grows to become emotionally distant from and indifferent to his mother.

Reference: Puri BK, Hall A, Ho R (2014). *Revision Notes in Psychiatry*. London: CRC Press, p. 64.

Question 23 Answer: e, Mental retardation not otherwise specified

Explanation: In the ICD-10 classification system, the following are included under mental retardation: F70 Mild Mental Retardation, F71 Moderate Mental Retardation, F72 Severe Mental Retardation, F73 Profound mental retardation, F78 Other mental retardation and F79 Unspecified mental retardation.

Reference: Puri BK, Hall A, Ho R (2014). *Revision Notes in Psychiatry*. London: CRC Press, p. 19.

Question 24 Answer: b, Depression regularly worse in the evening

Explanation: In melancholia, depression should be regularly worse in the morning but not in the evening. Patients can display marked psychomotor retardation or agitation. Core features of melancholia include loss of pleasure in almost all activities and lack of reactivity to usually pleasurable stimuli.

Reference and Further Reading: American Psychiatric Association (2000). *Diagnostic Criteria from DSM-IV-TR*. Washington, DC: American Psychiatric Association; Puri BK, Treasaden I (eds) (2010). *Psychiatry: An Evidence-Based Text*. London: Hodder Arnold, pp. 8, 613.

Question 25 Answer: a, Check serum free thyroxine (FT4) and free triiodothyronine (FT3)

Explanation: The next step is to check serum FT4 and FT3 to exclude overt hyperthyroidism if the serum TSH level is less than 0.4 mU/L. This woman is confirmed to suffer from subclinical hyperthyroidism if FT4 and FT3 are within the *Reference* range but TSH is suppressed.

Reference and Further Reading: Puri BK, Treasaden I (eds) (2010). *Psychiatry: An Evidence-Based Text*. London: Hodder Arnold, pp. 575–576, 681.

Question 26 Answer: d, Last 12 months

Explanation: In order for the diagnosis to be made, the schizophrenia must have occurred within the last 12 months, with some symptoms still being present. The depressive symptoms must fulfil at least the criteria for a depressive episode and must be present for at least 2 weeks.

Reference: Puri BK, Hall A, Ho R (2014). *Revision Notes in Psychiatry*. London: CRC Press, p. 355.

Question 27 Answer: c, Hyponatraemia

Explanation: Hyponatraemia is common in old people receiving SSRI treatment. They present with lethargy, muscle ache and nausea. More severe cases present with cardiac failure, confusion and seizure.

Reference and Further Reading: Puri BK, Treasaden I (eds) (2010). *Psychiatry: An Evidence-Based Text*. London: Hodder Arnold, pp. 1110, 1112.

Question 28 Answer: d, Thought broadcasting
Explanation: The psychopathology that the prisoner is experiencing is known as thought broadcasting. Thought broadcasting reefers to the delusion that one's thoughts are being broadcast out loud so that they could be perceived by others around.

Reference: Puri BK, Hall A, Ho R (2014). *Revision Notes in Psychiatry*. London: CRC Press, p. 7.

Question 29 Answer: c, Patients with Huntington's disease will die in 5–10 years after the onset of visible symptoms.
Explanation: Patients with Huntington's disease will die in 20 years after the onset of visible symptoms.

Reference and Further Reading: Puri BK, Treasaden I (eds) (2010). *Psychiatry: An Evidence-Based Text*. London: Hodder Arnold, pp. 546–547, 1101; Walker FO (2007). Huntington's disease. *Lancet,* 369: 219.

Question 30 Answer: d, Construction apraxia
Explanation: The concept tested is constructional apraxia. The patient usually would have difficulties with reproduction of simple geometric patterns and demonstrate inability to connect the separate parts together. This might be due to lesions involving the nondominant parietal lobe.

Reference: Puri BK, Hall A, Ho R (2014). *Revision Notes in Psychiatry*. London: CRC Press, p. 108.

Question 31 Answer: e, Object permanence
Explanation: Babies between the ages of 8 and 12 months develop the ability to find hidden objects. This ability is known as object permanence, the understanding that objects continue to exist even when they are out of sight. This is one of the most important developments during the sensorimotor stage as the baby displays goal-directed behaviour, which, according to Piaget, is the foundation of problem solving.

Reference and Further Reading: Puri BK, Treasaden I (eds) (2010). *Psychiatry: An Evidence-Based Text*. London: Hodder Arnold, pp. 113115.

Question 32 Answer: e, Worthlessness
Explanation: Based on the DSM-IV-TR diagnostic criteria, the presence of the following symptoms would suggest major depressive episode:

1. Guilt about things other than actions taken or not taken by the survivor at the time of the death

2. Thought of death other than the survivor feeling that he or she would be better off dead or should have died with the deceased person
3. Morbid preoccupation with worthlessness
4. Marked psychomotor retardation
5. Prolonged and marked functional impairment
6. Hallucinatory experiences other than thinking that he or she hears the voice of, or transiently sees the image of, the deceased person.

Reference and Further Reading: American Psychiatric Association (2000). *Diagnostic Criteria from DSM-IV-TR*. Washington, DC: American Psychiatric Association; Puri BK, Treasaden I (eds) (2010). *Psychiatry: An Evidence-Based Text*. London: Hodder Arnold, pp. 110, 111, 123, 881–887.

Question 33 Answer: e, Imposing the appropriate cost
Explanation: All of the aforementioned are correct, with the exception of imposing an appropriate cost. The role of the doctor includes defining the illness, legitimizing the illness, imposing an illness diagnosis if necessary and offering appropriate help. Doctors therefore control access to the sick role, and they and patients have reciprocal obligations and rights.

Reference: Puri BK, Hall A, Ho R (2014). *Revision Notes in Psychiatry*. London: CRC Press, p. 119.

Question 34 Answer: a, Critical comments, hostility, emotional over-involvement
Explanation: The Camberwell Family Interview includes five scales; Critical Comments, Hostility, Emotional over-involvement, Warmth and Positive remarks. The first three scales have been associated with high expressed emotions and are predictive of relapse.

Reference: Puri BK, Hall A, Ho R (2014). *Revision Notes in Psychiatry*. London: CRC Press, p. 121.

Question 35 Answer: a, Marital separation
Explanation: Death of spouse, divorce and marital separation are rated high on the life change value. Martial separation is associated with a life change value of 65, marriage with a life change value of 50, pregnancy with a value of 40, birth of a child with a value of 39 and problems with boss with a value of 23.

Reference: Puri BK, Hall A, Ho R (2014). *Revision Notes in Psychiatry*. London: CRC Press, p. 122.

Question 36 Answer: d, Depressive pseudo-dementia
Explanation: The biological symptoms such as sleep disturbance, poor appetite and weight loss are equally common in both the young and the old. The presence of mood symptoms in association with memory difficulties would be more prevalent in the old.

Reference: Puri BK, Hall A, Ho R (2014). *Revision Notes in Psychiatry*. London: CRC Press, p. 710.

Question 37 Answer: e, Top-down processing
Explanation: In top-down (conceptually driven) perceptual processing, perception is the end result of an indirect process that involves making inferences about the world based on the observer's knowledge and expectations. In suboptimal viewing condition, knowledge of the world and past experience allow the observer to make inferences about identity of the stimuli.

Reference and Further Reading: Puri BK, Treasaden I (eds) (2010). *Psychiatry: An Evidence-Based Text*. London: Hodder Arnold, pp. 229, 238, 243.

Question 38 Answer: c, Waxy flexibility
Explanation: The psychopathology that the patient has is waxy flexibility. There is a feeling of plastic resistance resembling the bending of a soft wax rod as the examiner moves part of the person's body, and that body part remains 'moulded' by the examiner in the new position.

Reference: Puri BK, Hall A, Ho R (2014). *Revision Notes in Psychiatry*. London: CRC Press, p. 3.

Question 39 Answer: c, Obsession with alcohol
Explanation: Based on the ICD-10 criteria, his repeated thoughts should be described as preoccupation with alcohol rather than obsession with alcohol.

Reference: World Health Organisation (1994). *ICD-10 Classification of Mental and Behavioural Disorders*. Edinburgh, UK: Churchill Livingstone.

Question 40 Answer: e, Asomatognosia
Explanation: Asomatognosia, which is the lack of awareness of the condition of all or part of the body, occurs usually when there is an inherent insult to the nondominant parietal lobe of the body. Other associated signs and symptoms that might occur due to an insult to the dominant parietal lobe include dysgraphesthesia and Wernicke's or Broca's aphasia.

Reference: Puri BK, Hall A, Ho R (2014). *Revision Notes in Psychiatry*. London: CRC Press, p. 114.

Question 41 Answer: b, 2 months
Explanation: In DSM-IV-TR, the category of uncomplicated bereavement is designated for virtually all symptoms of depression experienced during the first 2 months after the loss, with the exception of extreme feelings of worthlessness or active suicidal ideation. If the duration is longer than 2 months, the patient is considered to suffer from major depression and warrants antidepressant treatment.

Reference and Further Reading: American Psychiatric Association (2000). *Diagnostic Criteria from DSM-IV-TR*. Washington, DC: American Psychiatric Association; Puri BK, Treasaden I (eds) (2010). *Psychiatry: An Evidence-Based Text*. London: Hodder Arnold, pp. 110, 111, 123, 881–887.

Question 42 Answer: b, 40 areas are being probed during the interview
Explanation: The LEDS assessment tool looks into only 38 areas and not 40 areas. The LEEDS is a semi-structured interview schedule, with 38 areas being probed. It comprises detailed narratives collected about events, including their circumstances. It has high reliability and high validity.

Reference: Puri BK, Hall A, Ho R (2014). *Revision Notes in Psychiatry*. London: CRC Press, p. 122.

Question 43 Answer: b, Halstead–Reitan Battery
Explanation: The Halstead–Reitan Battery is a comprehensive test battery that could detect damage to the brain and whether the damage is lateralized, and if so, which hemisphere has been affected. It could also determine whether this is associated with an acute or a chronic disorder. It also determines whether the damage is focal in nature or more diffuse.

Reference: Puri BK, Hall A, Ho R (2014). *Revision Notes in Psychiatry*. London: CRC Press, p. 92.

Question 44 Answer: a, In the preoperational stage, rules are believed to be inviolable.
Explanation: The preoperational stage occurs between ages 2 and 7. At this stage, the child believes that rules are inviolable. This is known as authority morality. Circular reactions are repeated voluntary motor actions (e.g. imitation of familiar behaviours), which provide the child a means of adapting their first schemas. This occurs in the sensorimotor stage. Conservation is achieved in the concrete operational stage, and object permanence is fully developed by the age of 18 months, during the sensorimotor stage.

Reference and Further Reading: Puri BK, Hall AD (2002). *Revision Notes in Psychiatry*. London: Arnold, pp. 70–71.

Question 45 Answer: b, 1–4 units
Explanation: The Royal College of Obstetricians and Gynaecologists recommend that small amounts of alcohol during pregnancy (not more than one to two units, not more than once or twice a week) have not been shown to be harmful. Alcohol is measured in units. One unit of alcohol is the equivalent of a half a pint of lager or beer, a glass of wine or a single shot of a spirit (gin, vodka, rum).

Reference: Royal College of Obstetricians and Gynaecologists (1999). Alcohol Consumption and the Outcomes of Pregnancy (RCOG Statement 5). http://www.rcog.org.uk /womens-health/clinical-guidance/alcohol-and-pregnancy-information-you.

Question 46 Answer: c, Conduct disorder

Explanation: The clinical diagnosis in this case would be conduct disorder. Based on the ICD-10 classification system, there must be a repetitive and persistent pattern of behaviour in which either the rights of others or of age-appropriate societal norms are violated. Based on the ICD-10, these symptoms must have lasted for the past 6 weeks.

Reference: Puri BK, Hall A, Ho R (2014). *Revision Notes in Psychiatry*. London: CRC Press, p. 637.

Question 47 Answer: c, Mirtazapine

Explanation: Mirtazapine is a noradrenaline and specific serotonin antagonist.

Reference and Further Reading: Puri BK, Treasaden I (eds) (2010). *Psychiatry: An Evidence-Based Text*. London: Hodder Arnold, pp. 426, 661, 907, 1110–1111.

Question 48 Answer: e, Running commentary

Explanation: Samuel is experiencing auditory hallucinations (second person) as well as running commentary (he could hear them commenting about his actions). Running commentaries are classified as part of mood-incongruent complex auditory hallucinations. This might include voices discussing the person in third person as well as thoughts spoken out loud (thought echo).

Reference: Puri BK, Hall A, Ho R (2014). *Revision Notes in Psychiatry*. London: CRC Press, p. 7.

Question 49 Answer: a, Bottom-up processing

Explanation: In bottom-up (data-driven) perceptual processing, perception is a direct process and determined by the information presented to the sensory receptors of the observer. In suboptimal viewing condition, raw sensory information is analysed into basic features such as colour or movement. These features are then recombined at higher brain centres, where they are compared to stored images.

Reference and Further Reading: Puri BK, Treasaden I (eds) (2010). *Psychiatry: An Evidence-Based Text*. London: Hodder Arnold, pp. 229, 238, 243.

Question 50 Answer: c, Alcoholic hallucinosis

Explanation: This is a particular disorder that usually presents or recurs in those who are still drinking. This condition is characterized largely by auditory hallucinations in clear consciousness. They tend to show good prognosis and usually have a good response to antipsychotics.

Reference: Puri BK, Hall A, Ho R (2014). *Revision Notes in Psychiatry*. London: CRC Press, p. 518.

Question 51 Answer: b, Huntington's disease

Explanation: This man presents with chorea, and the most likely diagnosis is Huntington's disease in this age group supported by family history. Option (e) is possible but unlikely to start at this age. Option (a) causes neuropathy or myelopathy. Option (c) causes back and leg pain.

Reference and Further Reading: Ward N, Frith P, Lipsedge M (2001). *Medical Master-class Neurology, Ophthalmology and Psychiatry*. London: Royal College of Physicians; Puri BK, Treasaden I (eds) (2010). *Psychiatry: An Evidence-Based Text*. London: Hodder Arnold, pp. 523, 546–547, 1101.

Question 52 Answer: b, Social-order-maintaining orientation
Explanation: According to Kohlberg, at the pre-conventional level, morality is externally controlled by punishment and rewards. At the conventional level, societal laws cannot be disobeyed as they ensure societal order (i.e. social-order-maintaining orientation) and interpersonal cooperation (i.e. good-boy/good-girl orientation). At the post-conventional level, morality is defined in terms of abstract principles (i.e. social-contract and universal ethical principle orientations).

Reference and Further Reading: Berk LE (2006). *Child Development* (7th edition). Boston: Pearson, pp. 488–492; Puri BK, Treasaden I (eds) (2010). *Psychiatry: An Evidence-Based Text*. London: Hodder Arnold, pp. 118–119.

Question 53 Answer: d, 48 hours
Explanation: Based on the ICD-10 criteria for acute stress disorder. For transient stress which can be relieved, the symptoms begin to diminish after 8 hours.

Reference and Further Reading: World Health Organisation (1994). *ICD-10 Classification of Mental and Behavioural Disorders*. Edinburgh, UK: Churchill Livingstone; Puri BK, Treasaden I (eds) (2010). *Psychiatry: An Evidence-Based Text*. London: Hodder Arnold, p. 660.

Question 54 Answer: e, He does not have specific phobia, as there is no avoidance behaviour in his case.
Explanation: In this clinical situation, he does not have a specific phobia, as in order for the diagnosis to be made, the fear he experienced needs to be out of proportion to the norm, and cannot be reasons or explained away, and be beyond voluntary control and must have led to avoidance.

Reference: Puri BK, Hall A, Ho R (2014). *Revision Notes in Psychiatry*. London: CRC Press, p. 405.

Question 55 Answer: e, Topiramate
Explanation: Topiramate has the least prophylactic effects against future manic episodes.

Reference and Further Reading: Puri BK, Treasaden I (eds) (2010). *Psychiatry: An Evidence-Based Text*. London: Hodder Arnold, pp. 538, 699, 905, 910.

Question 56 Answer: e, Memory disturbances
Explanation: All of the aforementioned are classical clinical signs and symptoms of mania, with the exception of memory impairment. The core symptoms for mania include increased self-esteem, decreased need for sleep, being more talkative than usual, having flights of ideas, been easily distracted and having an increase in goal-directed activity or psychomotor agitation. There might also be excessive involvement in activities that have a high potential for painful and sexual consequences.

Reference: Puri BK, Hall A, Ho R (2014). *Revision Notes in Psychiatry*. London: CRC Press, p. 378.

Question 57 Answer: a, Hypercalcaemia
Explanation: Hypercalcaemia causes constipation, bone pain, nephrolithiasis and psychiatric symptoms. On the other hand, hypocalcaemia causes Trousseau sign (inflating the blood pressure cuff and maintaining the cuff pressure above systolic will cause carpal spasms) and Chvostek's sign (tapping of the inferior portion of the zygoma will produce facial spasms). Option (b) to (e) can present acutely with movement disorder and confusion.

Further Reading: Puri BK, Treasaden I (eds) (2010). *Psychiatry: An Evidence-Based Text*. London: Hodder Arnold, p. 523.

Question 58 Answer: d, Rey–Osterrieth Test
Explanation: The Rey–Osterrieth Test would be capable of picking up these deficits. In this visual memory test, the subject is presented with a complex design. The subject is asked to copy the design, and then, 40 minutes later, without previous notification that this will occur, the subject is asked to draw the same design again from memory. Nondominant temporal lobe damage could lead to impaired performance on this test, whereas domain temporal lobe damage tends not to (but is associated with verbal memory difficulties).

Reference: Puri BK, Hall A, Ho R (2014). *Revision Notes in Psychiatry*. London: CRC Press, p. 95.

Question 59 Answer: b, Afro-Caribbean immigrants to the United Kingdom have a higher risk of schizophrenia.
Explanation: The option (b) is true. This phenomenon is seen in the second generation of immigrants. The higher prevalence of schizophrenia in urban areas is a result of the interaction of genetic factors, migration, higher rates of social deprivation and social problems in the inner city.

Reference: Puri BK, Hall A, Ho R (2014). *Revision Notes in Psychiatry*. London: CRC Press, p. 358.

Question 60 Answer: a, Tryptophan hydroxylase gene
Explanation: The aforementioned gene has been implicated in the aetiology of predisposing individuals towards bipolar disorders.

Reference: Puri BK, Hall A, Ho R (2014). *Revision Notes in Psychiatry*. London: CRC Press, p. 263.

Question 61 Answer: a, Narcolepsy
Explanation: The core symptom would be excessive daytime sleepiness. There would also be other symptoms such as hypersomnia, sleep attacks, cataplexy, hypnagogic hallucinations and sleep paralysis.

Reference: Puri BK, Hall A, Ho R (2014). *Revision Notes in Psychiatry*. London: CRC Press, p. 616.

Question 62 Answer: d, Post-schizophrenia depression
Explanation: Post-schizophrenia depression has been associated with an increased risk of suicide. Post-schizophrenic depression is diagnosed when there is prolonged depressive symptom when the psychotic symptoms have subsided and depression then occurs within 12 months of the schizophrenic episode.

Reference: Puri BK, Hall A, Ho R (2014). *Revision Notes in Psychiatry*. London: CRC Press, p. 354.

Question 63 Answer: d, Sertraline
Explanation: Sertraline causes most intense gastrointestinal side effects.

Reference and Further Reading: Puri BK, Treasaden I (eds) (2010). *Psychiatry: An Evidence-Based Text*. London: Hodder Arnold, pp. 425–427, 603.

Question 64 Answer: e, Facial expression can affect emotional response.
Explanation: Option (e) is true. Laird tested the facial feedback hypothesis in his study on the effects of facial expression on the quality of emotional experience. It was found that participants rated cartoon slides as funnier when they had a 'smiling' expression, than while they were 'frowning'. They also described feeling angrier when 'frowning' and happier when 'smiling'.

According to the James–Lange theory, physiological changes occur before emotions. It is the interpretation of these physiological changes that give rise to the experience of emotions.

Distress is not a primary emotion. Ekman identified six primary emotions: happiness, surprise, anger, disgust, fear and sadness.

According to the Cannon–Bard theory, the thalamus processes the emotion-arousing stimulus and then sends the signals to the cortex, where emotion is consciously experienced, and to the hypothalamus, where physiological changes are activated.

According to Lazarus, some degree of cognitive processing is a prerequisite for an emotional response to a stimulus. He proposed that such cognitive appraisal does not have to involve conscious processing and can be fairly automatic.

Reference and Further Reading: Laird JD (1974). Self-attribution of emotion: the effects of facial expression on the quality of emotional experience. *Journal of Personality and Social Psychology*, 29: 475–485; Lazarus RS (1982).Thoughts on the relations between emotions and cognition. *American Physiologist*, 37: 1019–1024; Puri BK, Treasaden I (eds) (2010). *Psychiatry: An Evidence-Based Text*. London: Hodder Arnold, pp. 166–176.

Question 65 Answer: e, Delusional perception
Explanation: Delusional perception refers to the delusional theme that events, objects or other people in one's immediate environment have a particular and unusual significance.

Reference: Puri BK, Hall A, Ho R (2014). *Revision Notes in Psychiatry*. London: CRC Press, p. 6.

Question 66 Answer: c, Daytime sleep attacks, cataplexy, hypnogogic hallucination
Explanation: Narcolepsy refers to the daytime sleep attacks without warning. Cataplexy are episodes of partial (often face or jaw) or complete loss of muscle tone that result in the patient falling to the ground. Hypnogogic hallucinations are pre-sleep dreams associated with sleep-onset REM activity. Catalepsy refers to waxy flexibility and is found in catatonia.

Reference and Further Reading: Ward N, Frith P, Lipsedge M (2001). *Medical Masterclass Neurology, Ophthalmology and Psychiatry*. London: Royal College of Physicians; Puri BK, Treasaden I (eds) (2010). *Psychiatry: An Evidence-Based Text*. London: Hodder Arnold, pp. 845, 847–848, 851.

Question 67 Answer: d, Based on the ICD-10, panic disorder is classified into panic disorder with agoraphobia and panic disorder without agoraphobia.
Explanation: Only the DSM-IV-TR but not the ICD-10 classifies panic disorder into panic disorder with agoraphobia and panic disorder without agoraphobia.

Reference and Further Reading: American Psychiatric Association (2000). *Diagnostic Criteria from DSM-IV-TR*. Washington, DC: American Psychiatric Association; World Health Organisation (1994). ICD-10 Classification of Mental and Behavioural Disorders. Edinburgh, UK: Churchill Livingstone; Puri BK, Treasaden I (eds) (2010). *Psychiatry: An Evidence-Based Text*. London: Hodder Arnold, pp. 649–650.

Question 68 Answer: d, It cannot be used to differentiate between dementia and delirium.
Explanation: The MMSE could help to differentiate between dementia and delirium. The MMSE is a brief test that can be routinely used to rapidly detect possible dementia, to estimate the severity of cognitive impairment and to follow the course of cognitive changes over time. It can be used to differentiate between delirium and dementia.

Reference: Puri BK, Hall A, Ho R (2014). *Revision Notes in Psychiatry*. London: CRC Press, p. 98.

Question 69 Answer: a, Blessed Dementia Scale
Explanation: The Blessed Dementia Scale is a questionnaire that can be given to a care-giver or relative for administration. There are three sets of questions within the questionnaire. The first set of questions deals with activities of daily living. The second set of questions deals with further activities of daily living. The third set of questions assesses changes in personality, interest as well as drive.

Reference: Puri BK, Hall A, Ho R (2014). *Revision Notes in Psychiatry*. London: CRC Press, p. 99.

Question 70 Answer: b, 0.05
Explanation: The prevalence of recent aggressive behaviour among outpatients with schizophrenia has been estimated to be around 5%.

Reference: Puri BK, Hall A, Ho R (2014). *Revision Notes in Psychiatry*. London: CRC Press, p. 370.

Question 71 Answer: e, This condition is a perceptual rather than ideational or cognitive disturbance.
Explanation: This condition is Doppelganger. The Doppelgänger phenomenon is the subjective feeling of doubling, where the person feels like his exact 'double' is present both outside alongside and inside oneself. Statement (e) is false because Doppelganger is an ideational or cognitive rather than perceptual disturbance.

Reference and Further Reading: Sims A (2003). *Symptoms of the Mind: An Introduction to Descriptive Psychopathology*. London: Saunders, pp. 217–220, 221, 400.

Question 72 Answer: d, Overt behaviour can lead to emotions without visceral changes.
Explanation: Two studies by Valins and Laird suggested that overt behaviour could lead to emotions without visceral changes. These two studies support the James–Lange theory. According to the James–Lange theory, the experience of emotion is based on the interpretation of bodily changes by the cortex. It is argued that the James–Lange theory emphasizes skeletal changes rather than visceral changes.

References and Further Reading: Puri BK, Treasaden I (eds) (2010). *Psychiatry: An Evidence-Based Text*. London: Hodder Arnold, pp. 168–169; Puri BK, Hall AD. 2002: *Revision Notes in Psychiatry*. London: Arnold, p. 42; Valins S (1966). Cognitive effects of false heart-rate feedback. *Journal of Personality and Social Psychology*, 4: 400–408; Laird JD (1974). Self-attribution of emotion: The effects of facial expression on the quality of emotional experience. *Journal of Personality and Social Psychology*, 29: 475–485.

Question 73 Answer: a, Verbal aggression
Explanation: Amongst schizophrenic patients, the most common type of violence would be verbal aggression. It has a prevalence rate of around 45%.

Reference: Puri BK, Hall A, Ho R (2014). *Revision Notes in Psychiatry*. London: CRC Press, p. 370.

Question 74 Answer: b, Iron deficiency

Explanation: In restless leg syndrome, the patient has an irresistible urge to move his or her body to stop uncomfortable or odd sensation. One in five patients have iron deficiency but three in four patients may have increased iron stores. Nevertheless, restless leg syndrome is associated with iron deficiency but not other mineral or electrolyte deficiency.

Further Reading: Puri BK, Treasaden I (eds) (2010). *Psychiatry: An Evidence-Based Text*. London: Hodder Arnold, pp. 682, 850, 851.

Question 75 Answer: b, Cambridge Examination for Mental Disorders

Explanation: The CAMDEX involves a structured clinical interview with the patient to obtain necessary information about his current condition as well as past history. In addition, a series of neuropsychological tests are also done. A structured interview with a relative or other informant to obtain further information is also conducted. It also includes a range of objective cognitive tests that constitute a mini-neuropsychological battery, known as the CAMCOG (Cambridge Cognitive Examination).

Reference: Puri BK, Hall A, Ho R (2014). *Revision Notes in Psychiatry*. London: CRC Press, p. 99.

Question 76 Answer: b, It occurs only in Malays and there has not been reports of Amok from any other countries.

Explanation: Reports of Amok from other countries do exist, thus questioning its position as a culture bound syndrome.

Reference: Puri BK, Hall A, Ho R (2014). *Revision Notes in Psychiatry*. London: CRC Press, p. 461.

Question 77 Answer: b, The DSM-IV-TR and ICD-10 specify PTSD with delayed onset.

Explanation: The DSM-IV-TR and ICD-10 specify PTSD with delayed onset if onset of symptoms is at least 6 months after the stressor. Options (a) and (e) are incorrect because the DSM-IV-TR but not the ICD-10 specifies acute and chronic PTSD. Option (d) is incorrect because acute PTSD is defined as the duration of symptoms is less than 3 months by the DSM-IV-TR.

References and Further Reading: American Psychiatric Association (2000). *Diagnostic Criteria from DSM-IV-TR*. Washington, DC: American Psychiatric Association; World Health Organisation (1994). *ICD-10 Classification of Mental and Behavioural Disorders*. Edinburgh, UK: Churchill Livingstone; Puri BK, Treasaden I (eds) (2010). *Psychiatry: An Evidence-Based Text*. London: Hodder Arnold, pp. 643, 660.

Question 78 Answer: c, Echolalia

Explanation: The correct answer should be echolalia. Echolalia refers to the automatic imitation by the person of another person's speech. It can occur even when the person does not understand the speech form. Vorbeireden refers to approximate answers and usually occurs in Ganser syndrome. Cryptolia refers to speech that is in a language which no one could comprehend. Neologism refers to a new word that is being constructed by the person or an everyday word which is now being used in a special way by the person. Perseveration differs from the answer (echolalia), in that in perseveration, usually both speech and movement are affected. Mental operations are continued usually beyond the point at which they are considered relevant.

Reference: Puri BK, Hall A, Ho R (2014). *Revision Notes in Psychiatry*. London: CRC Press, p. 4.

Question 79 Answer: e, Schachter–Singer theory

Explanation: According to the Schachter–Singer theory, the experience of emotion is a function of physiological arousal and the cognitive appraisal of that arousal in light of situational cues. Schachter states that the type of physiological arousal is immaterial; it is the cognitive labelling of the particular emotion that influences its conscious experience. This theory is also called Schachter's cognitive labelling theory.

Reference and Further Reading: Puri BK, Treasaden I (eds) (2010). *Psychiatry: An Evidence-Based Text*. London: Hodder Arnold, pp. 171–175.

Question 80 Answer: b, Length of QRS interval

Explanation: Amitriptyline is associated with an increase in length of QRS interval.

Reference and Further Reading: Puri BK, Treasaden I (eds) (2010). *Psychiatry: An Evidence-Based Text*. London: Hodder Arnold, p. 907.

Question 81 Answer: c, Normal-pressure hydrocephalus

Explanation: The triad of normal-pressure hydrocephalus is classically defined as memory loss, urinary incontinence and gait disturbance. Subdural haematoma is associated with a history of head injury. Neurosyphilis causes general paresis and is now extremely rare.

Reference and Further Reading: Ward N, Frith P, Lipsedge M (2001). *Medical Masterclass Neurology, Ophthalmology and Psychiatry*. London: Royal College of Physicians; Puri BK, Treasaden I (eds) (2010). *Psychiatry: An Evidence-Based Text*. London: Hodder Arnold, p. 583.

Question 82 Answer: e, The patient tries to resist his thoughts

Explanation: Resistance is seen in people with obsessive-compulsive disorder but not delusional disorder.

Reference and Further Reading: Puri BK, Treasaden I (eds) (2010). *Psychiatry: An Evidence-Based Text*. London: Hodder Arnold, pp. 656–659.

Question 83 Answer: d, Mirtazapine

Explanation: According to the NICE guidelines, mirtazapine should be the antidepressant of choice if a patient takes heparin or warfarin on a daily basis.

Reference: NICE Clinical Guidelines 9, 2010. www.nice.org.uk.

Question 84 Answer: b, Loss of alpha activity and increase in diffuse slow waves

Explanation: In Alzheimer's disease, there is loss of high-frequency (e.g. alpha or beta) activity and increase in diffuse slow waves. There is an increase in low-frequency (delta and theta) activity.

Reference and Further Reading: Ward N, Frith P, Lipsedge M (2001). *Medical Masterclass Neurology, Ophthalmology and Psychiatry*. London: Royal College of Physicians; Puri BK, Treasaden I (eds) (2010). *Psychiatry: An Evidence-Based Text*. London: Hodder Arnold, pp. 405, 1103–1104.

Question 85 Answer: b, This is a condition that strictly affects individuals of the Indian culture.

Explanation: It was previously also prevalent in Europe before masturbation was prohibited by religion and emission was considered as sin.

Reference: Puri BK, Hall A, Ho R (2014). *Revision Notes in Psychiatry*. London: CRC Press, p. 462.

Question 86 Answer: d, Piblotoq

Explanation: This is a dissociative state seen amongst Eskimo women. The patient would tear off her clothing, scream, cry and run about wildly. It might result in suicidal or homicidal behaviour.

Reference: Puri BK, Hall A, Ho R (2014). *Revision Notes in Psychiatry*. London: CRC Press, p. 462.

Question 87 Answer: e, Sertraline

Explanation: According to the NICE guidelines, sertraline should be the antidepressant of choice if a patient has history of cardiac diseases.

Reference: NICE Clinical Guidelines 9, 2010. www.nice.org.uk.

Question 88 Answer: c, This phenomenon is increased by attention.

Explanation: This phenomenon is pareidolic illusion. Pareidolic illusion refers to the type of intense imagery ('Monkey God') that persists even when the person looks at a real object (callus of a tree) in the external environment. The image and percept occur together and the image is recognized as unreal. Pareidolic illusion is increased by attention as the image becomes more detailed.

Reference and Further Reading: Sims A (2003). *Symptoms of the Mind: An Introduction to Descriptive Psychopathology*. London: Saunders, pp. 96–97.

Question 89 Answer: d, Imipramine
Explanation: This patient presents with metabolic acidosis and prolonged QTc. This clinical picture is classically related to tricyclic antidepressant overdose. Hence, the best answer is (d).

Reference and Further Reading: Puri BK, Treasaden I (eds) (2010). *Psychiatry: An Evidence-Based Text*. London: Hodder Arnold, p. 907.

Question 90 Answer: e, Meniere's disease
Explanation: A history of tinnitus and deafness in the context of episodic vertigo points towards Meniere's disease. If ataxia and/or facial weakness is also present, it points towards a cerebello-pontine angle lesion, e.g. acoustic neuroma.

Reference and Further Reading: Ward N, Frith P, Lipsedge M (2001). *Medical Masterclass Neurology, Ophthalmology and Psychiatry*. London: Royal College of Physicians; Puri BK, Treasaden I (eds) (2010). *Psychiatry: An Evidence-Based Text*. London: Hodder Arnold, pp. 559, 646.

Question 91 Answer: a, Transference
Explanation: Transference is likely to be what is hindering the progress of the therapeutic relationship between the patient and the therapist. Transference is an unconscious process in which the patient transfers to the therapist feelings, emotions and attitudes that have been experienced previously. This in turn would have an effect on the way the new relationship has developed.
Reference:
Puri BK, Hall A, Ho R (2014). *Revision Notes in Psychiatry*. London: CRC Press, p. 132.

Question 92 Answer: e, 16 weeks
Explanation: These maternal serum markers have been known to be elevated at around 16 weeks of gestational age.

Reference: Puri BK, Hall A, Ho R (2014). *Revision Notes in Psychiatry*. London: CRC Press, p. 665.

Question 93 Answer: d, 15%–20% increment
Explanation: Previous studies have indicated that there is up to 18% incidence of inheriting bipolar disorder.

Reference: Puri BK, Hall A, Ho R (2014). *Revision Notes in Psychiatry*. London: CRC Press, p. 285.

Question 94 Answer: d, Stagnant phase
Explanation: The stages of psychosexual development proposed include oral, anal, phallic, latency and also the genital phase.

Reference: Puri BK, Hall A, Ho R (2014). *Revision Notes in Psychiatry*. London: CRC Press, p. 133.

Question 95 Answer: b, Autistic disorder
Explanation: Based on the current DSM-5 criteria, two main symptom clusters should exist. This should include persistent deficits in social communication, social interaction across contexts and the ability to maintain relationships; as well as restricted, repetitive patterns of behaviour, interests or activities.

Reference: Puri BK, Hall A, Ho R (2014). *Revision Notes in Psychiatry*. London: CRC Press, p. 625.

Question 96 Answer: b, 5–6 years
Explanation: The peak age of onset of the aforementioned disorder is usually between 5 and 6 years.

Reference: Puri BK, Hall A, Ho R (2014). *Revision Notes in Psychiatry*. London: CRC Press, p. 639.

Question 97 Answer: d, Focused (selective) attention
Explanation: Selective attention is the ability to attend to one type of information while ignoring other distracting information. The unattended information is still being processed simultaneously and the listener can rapidly switch channels if appropriate, which is why Lucy can recognize her name being called.

Reference and Further Reading: Puri BK, Treasaden I (eds) (2010). *Psychiatry: An Evidence-Based Text*. London: Hodder Arnold, pp. 179–186; Puri BK, Hall AD (2002). *Revision Notes in Psychiatry*. London: Arnold, p. 16.

Question 98 Answer: e, The hallucinations respond favourably to antipsychotics.
Explanation: The hallucinations respond poorly to antipsychotics. The hallucinations may lead to persecutory delusions and it is termed as substance-induced psychotic disorder with hallucinations in DSM-IV. Auditory hallucinations are more common than visual hallucinations. The auditory hallucinations are well-localized, derogatory and in second person. The voices are called phonemes, which are fragmented words or short sentences.

Reference and Further Reading: Campbell RJ (1996). *Psychiatric Dictionary*. Oxford, UK: Oxford University Press; Sims A (2003). *Symptoms of the Mind: An Introduction to Descriptive Psychopathology*. London: Saunders, p. 100.

Question 99 Answer: d, Trazodone
Explanation: Trazodone is associated with priapism at high doses. It can be used as a hypnotic between 25 and 150 mg/day without causing tolerance, dependence or rebound insomnia.

Reference and Further Reading: Puri BK, Treasaden I (eds) (2010). *Psychiatry: An Evidence-Based Text*. London: Hodder Arnold, pp. 744, 912.

Question 100 Answer: c, Hyperkinetic disorder
Explanation: The diagnostic criteria for hyperkinetic disorder state that there must be a persistent pattern of inattention, hyperactivity and impulsivity across two different settings and this must have resulted in significant functional impairments. The diagnostic criteria also state that the onset should be prior to the age of 7.

Reference: Puri BK, Hall A, Ho R (2014). *Revision Notes in Psychiatry*. London: CRC Press, p. 631.

Question 101 Answer: d, Latency phase
Explanation: The sexual drive remains relatively latent during the latency stage, which typically occurs around the age of 5–6 years.

Reference: Puri BK, Hall A, Ho R (2014). *Revision Notes in Psychiatry*. London: CRC Press, p. 133.

Question 102 Answer: d, Narcissistic personality disorder
Explanation: All of the aforementioned could be located on both the ICD-10 and DSM-5, with the exception of narcissistic personality disorder.

Reference: Puri BK, Hall A, Ho R (2014). *Revision Notes in Psychiatry*. London: CRC Press, p. 439.

Question 103 Answer: a, Death of a close spouse
Explanation: Death of a close spouse has been considered to be the most stressful event with 100 life change units.

Reference: Holmes TH, Rahe RH (1967). The social readjustment scale. *Journal of psychosomatic research*, 11: 213–218.

Question 104 Answer: e, Temporal lobe
Explanation: This man is hallucinating a panoramic view which involves seeing a wide area. This is a form of complex hallucination and is found in people with temporal lobe epilepsy.

Reference: Nožica T, Marković D, Maračić L, Franko A, Gregorović E, Radolović-Prenc L (2006). Temporal lobe epilepsy with panorama hallucination. *Journal of Hospital Pula*, 3(3): 75–77.

Question 105 Answer: e, Being of high birth wright
Explanation: All of the aforementioned are factors that are deemed responsible for someone to develop schizophrenia. Low birth weight and urban birth have been known to be risk factors for schizophrenia.

Reference: Puri BK, Hall A, Ho R (2014). *Revision Notes in Psychiatry*. London: CRC Press, p. 360.

Question 106 Answer: b, Animus

Explanation: Based on his theory, the animus correctly describes the masculine prototype that is present within every individual.

Reference: Puri BK, Hall A, Ho R (2014). *Revision Notes in Psychiatry*. London: CRC Press, p. 133.

Question 107 Answer: d, It does not result in the subsequent avoidance of similar situations.

Explanation: In order to fulfil the diagnostic criteria, the onset of the panic disorder usually would result in a hurried exit and a subsequent avoidance of similar situations.

Reference: Puri BK, Hall A, Ho R (2014). *Revision Notes in Psychiatry*. London: CRC Press, p. 413.

Question 108 Answer: b, Charles Bonnet syndrome

Explanation: Charles Bonnet syndrome is characterized by the presence of complex visual hallucinations occurring in persons with visual impairment and no demonstrable psychopathology. The hallucinations vary from elementary (geometric figures) to complex hallucinations (seeing human figures or animals) and are more vivid than the limits of their impaired vision. There is usually insight that the hallucinations are not 'real' and the percepts may be modified by voluntary control. The syndrome is also associated with some fears of developing a mental illness.

Reference and Further Reading: Sims A (2003). *Symptoms of the Mind: An Introduction to Descriptive Psychopathology*. London: Saunders, pp. 104–105.

Question 109 Answer: a, Bupropion

Explanation: Bupropion is contraindicated because of seizure risk in bulimia nervosa. Fluoxetine has the best evidence to reduce binge eating, purging and psychological problems of bulimia nervosa. Higher doses of fluoxetine are required to treat bulimia nervosa compared with severe depressive disorder.

Reference and Further Reading: Puri BK, Treasaden I (eds) (2010). *Psychiatry: An Evidence-Based Text*. London: Hodder Arnold, pp. 611, 907, 913.

Question 110 Answer: b, Biological factors include the presence of elevated plasma dopamine levels.

Explanation: Biological factors include the presence of low plasma dopamine levels instead of elevated levels. It is true that conduct disorder is associated with the inheritance of antisocial traits from parents who have demonstrated criminal activities. Previous research has demonstrated an association with parental criminality as well as with repeated physical and sexual abuse.

Reference: Puri BK, Hall A, Ho R (2014). *Revision Notes in Psychiatry*. London: CRC Press, p. 635.

Question 111 Answer: d, Lack of control of the accident
Explanation: The aforementioned options are predisposing factors for PTSD, except option (d).

Reference and Further Reading: Puri BK, Treasaden I (eds) (2010). *Psychiatry: An Evidence-Based Text*. London: Hodder Arnold, pp. 660–661.

Question 112 Answer: c, Episiotomy during vaginal delivery
Explanation: This woman suffers from postnatal depression. Episiotomy during vaginal delivery or vaginal delivery is not an established risk factor for postnatal depression. Old age is an aetiological factor for postnatal depression.

Reference and Further Reading: Puri BK, Treasaden I (eds) (2010). *Psychiatry: An Evidence-Based Text*. London: Hodder Arnold, pp. 635–636, 722–724.

Question 113 Answer: c, Personality is not shaped by culture.
Explanation: Option (c) is false. Personality is shaped by culture and associated values and norms. Culture has a great impact on child-rearing patterns and this will ultimately shape personality. The term 'personality disorder' is culturally biased.

Option (b) is true. Culture has a pathoplastic effect on psychopathology because culture can influence overall psychopathology as well as individual symptoms. The contents of delusions and hallucinations can be modified according to cultural and prevalent social norms. For example, mustard gas formed a key component of delusions immediately after the Second World War, and attacks by terrorists formed a key component of delusions after the Iraq War.

Option (d) is true. Both hallucinations and paranoid thoughts are said to be more common in ethnic-minority groups who may feel persecuted by the mainstream culture. Ethnic-minority patients may not wish to reveal their true mental state to psychiatrists who are from the mainstream culture.

Option (e) is true. The nosological systems employed by psychiatry are largely anglocentric (e.g. DSM-IV-TR) and eurocentric (e.g. ICD-10). The DSM-IV-TR and ICD-10 diagnostic criteria assume that the mental illnesses commonly found in European patients present in the similar way in the non-European patients.

Reference and Further Reading: Bhugra D, Bhui K (2001). *Cross-Cultural Psychiatry: A Practical Guide*. London: Arnold.

Question 114 Answer: a, Alcohol dependence
Explanation: The usage of alcohol in an individual with anorexia nervosa is known to increase the incidence of mortality.

Reference: Puri BK, Hall A, Ho R (2014). *Revision Notes in Psychiatry*. London: CRC Press, p. 581.

Question 115 Answer: c, 5-HT2A/2C receptors
Explanation: The stimulation of 5-HT2A/2C receptors by SSRI would lead to sexual side effects. This is also associated with circadian rhythm disturbances.

Reference: Puri BK, Hall A, Ho R (2014). *Revision Notes in Psychiatry*. London: CRC Press, p. 230.

Question 116 Answer: a, Bruising
Explanation: Fluoxetine inhibits the metabolism of warfarin and increases bleeding tendency. This will lead to bruising.

Reference and Further Reading: Puri BK, Treasaden I (eds) (2010). *Psychiatry: An Evidence-Based Text*. London: Hodder Arnold, pp. 698, 708, 724, 762.

Question 117 Answer: e, This phenomenon is more common in women.
Explanation: This phenomenon is autoscopy. Autoscopy is a visual hallucination of seeing an image of oneself viewed from within one's physical body. The double imitates the movement and facial expressions of the original, as if being a reflection in a mirror, and typically appears as semi-transparent. Associated auditory, kinaesthetic and emotional perceptions are frequent. The autoscopic episode usually lasts for a few seconds with the subject seeing his own face, mostly occurs when lying in bed and is often accompanied by distress, fear, anxiety and depression. Autoscopy is more common in men with M:F ratio = 2:1. It also occurs in organic disorders such as parietooccipital lesions, temporoparietal lobes, epilepsy, schizophrenia and substance misuse. Neurological and psychiatric disorder can occur in 60% of cases.

Reference and Further Reading: Sims A (2003). *Symptoms of the Mind: An Introduction to Descriptive Psychopathology*. London: Saunders, pp. 105–106.

Question 118 Answer: c, Cocaine withdrawal
Explanation: Cocaine intoxication typically causes olfactory hallucination. Cocaine withdrawal causes depression, insomnia, anorexia, fatigue, irritability, restlessness and craving. Olfactory hallucinations are associated with the sense of smell and strong emotional component. The smell may or may not be pleasant and has a unique significance to the person.

Reference and Further Reading: Sims A (2003). *Symptoms of the Mind: An Introduction to Descriptive Psychopathology*. London: Saunders, p. 107.

Question 119 Answer: a, Family members did not agree with the premature discharge and their opinions were not sought.
Explanation: Negligence causes direct damage. Negligence occurs when a doctor deviates from fiduciary duty and dereliction. Option (b) refers to dereliction which means that a doctor must exercise a reasonable degree of knowledge and skills exercised by other members of the profession in similar circumstances. For option (c), damages include both physical and psychological harm. Option (e) refers to fiduciary duty which means that a doctor must act in the patient's best interests.

Reference and Further Reading: Puri BK, Treasaden I (eds) (2010). *Psychiatry: An Evidence-Based Text*. London: Hodder Arnold, pp. 1221–1222.

Question 120 Answer: e, Benjamin Rush

Explanation: Benjamin Rush and Samuel Merrit published the first textbook in psychiatry in 1812.

Reference: Puri BK, Hall A, Ho R (2014). *Revision Notes in Psychiatry*. London: CRC Press, p. 139.

Question 121 Answer: d, Bleuler

Explanation: It was in 1911 that Bleuler introduced the term schizophrenia, applied it to Kraepelin's cases of dementia praecox and expanded the concept to include what today may be considered schizophrenia spectrum disorders. He considered the symptoms of ambivalence, autism, affective incongruity and disturbance of association of thought to be fundamental, with delusions and hallucinations assuming secondary status.

Reference: Puri BK, Hall A, Ho R (2014). *Revision Notes in Psychiatry*. London: CRC Press, p. 351.

Question 122 Answer: b, Karl Ludwig Kalbaum

Explanation: Karl Ludwig Kahlbaum was responsible for coining the term 'catatonia'.

Reference: Puri BK, Hall A, Ho R (2014). *Revision Notes in Psychiatry*. London: CRC Press, p. 140.

Question 123 Answer: a, Autonomy, nonmaleficence, beneficence, justice

Explanation: The four core ethical principles are autonomy, non-maleficence, beneficence and justice. Autonomy refers to the obligation of a doctor to respect his or her patients' rights to make their own choice in accordance with their beliefs and responsibilities. Non-maleficence refers to the obligation of a doctor to avoid harm to his or her patients. Beneficence refers to the fundamental commitment of a doctor to provide benefits to patients and to balance benefits against risk when making such a decision. Justice refers to fair distribution of medical services or resources.

Reference: Puri BK, Hall A, Ho R (2014). *Revision Notes in Psychiatry*. London: CRC Press, p. 146.

Question 124 Answer: c, Munchausen syndrome

Explanation: In such a disorder, the patient would intentionally produces physical or psychological symptoms but the patient is unconscious about his or her underlying motives. Most of the time, the patient would have some prior working experience in the healthcare setting. Common presenting signs would include bleeding, diarrhoea, hypoglycaemia, infection, impaired wound healing, vomiting and rashes.

Reference: Puri BK, Hall A, Ho R (2014). *Revision Notes in Psychiatry*. London: CRC Press, p. 471.

Question 125 Answer: c, Sodium valproate
Explanation: In general, new anticonvulsants are more likely to cause visual side effects than the older anticonvulsants. For example, carbamazepine causes visual hallucination but relatively rarely. Gabapentin causes visual-field defects, photophobia, bilateral or unilateral ptosis and ocular haemorrhage. Topiramate causes acute onset of decreased visual acuity and/or ocular pain. Vigabatrin causes concentric visual-field defects.

Reference and Further Reading: Puri BK, Treasaden I (eds) (2010). *Psychiatry: An Evidence-Based Text*. London: Hodder Arnold, pp. 532, 538.

Question 126 Answer: e, Suggestive probes
Explanation: Open-ended questioning, reflective listening, summarizing and allowing for silence would be appropriate. Suggestive probes would not be appropriate as they tend to mislead the patient, and in this case (suicide risk assessment), it would be of importance to gather a precise and accurate history.

Reference: Puri BK, Hall A, Ho R (2014). *Revision Notes in Psychiatry*. London: CRC Press, p. 332.

Question 127 Answer: d, Mood refers to a static unidimensional emotion on a depression-mania spectrum with depression and mania at the extremes and euthymia in the middle.
Explanation: Option (d) is incorrect because mood is a dynamic and multidimensional emotion which includes normal variation such as happiness and reactivity to environments.

Reference and Further Reading: Poole R, Higgo R (2006). *Psychiatric Interviewing and Assessment*. Cambridge, UK: Cambridge University Press; Puri BK, Treasaden I (eds) (2010) *Psychiatry: An Evidence-Based Text*. London: Hodder Arnold, pp. 985–986.

Question 128 Answer: d, Emil Kraepelin
Explanation: In 1896, it was Emil Kraepelin who grouped together catatonia, hebephrenia, and the deteriorating paranoid psychosis under the name of dementia praecox. Dementia praecox has a poorer prognosis compared with manic-depressive psychosis, which has a better prognosis.

Reference: Puri BK, Hall A, Ho R (2014). *Revision Notes in Psychiatry*. London: CRC Press, p. 351.

Question 129 Answer: a, Admit own feelings and inform the patient that the staff are frightened of his aggression and anger.
Explanation: Option (a) may confuse the patient and give the wrong impression to the patient that the staff are incompetent in handling his aggression and anger. Patients with antisocial personality disorder may see this as weakness of the team and manipulate the situation by escalating his aggression and anger. Psychiatrist

in this situation should deliver a clear and correct message to inform the patient that physical violence is not acceptable and there are chemical and physical interventions to help him to calm down.

Reference: Poole R, Higgo R (2006). *Psychiatric Interviewing and Assessment*. Cambridge, UK: Cambridge University Press.

Question 130 Answer: a, The theory emphasized that a doctor needs to be caring, compassionate, committed and conscientious in nature.
Explanation: The virtue theory emphasizes on the key personality qualities that a doctor would need. Plato and Aristotle emphasized that a doctor needs to be caring, compassionate, committed and conscientious in nature.

Reference: Puri BK, Hall A, Ho R (2014). *Revision Notes in Psychiatry*. London: CRC Press, p. 146.

Question 131 Answer: b, Oppositional defiant behaviour
Explanation: The ICD-10 classification system states that there must be a repetitive and persistent pattern of behaviour in which either the basic rights of others or major age-appropriate social rules are being violated. The minimum duration of the symptoms should last at least 6 months. It is important to note that children with oppositional defiant disorder tend to have temper tantrums, be very angry and spiteful, initiate arguments with adults, defy rules and blame others for it. It is crucial to note that children with oppositional defiant disorder should not have more than two symptoms related to physical assault, damage of properties and running away from school or home.

Reference: Puri BK, Hall A, Ho R (2014). *Revision Notes in Psychiatry*. London: CRC Press, p. 637.

Question 132 Answer: c, Amphetamines
Explanation: Amphetamines could cause excessive release of dopamine and this would usually lead to a hyper-excitable state. This might lead to symptoms such as tachycardia, arrhythmia, hyperthermia and irritability.

Reference: Puri BK, Hall A, Ho R (2014). *Revision Notes in Psychiatry*. London: CRC Press, p. 542.

Question 133 Answer: d, 5–14 days
Explanation: Lithium remains a first-line treatment for bipolar disorder. It has equal effectiveness in mania to valproate, carbamazepine, risperidone, quetiapine and first-generation antipsychotics. Its onset of action is around 5–14 days. Its antimanic effects are proportional to a plasma level between 0.6 and 1.2 mEq/L. Lithium shows a superior effect to placebo in acute bipolar depression.

Reference and Further Reading: Puri BK, Treasaden I (eds) (2010). *Psychiatry: An Evidence-Based Text*. London: Hodder Arnold, pp. 613, 623, 630, 632, 633, 909–910.

Extended Matching Items (EMIs)

Theme: Psychosexual development

Question 134 Answer: b, Anal phase
Explanation: The anal phase occurs from around 15–18 months to around 30–36 months of age. Erotogenic pleasure is derived from stimulation of the anal mucosa, initially through faecal excretion and later also through faecal retention.

Question 135 Answer: c, Phallic phase
Explanation: This phase takes place from around 3 years of age to around the end of the fifth year. Boys pass through the Oedipal complex. Girls develop penis envy and pass through the Electra complex.

Question 136 Answer: d, Latency period
Explanation: This is a phase that occurs from 5–6 years to the onset of puberty. The sexual drive remains relatively latent during this period.

Question 137 Answer: e, Genital phase
Explanation: It should be noted that from the onset of puberty to young adulthood, a strong resurgence in the sexual drive takes place. Successful resolution of conflicts from this and previous psychosexual stages leads to a mature well-integrated adult identity.

Reference: Puri BK, Hall A, Ho R (2014). *Revision Notes in Psychiatry*. London: CRC Press, p. 133.

Theme: Psychodynamic theory of defence mechanisms

Question 138 Answer: j, Turning against the self
Explanation: Turning against the self refers to how an impulse which is meant to express to another is now turned against oneself.

Question 139 Answer: l, Sublimation
Explanation: Sublimation refers to the process that utilizes the force of a sexual instinct in drives, affects and memories in order to motivate creative activities having no apparent connection with sexuality.

Question 140 Answer: m, Regression
Explanation: Transition, at times of stress and threat, to moods of expression and functioning that are on a lower level of complexity, so that one returns to an earlier level of maturity and functioning.

Question 141 Answer: e, Projection
Explanation: In projection, unacceptable qualities, feelings and thoughts or wishes are projected onto another person or thing. This is very often seen in paranoid patients.

Question 142 Answer: d, Undoing
Explanation: This refers to an attempt that is made to negate or atone for forbidden thoughts, affects or memories. This defence mechanism is seen, for example, in the compulsion of magic in patients with obsessive-compulsive disorders.

Reference: Puri BK, Hall A, Ho R (2014). *Revision Notes in Psychiatry*. London: CRC Press, p. 136.

Theme: Competency and capacity

Question 143 Answer: c, Testamentary capacity
Explanation: To make a will, a person must be of sound disposing mind. This means that the person must understand to whom he or she is giving personal property, understand and recollect the extent of personal property and understand the nature and extent of the claims upon the person, both of those included and of those excluded from the will.

Question 144 Answer: d, Capacity for informed consent
Explanation: It is the responsibility of the doctor to judge whether a patient has the capacity to give a valid consent. The doctor has a duty to provide information in a language understandable by a lay person about a condition, the benefits and the risks of a proposed treatment and alternatives to a treatment. The high court has held that an adult has capacity to consent to a medical or surgical treatment if he or she can (a) understand and retain the information relevant to the decision in question, (b) believe in the information and (c) weigh the information in balance to arrive at a choice.

Question 145 Answer: a, Capacity
Explanation: Competence is a legal concept and refers to the capacity to act and understand. Competence is determined only by the legal system, such as the competence to adopt a child.

Question 146 Answer: e, Advocacy
Explanation: An advocate enters into a relationship with the patient, to speak on his or her behalf and to represent the patient's wishes to stand up for his or her rights. An advocate has no legal status: the patient should have an idea of personal p*Reference*: s so that the advocate truly represents the patient's wishes.

Question 147 Answer: f, Appointeeship
Explanation: An appointee is someone authorized by the Department of Social Security to receive and administer benefits on the behalf of someone else who is not able to administer money derived from social security and cannot be used to administer any other income or assets. If benefits accumulate, application may need to be made to the Public Trust Office or the Court of Protection to gain access to the accumulated capital.

Reference: Puri BK, Hall A, Ho R (2014). *Revision Notes in Psychiatry*. London: CRC Press, p. 148.

Question 148 Answer: c, Naivety
Explanation: This refers to naivety because colour of skin, ethnicity and cultural identity play no role in this person's life.

Question 149 Answer: a, Acceptance
Explanation: This can be passive or active acceptance. This may also create conflict within oneself.

Question 150 Answer: e, Resistance and naming
Explanation: Although the full meaning of one's own cultural identity in the broader society is understood, this understanding may lead to anger and frustration.

Question 151 Answer: d, Redefinition and reflection
Explanation: Redefinition and reflection refer to the establishment of cultural identity in a person's own right.

Question 152 Answer: b, Multi-perspective internalization
Explanation: Multi-perspective internalization is the final stage when a person can appreciate his or her own cultural identity with pride.

Reference and Further Reading: Bhugra D, Bhui K (2001). *Cross-cultural Psychiatry: a Practical Guide*. Arnold: London.

Theme: Abnormal experiences

Question 153 Answer: g, Running commentary, i, Third person hallucination
Explanation: Running commentary is an auditory hallucination consisting of voices commenting on the patient's behaviour.

Question 154 Answer: c, Command hallucination, h, Second person hallucination
Explanation: Command hallucination is an auditory hallucination in which the voices command the person to perform certain acts.

Question 155 Answer: b, Hearing voices arguing, i, Third person hallucination
Explanation: The third person auditory hallucinations involve two voices arguing.

Question 156 Answer: e, Hygric hallucination
Explanation: Hygric hallucination is a superficial hallucination in which the person feels the presence of fluid in his or her body.

Question 157 Answer: d, Haptic hallucination
Explanation: Haptic hallucinations are superficial sensations of touch on or under the skin.

Question 158 Answer: j, Reduplicative hallucination
Explanation: Reduplicative hallucination refers to the sensation of the presence of a duplication of a certain body part.

Reference and Further Reading: Puri BK, Hall AD (2002). *Revision Notes in Psychiatry*. London: Arnold, p. 154.

Question 159 Answer: c, Illusion
Explanation: Illusion. It is an involuntary false perception in which a transformation of a real object (i.e. curtain) takes place.

Question 160 Answer: j, Visual hyperaesthesia
Explanation: Visual hyperaesthesia refers to changes in sensory perception in which there is an increased intensity of visual stimuli.

Question 161 Answer: b, Dysmegalopsia
Explanation: Dysmegalopsia (also known as the Alice in Wonderland effect); illusory change in the size and shape (both reduction and increase in size).

Question 162 Answer: d, Macropsia
Explanation: Macropsia refers to visual sensation of objects being larger than their actual size.

Question 163 Answer: f, Pareidolia
Explanation: Pareidolia refers to the type of intense imagery (i.e. Jesus' face) that persists even when the person looks at a real object (callus of a tree) in the external environment.

Question 164 Answer: g, Peduncular hallucination
Explanation: Peduncular hallucination is a form of vivid and colourful visual hallucination.

Reference and Further Reading: Puri BK, Treasaden I (eds) (2010). *Psychiatry: An Evidence-Based Text*. London: Hodder Arnold, pp. 234–237.

Theme: Type of prevention
Question 165 Answer: b, Secondary prevention
Explanation: Secondary prevention is usually directed at people who show early signs of disorder and the goal is to shorten the duration of the disorder by early and prompt treatment.

Question 166 Answer: a, Primary prevention
Explanation: Primary prevention efforts are directed at people who are essentially normal, but believed to be 'at risk' from the development of a particular disorder.

Question 167 Answer: c, Tertiary prevention
Explanation: Tertiary prevention is designed to reduce the severity and disability associated with a particular disorder.

Reference: Paykel ES, Jenkins R (1994). *Prevention in Psychiatry*. London: Gaskell.

Theme: Prevention strategies in schizophrenia

Question 168 Answer: d, Reduction in perinatal trauma, e, Reduction in stress associated with migration, f, Successful treatment of middle ear disease in childhood

Explanation: Primary prevention targets at people before the onset of schizophrenia and it includes reduction of schizophrenia-like psychosis, prevention of perinatal trauma and targeting at adverse social factors (e.g. stress associated with migration). Successful treatment of middle ear disease in childhood may reduce the risk of temporal lobe epilepsy and schizophrenia-like psychosis.

Question 169 Answer: b, Maintenance in antipsychotic treatment, c, Psychoeducation about schizophrenia

Explanation: Secondary prevention targets at people who have developed schizophrenia. Secondary prevention strategies include drug treatment and social treatment (e.g. psychoeducation of schizophrenia).

Question 170 Answer: a, Listen to loud stimulating music to drown out the auditory hallucinations not responding to antipsychotic treatment

Explanation: Tertiary prevention is designed to reduce the severity and disability associated with schizophrenia such as auditory hallucination not responding to treatment.

Reference: Paykel ES, Jenkins R (1994). *Prevention in Psychiatry*. London: Gaskell.

Question 171 Answer: a, Classical migraine

Explanation: Classical migraine may be associated with visual phenomena (fortification spectra) and most patients feel nauseated. Additional features such as weakness, paresthesia, aphasia, diplopia and visual loss are often worrying but can all happen as part of migraine aura.

Question 172 Answer: e, Orbital onset migraine

Explanation: Orbital onset migraine starts in and around the orbit.

Question 173 Answer: f, Occipital onset migraine

Explanation: Occipital onset migraine starts in the occipital area.

Question 174 Answer: h, Tension headache

Explanation: Tension headache

Reference and Further Reading: Ward N, Frith P, Lipsedge M (2001). *Medical Masterclass Neurology, Ophthalmology and Psychiatry*. London: Royal College of Physicians; Puri BK, Treasaden I (eds) (2010). *Psychiatry: An Evidence-Based Text*. London: Hodder Arnold, pp. 519–520.

Question 175 Answer: c, 9–11 years
Explanation: Children aged 9–11 years need more information and facts to gain control. They also try to avoid negative emotions by preoccupying themselves with activities.

Question 176 Answer: a, 3–5 years
Explanation: Children aged 3–5 years are usually confused and ask repetitive Questions regarding the deceased. They may display inappropriate reactions and have difficulty to understand abstract concept of death.

Question 177 Answer: b, 6–8 years
Explanation: Children aged 6–8 years understand death. They do not have ego-strength to cope and may blame themselves for the death. They may have magical thinking.

Question 178 Answer: e, 15–17 years
Explanation: Adolescents aged 15–17 years have grief reactions most similar to adults.

Theme: Clinical diagnosis
Question 179 Answer: f, Catatonic schizophrenia
Explanation: This person suffers from catatonic schizophrenia. When he was in the catatonic state, he exhibited waxy flexibility. Hence, he was described as still as a 'statue'.

Reference and Further Reading: Puri BK, Treasaden I (eds) (2010). *Psychiatry: An Evidence-Based Text*. London: Hodder Arnold, pp. 579, 925.

Question 180 Answer: k, Malignant catatonia
Explanation: This solider suffers from malignant catatonia.

Question 181 Answer: g, Depressive episode
Explanation: This woman suffers from moderate-to-severe depressive episode. The childbirth is a distractor because this patient does not meet the diagnostic criteria for postnatal depression as the onset of depression is too late. Her checking behaviour is secondary to low mood and pessimism.

Reference and Further Reading: Puri BK, Treasaden I (eds)(2010). *Psychiatry: An Evidence-Based Text*. London: Hodder Arnold, pp. 614–624.

Question 182 Answer: e, Bipolar disorder – manic episode
Explanation: This man is in the manic phase as evidenced by grandiosity (pursuing a PhD degree, advising the Prime Minister), delusion of persecution as a result of grandiosity (probably he thought that he was a celebrity and chased by paparazzi), dangerous driving and foolhardy investment in the food business. The patient

firmly believes that he suffers from schizophrenia but this is a distractor as he may hear mood-congruent auditory hallucination. The antidepressant was stopped as a result of antidepressant-induced mania.

Reference and Further Reading: Puri BK, Treasaden I (eds) (2010). *Psychiatry: An Evidence-Based Text*. London: Hodder Arnold, pp. 624–634.

Question 183 Answer: s, Psychotic depression
Explanation: This 50-year-old man exhibits nihilistic delusion and it is considered to be a mood-congruent delusion in patients with severe depressive episode.

Theme: Defence mechanisms
Question 184 Answer: c, Displacement
Explanation: This is displacement. Negative emotions are transferred from their original object to a less threatening substitute.

Question 185 Answer: i, Denial
Explanation: This is denial. The external reality of an unwanted or unpleasant piece of information is denied.

Question 186 Answer: b, Intellectualization
Explanation: He avoids disturbing feelings by engaging in excessive abstract thinking. This is intellectualization.

Reference and Further Reading: Puri BK, Hall AD (2002). *Revision Notes in Psychiatry*. London: Arnold, p. 168–169.

Theme: Concepts of dynamic psychotherapy
Question 187 Answer: k, Resistance
Explanation: This man is exhibiting resistance and the trainee cannot probe further.

Reference and Further Reading: Puri BK, Treasaden I (eds) (2010). *Psychiatry: An Evidence-Based Text*. London: Hodder Arnold, pp. 948–949.

Question 188 Answer: j, Process interpretation
Explanation: The trainee has performed process interpretation and attributed client's anger to his leave.

Reference and Further Reading: Puri BK, Treasaden I (eds) (2010). *Psychiatry: An Evidence-Based Text*. London: Hodder Arnold, pp. 947–953.

Question 189 Answer: b, Affirmation
Explanation: This process is known as affirmation.

Theme: General adult psychiatry

Question 190 Answer: a, Allport's theory

Explanation: Common traits are basic modes of adjustment applicable to all members of a society (e.g. the level of aggression of each member of a society can be assessed by a scale of aggression). Individual traits are unique sets of personal dispositions and ways of organizing the world based on life experiences.

Question 191 Answer: c, Eysenck's theory

Explanation: This is Eysenck's theory.

Question 192 Answer: b, Cattell's theory

Explanation: L-data (L stands for life) refer to ratings made by the observers. Q-data (Q stands for questionnaires) refer to the scores on personality questionnaires. T-data (T stands for tests) refer to the objective tests that are specifically designed to measure personality.

Question 193 Answer: d, Type A personality

Explanation: Type A personality is associated with increased systolic blood pressure, heart rate, plasma adrenaline, noradrenaline levels and cortisol levels.

Reference and Further Reading: Puri BK, Treasaden I (eds) (2010). *Psychiatry: An Evidence-Based Text*. London: Hodder Arnold, pp. 278–284.

INDEX

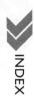